Advances in Analytical Techniques for Forensic Investigation

Scrivener Publishing
100 Cummings Center, Suite 541J
Beverly, MA 01915-6106

Publishers at Scrivener
Martin Scrivener (martin@scrivenerpublishing.com)
Phillip Carmical (pcarmical@scrivenerpublishing.com)

Advances in Analytical Techniques for Forensic Investigation

Edited by

Priyanka Chhabra

Divya Bajpai Tripathy

Anjali Gupta

Rajeev Kumar

Kajol Bhati

and

Shruti Shukla

Scrivener Publishing

WILEY

This edition first published 2024 by John Wiley & Sons, Inc., 111 River Street, Hoboken, NJ 07030, USA and Scrivener Publishing LLC, 100 Cummings Center, Suite 541J, Beverly, MA 01915, USA

For more information about Scrivener publications please visit www.scrivenerpublishing.com.

Wiley Global Headquarters
111 River Street, Hoboken, NJ 07030, USA

For details of our global editorial offices, customer services, and more information about Wiley products visit us at www.wiley.com.

Library of Congress Cataloging-in-Publication Data

ISBN 978-1-394-16631-2

Front cover images supplied by Adobe Firefly
Cover design by Russell Richardson

Set in size of 11pt and Minion Pro by Manila Typesetting Company, Makati, Philippines

Printed in the USA

10 9 8 7 6 5 4 3 2 1

Contents

Preface **xvii**

1 Introduction to Analytical Techniques for Forensic Analysis **1**
Megha Walia, Bhoopesh Kumar Sharma and Faray Jamal
1.1 Introduction 2
1.1.1 Forensic Analysis 2
1.1.2 Introduction to Instrumentation in Forensic Science 3
1.1.2.1 Validation of Instrument 4
1.1.2.2 Instrumentation for Organic Evidence 5
1.1.2.3 Instrumentation for Inorganic Evidence 5
1.1.2.4 Instrumentation for Biological Evidence 6
1.1.2.5 Instrumentation for Chemical Evidences 7
1.1.2.6 Instrumentation for Physical Evidences 8
1.2 Analytical Techniques for Evidence Analysis 8
1.2.1 Spectroscopy 8
1.2.1.1 Infrared Spectroscopy 10
1.2.1.2 UV-Visible Spectroscopy 10
1.2.1.3 Nuclear Magnetic Resonance Spectroscopy (NMR) 11
1.2.1.4 Mass Spectrometer (MS) 13
1.2.2 Chromatographic Techniques 16
1.2.2.1 Gas Chromatography (GC) 17
1.2.2.2 High Performance Liquid Chromatography (HPLC) 18
1.2.2.3 High Performance Thin Layer Chromatography (HPTLC) 18
1.2.3 Hyphenated Techniques 19
1.2.4 Microscopic Techniques 20
1.2.4.1 Optical Microscope 21
1.2.4.2 Electron Microscope 22
1.2.4.3 Stereomicroscope 24

1.2.4.4 Comparison Microscope 25
1.2.4.5 Energy Dispersive X-Ray Coupled Microscopy in Forensic Science 26
1.2.5 X-Ray Diffraction (XRD) 26
1.2.6 Nanotechnology 27
1.3 Conclusion 28
References 29

2 Forensic Sample Collection and Preparation 35
Anuj Sharma, Poonam Kumari, Abhishek R. Rai, Varad Nagar, Vaibhav Sharma, Archana Gautam, Tina Sharma, Rajeev Kumar and Mahipal Singh Sankhla
2.1 Introduction 36
2.2 Collection and Preservation of Evidence at the Crime Scene 37
2.2.1 Physical Evidence 37
2.2.2 Biological Evidences 37
2.2.3 Trace Evidences 40
2.2.4 Impression Evidence 41
2.2.5 Explosives 42
2.2.6 Hair and Fibers 43
2.2.7 Documentary Evidence 45
2.2.8 Digital Evidences 46
2.3 Legal Considerations 47
2.4 Chain of Custody 47
2.4.1 Importance and Significance of Chain of Custody in Forensic Science 47
2.5 Admissibility in Court 48
2.6 Forensic Laboratory Analysis 48
2.7 DNA Analysis 49
2.7.1 Types of Crime Scenes Where an Expert Can Find DNA 49
2.7.2 Techniques Used 49
2.8 Fingerprint Analysis 50
2.8.1 Collection 50
2.8.2 Development 50
2.8.3 Lifting 51
2.8.4 Analysis 51
2.8.5 Evaluation 52
2.9 Ballistic Analysis 52
2.9.1 Visual Examination 52
2.9.2 Gunshot Residue Analysis 52

2.9.3 Trajectory Analysis 53
2.10 Toxicology Analysis 53
2.10.1 Spectroscopy 53
2.10.2 Chromatography 53
2.10.3 Immunoassays 54
2.10.4 Mass Spectrometry 54
2.11 Quality Control Measures 54
2.11.1 Validation of Methods 54
2.11.2 Calibration 55
2.11.3 Quality Assurance Programs 55
2.11.4 Documentation and Record Keeping 55
2.11.5 Documentation and Reporting of Evidences 55
2.12 Challenges and Emerging Technologies 55
2.12.1 Contamination 56
2.12.2 Microbial Contamination 56
2.12.3 Packaging and Storage Contamination 56
2.12.4 Preservation Difficulties 56
2.13 Handling Digital Evidence 56
2.14 Emerging Technologies 57
2.15 Advances in DNA Analysis 58
2.16 AI and Machine Learning in Forensic Analysis 58
2.17 Cyber Forensics Techniques 59
2.18 Conclusion 59
References 60

3 Vibrational Spectroscopy in Forensic Sample Analysis 69
Harjeet Singh, Noble George, Deepti Attitiniti and Shivani R. Pandya
3.1 Fundamentals of Vibrational Spectroscopy (VS) 70
3.2 General Forms of Vibrational Spectroscopy 70
3.2.1 Raman Spectroscopy: Science of Elastic and Inelastic Scattering of Photons 71
3.2.2 IR Spectroscopy: Technique Based on Interaction of Infrared Radiation with Matter 72
3.2.3 Chemometrics: Data Driven Science to Extract Chemical Information 73
3.3 The Deployment of Vibrational Spectroscopy in Forensics and Criminal Investigations 74
3.3.1 Biological Fluids 75
3.3.2 Ballistics 79
3.3.3 Document and Ink Evidences 81

3.3.4 Trace Evidences 81
3.3.5 Controlled Substances 84
3.4 Conclusions and Future Prospects 85
References 86

4 UV-Vis Spectroscopy in Forensic Sample Investigation 93
Ashita Anand, Palash Kumar Manna and Shruti Shukla
4.1 Introduction 94
4.2 Forensic Science 94
4.3 UV-Vis Spectroscopy 95
4.4 Applications of UV/Visible Spectroscopy in Forensic Science 97
4.4.1 Analysis of Narcotics and Drug Testing 97
4.4.2 Determination of Alcohol in Blood 98
4.4.3 Ink Analysis 99
4.4.4 Analysis of Carbon Monoxide Poisoning in Forensic Blood Samples 100
4.4.5 Forensic Determination of Metals by UV/Visible Spectroscopy 101
4.4.6 Examination of Blood Stains by UV/Visible Spectroscopy 103
4.4.7 Forensic Discrimination of Dyed Fiber Collected from the Incident Site 104
4.5 Future Perspective 105
4.6 Conclusion 105
Consent for Publication 106
Conflict of Interest 106
Acknowledgement 107
References 107

5 Nuclear Magnetic Resonance Spectroscopy: A Versatile Tool for Forensic Sample Analysis 113
Devi Deepti Attinti, Kwasi Kantanka Safo, M. Balakrishna, Noble George and Shivani Pandya
5.1 Introduction to NMR in Forensic Science 114
5.1.1 Overview of NMR Spectroscopy 114
5.1.2 Importance of NMR in Forensic Analysis 115
5.2 NMR Instrumentation and Sample Preparation 116
5.2.1 Types of NMR Spectrometers 116
5.2.1.1 Continuous-Wave NMR Spectrometer (CW-NMR) 116
5.2.1.2 Fourier-Transform NMR Spectrometer (FT-NMR) 117

5.2.2 Sample Preparation Techniques 118
5.2.3 Quantitative NMR (qNMR) Spectroscopy 118
5.3 NMR Spectroscopy Techniques 119
5.3.1 One Dimensional NMR Spectroscopy 119
5.3.2 Two-Dimensional NMR Spectroscopy (2D NMR) 120
5.3.3 Solid State NMR Spectroscopy 121
5.3.4 Dynamic Nuclear Polarization (DNP)-Enhanced NMR Spectroscopy 122
5.4 Forensic Applications of NMR Spectroscopy 123
5.4.1 Drug Analysis 123
5.4.2 Forensic Toxicology 124
5.4.3 Body Fluid Analysis 124
5.4.4 Fire Debris Analysis 126
5.4.5 Polymer and Paint Analysis 127
5.4.6 Fiber Analysis 128
5.5 Data Processing and Interpretation 128
5.5.1 Spectral Processing Techniques 128
5.5.2 Spectral Interpretation and Analysis 130
5.5.3 Chemometrics and Statistical Analysis 132
5.6 Conclusion 133
5.6.1 Challenges and Opportunities 133
5.6.2 Future Outlook and Potential Advancements 134
References 134

6 Forensic Aspects of Mass Spectroscopy and Isotope Ratio Mass Spectroscopy 149
Elipe Arjun, Priyanka Chhabra and Priyanka Singh
6.1 Introduction 149
6.1.1 Overview of Isotopes and Mass Spectroscopy 150
6.1.2 The Importance of Stable Isotope Analysis Assists Forensic Cases 152
6.1.3 Stable Isotope Abundances in Forensic Evidence 154
6.2 Mass Spectroscopy Principle Instrumentation 154
6.2.1 Mass Spectrometry 154
6.2.2 Principle 155
6.2.3 Instrumentation 155
6.3 Ion Source 155
6.3.1 Electron Impact (EI) 156
6.3.2 Electrospray Ionization (ESI) 156
6.3.3 Matrix-Assisted Laser Desorption/Ionization (MALDI) 157

6.3.4 Chemical Ionization 157
6.4 Mass Analyzer 157
6.4.1 Quadrupole Mass Analyzer 157
6.4.2 Time-of-Flight (TOF) Mass Analyzer 157
6.4.3 Magnetic Sector Mass Analyzer 158
6.5 Detector 158
6.5.1 Electron Multiplier Detector 158
6.5.2 Time-to-Digital Converter (TDC) Detector 158
6.5.3 Channeltron Detector 158
6.5.4 High Mass Detection Detectors 158
6.6 Applications of Mass Spectrometry in Forensics 159
6.6.1 Toxicology 159
6.6.2 Explosives 160
6.6.3 Environmental Forensics 161
6.6.4 DNA Sequencing and Proteomics 161
6.6.5 Forensic Geochemistry 162
6.6.6 Forensic Chemistry 163
6.7 Isotope Ratio Mass Spectrometry Principle and Instrumentation 164
6.7.1 Isotope Ratio Mass Spectrometry (IRMS) 164
6.7.2 Principle 165
6.7.3 Instrumentation 165
6.7.4 Ion Source 166
6.7.5 Types of Ion Sources in IRMS 166
6.7.5.1 Electron Impact Ionization (EI) 166
6.7.5.2 Chemical Ionization (CI) 167
6.7.5.3 Field Ionization (FI) 168
6.7.6 Mass Analyzer 168
6.7.7 Detector 169
6.7.8 Isotope Ratio Measurement System 169
6.7.9 Gas Handling System 170
6.8 Applications of Isotope Ratio Mass Spectroscopy in Forensics 170
6.8.1 Environmental Forensic Applications 170
6.8.2 Wildlife Forensic Applications 171
6.8.3 Illicit Drug Applications 172
6.8.4 Forensic Applications of Archaeology and Anthropology 173
6.8.5 Food Forensic Applications 175
6.8.6 Application of IRMS in Questioned Documents 176
6.8.7 Miscellaneous 176

6.9 Case Study 177
6.10 Challenges and Limitations of Mass Spectrometry in Forensics 178
6.11 Conclusion 179
References 180

7 Application of Plasma and Atomic Absorption Spectroscopy in Sample Analysis 189
Jyoti Singh and Shrutika Singla
7.1 Introduction 189
7.2 Absorption Spectroscopy 192
7.3 Atomic Absorption Spectroscopy (AAS) 192
7.3.1 Principle 194
7.3.2 Instrumentation 194
7.3.3 Working 197
7.4 Plasma Absorption Spectroscopy (PAS) 197
7.4.1 Principle 199
7.4.2 Instrumentation 199
7.4.3 Working 201
7.5 Analysis of Forensic Samples Using AAS and PAS 201
7.5.1 Biological Samples and Matrices 201
7.5.2 Drugs and Pharmaceutical Industry 203
7.5.3 Forensic Medicine 204
7.5.4 Soil 204
7.5.5 Explosives, Gunshot Residues, and Ammunition 205
7.5.6 Glass 206
7.5.7 Heavy Metals 206
7.5.8 Environmental Samples 207
7.5.9 Miscellaneous Samples 207
Consent for Publication 208
Conflict of Interest 208
Acknowledgement 208
References 208

8 Application of Gas Chromatography in Criminalistics 215
Ankit Singh and Namrata Singh
8.1 Introduction 216
8.1.1 Evolution of Gas Chromatography 216
8.2 Gas Chromatography 217
8.3 Principle of Gas Chromatography 218
8.4 Instrumentation of Gas Chromatography 219

8.5 Advancement in Gas Chromatography Technique 221
8.5.1 High-Resolution GC 221
8.5.2 Fast GC 222
8.5.3 Multidimensional GC 223
8.5.4 Mass Spectrometry (MS) Detection 224
8.6 Miniaturization and Automation in GC 225
8.6.1 Miniaturization 225
8.6.2 Automation 226
8.7 Application of Gas Chromatography in Criminalistics 226
8.7.1 Drug Analysis Using GC 227
8.7.2 Arson Investigation 229
8.7.3 Explosive Analysis 230
8.7.4 Toxin Analysis 232
8.7.5 Food and Beverage Analysis 233
8.7.6 Trace Evidences Analysis 233
8.8 Conclusion 236
References 236

9 HPLC and HP-TLC 241

Lovlish Gupta, Abhiramy S. Shenoy and Divya Bajpai Tripathy

9.1 Introduction 242
9.2 Principle 246
9.2.1 Basic Principle of HPLC 246
9.2.2 Basic Principle of HP-TLC 246
9.2.3 Basic Parameters and Steps Involved 247
9.3 Applications of HPLC and HP-TLC in Forensic Sciences 249
9.3.1 Forensic Examination of Samples Using HPLC 250
9.3.1.1 Forensic Examination of Toxicological Samples 250
9.3.1.2 Examination of Explosives and Explosives Substances 252
9.3.1.3 Examination of Textile and Fabrics 253
9.3.1.4 Examination of Questioned Documents and Variable Inks 254
9.3.1.5 Examination of Narcotics, Psychotropic Substances and Pharmaceutical Substances 255
9.3.1.6 Examination of Cosmetic Products 256
9.3.2 Forensic Examination of Samples Using HP-TLC 257
9.3.2.1 Forensic Examination of Toxicological Samples 257

9.3.2.2 HP-TLC Fingerprinting to Detect Medicinal Merits 258
9.3.2.3 Examination of Textile and Fabrics 259
9.3.2.4 Examination of Questioned Documents and Variable Inks 260
9.3.2.5 Examination of Narcotics, Psychotropic Substances and Pharmaceutical Substances 261
9.3.2.6 Examination of Cosmetic Products 262
9.4 Conclusion 262
Consent for Publication 263
Conflict of Interest 263
Acknowledgement 263
References 263

10 Forensic Aspects of Hyphenated Techniques 271
Nisha, Priyanka Singh and Priyanka Chhabra
10.1 Introduction to Hyphenated Techniques in Forensic Science 272
10.2 Hyphenated Techniques Used in Forensic Science 273
10.2.1 Gas Chromatography-Mass Spectrometry (GC-MS) 273
10.2.1.1 Principle and Instrumentation 273
10.2.1.2 Applications of GC-MS in Forensic Science 275
10.2.2 Head Space–Gas Chromatography (HS-GC) 278
10.2.2.1 Principle and Instrumentation 279
10.2.2.2 Applications of HS-GC in Forensic Science 281
10.2.3 Gas Chromatography-Infrared Spectroscopy (GC-IR) 282
10.2.3.1 Principle and Instrumentation 283
10.2.3.2 Applications of GC-IR in Forensic Science 284
10.2.4 Liquid Chromatography-Mass Spectrometry (LC-MS) 286
10.2.4.1 Principle and Instrumentation 286
10.2.4.2 Applications of LC-MS in Forensic Science 288
10.2.5 Fourier Transform Infrared Spectroscopy-Mass Spectrometry (FTIR-MS) 289
10.2.5.1 Principle and Instrumentation 289

10.2.5.2 Applications of FTIR-MS in Forensic Science 291
10.2.6 Liquid Chromatography-Tandem Mass Spectrometry (LC-MS/MS) 291
10.2.6.1 Principle and Instrumentation 292
10.2.6.2 Applications of LC-MS/MS in Forensic Science 294
10.2.7 Capillary Electrophoresis-Mass Spectrometry (CE-MS) 296
10.2.7.1 Principle and Instrumentation 296
10.2.7.2 Applications of CE-MS in Forensic Science 297
10.3 Conclusion 299
References 300

11 Microscopic Techniques and Their Application in Forensic Science 307
Vaishnavi M.A., Malavika Venu, Ravshish Kaur Kohli and Pooja Puri
11.1 Introduction to Microscopy 308
11.2 Types of Microscopes 309
11.2.1 Optical Microscope 309
11.2.2 Stereomicroscope 310
11.2.3 Bright Field Microscope 311
11.2.4 Confocal Microscope 314
11.2.5 Fluorescence Microscope 316
11.2.6 Polarizing Microscope 318
11.2.7 Electron Microscope 320
11.2.8 TEM 321
11.2.9 Scanning Electron Microscope (SEM) 323
11.2.10 Atomic Force Microscope (AFM) 324
11.3 Forensic Application of Microscopy 326
11.3.1 Biological Samples 326
11.3.2 Fibers 328
11.3.3 Explosives and Gunshot Residues Analysis 328
11.3.4 Glass 330
11.3.5 Paint 331
11.3.6 Questioned Document 332
11.3.7 Soil and Materials 333
11.3.8 Fingerprint Identification 334

Conclusion 334
References 335

12 EDX and X-Ray Technique in Forensic Science 339
Muskan Dhawan, Rhea Sharma and Gayatri Sharma
12.1 Introduction and Overview 339
12.2 Importance of XRD and EDX Technique in Forensic Science 341
12.2.1 Importance of XRD 341
12.2.2 Importance of EDX 342
12.3 Instrumentation for XRD and EDX Techniques 343
12.3.1 Principle, Working and Instrumentation for XRD 343
12.3.2 Principle, Working, and Instrumentation for EDX Spectroscopy 347
12.3.3 Sample Preparation 350
12.3.3.1 Sample Preparation for XRD 350
12.3.3.2 Sample Preparation for Biological Specimens Using EDX Technique 351
12.4 Applications of EDX and X-Ray Technique in Forensic Science 352
12.4.1 Drug Analysis 352
12.4.2 Fire Debris 353
12.4.3 Body Fluid Analysis 354
12.4.4 Paint and Polymer Analysis 355
12.4.5 Fiber Analysis 357
12.5 Future Aspects and Conclusion 357
References 358

13 Nanotechnology in Forensic Science 363
Bhoopesh Kumar Sharma, Megha Walia and Faray Jamal
13.1 Introduction 364
13.1.1 Exploring the Field of Nanotechnology 365
13.1.1.1 Classification of Nanomaterials 365
13.2.2 Characterization of Nanomaterials 366
13.2.2.1 UV-Visible Spectroscopy (Spectroscopic Analysis) 366
13.2.2.2 Transmission Electron Microscopy (TEM) 367
13.2.2.3 Dynamic Light Scattering (DLS) 368
13.2.2.4 Inductively Coupled Plasma Mass Spectrometry (ICP-MS) 369

13.2.2.5 Dark Field Microscopy (DFM) 370
13.3 Techniques for the Synthesis of Nanomaterials 371
13.3.1 Top-Down Approaches 371
13.3.1.1 Mechanical Milling 371
13.3.1.2 Electrospinning 371
13.3.1.3 Lithography 372
13.3.1.4 Sputtering 372
13.3.2 Bottom-Up Approaches 373
13.3.2.1 Chemical Vapor Deposition (CVD) 373
13.3.2.2 Solvothermal and Hydrothermal Methods 373
13.3.2.3 The Sol–Gel Method 374
13.3.2.4 Reverse Micelle Method 375
13.4 Role of Nanotechnology in Forensic Investigation 375
13.4.1 Explosive Residue Detection 375
13.4.2 Fire Debris Analysis 376
13.4.3 GSR Analysis 377
13.4.4 Detection of Fingerprints 378
13.4.5 DNA Analysis 379
13.4.6 Drug and Toxicology Testing 380
13.4.7 Detection of Food Adulteration 381
13.4.8 Counterfeiting Prevention and Homeland Security 382
13.4.9 Bio Sensors and Nano Trackers 383
13.4.10 Nanotechnology and Questioned Document 384
13.5 Conclusion 384
References 385

Index **395**

Preface

Forensic science is a multidisciplinary field that employs various scientific disciplines, such as chemistry, biology, and physics, to gather, examine, and interpret physical evidence associated with criminal activities. It serves as a crucial bridge between criminal actions and the legal system, guiding investigations through various stages, from scrutinizing crime scenes to preparing evidence for courtroom presentation. Analytical methods like spectroscopy, chromatography, and microscopy are essential tools in uncovering valuable information from physical evidence, ensuring precise analysis. Emerging technologies, such as nanotechnology and hybrid methods, also contribute to evidence examination. The importance of this field becomes apparent in its capacity to identify and decipher a wide range of evidence, including biological, chemical, and physical traces. Biological samples encompass materials like hair, blood, semen, and insects, while chemical evidence involves substances like poisons and explosives. Physical evidence includes items such as fingerprints, glass, fibers, and paints. Each type of evidence requires specific analytical techniques for accurate analysis. Forensic evidence analysed through these methods plays a pivotal role in criminal investigations. This comprehensive handbook addresses the use and applications of these techniques, catering to a diverse audience, including students, researchers, forensic scientists, medical professionals, educators, and law enforcement personnel.

The chapters presented within this book offer an in-depth description, theory, principal, sample preparation and analysis of various forensic evidence ranging from biological, chemical, and physical evidence through various conventional and advanced analytical techniques. Each chapter delves into specific applications of analytical instruments, highlighting their use in identification and analyzing forensic evidence.

Chapter 1 "Introduction to Analytical Techniques for Forensic Analysis" This chapter provides a comprehensive discussion regarding various analytical techniques and their application in the forensic analysis of diverse samples encountered at crime scenes. These samples encompass blood, semen, saliva, DNA, explosives, paints, glass, inks, urine, drugs, poisons, and questioned documents.

Chapter 2: "Forensic Sample Collection and Preparation" In this chapter, cutting-edge techniques employed in the collection, sampling, and preparation of forensic samples for subsequent analysis using different analytical methods are explored.

Chapter 3 "Vibrational Spectroscopy in Forensic Sample Analysis" delves into the realm of vibrational spectroscopy, including FT-IR, Raman spectroscopy, and vibrational circular dichroism, elucidating their application in the analysis of a broad spectrum of biological, chemical, and toxicological samples.

Chapter 4 "UV-Vis Spectroscopy in Forensic Sample Investigation" investigates the extensive utility of UV-visible spectroscopy across various domains of forensic science. Encompassing drug identification, chemical analysis, and quantification, this section provides insights into the principles, theories, and applications of UV-Vis spectroscopy.

Chapter 5 "Forensic Application of Nuclear Magnetic Resonance (NMR) Spectroscopy" sheds light on the forensic applications of Nuclear Magnetic Resonance (NMR) spectroscopy. The focus is on its role in elucidating the molecular structure of diverse body fluids, drug analysis, and identification of counterfeit samples, enhancing the accuracy of forensic investigations.

Chapter 6 "Forensic Aspects of Mass Spectrometry and Isotope Ratio Mass Spectrometry" underscores the significance of Mass Spectrometry and Isotope Ratio Mass Spectrometry in forensic science. Notably effective in identifying and analyzing chemicals, especially in drug analysis, this section explores their widespread applications.

Chapter 7 "Application of Plasma and Atomic Absorption Spectroscopy in Sample Analysis" concentrates on elemental analysis at minute concentrations, pivotal in forensic science for confirming the elemental composition of forensic evidence. The discussion revolves around the forensic use of plasma and atomic absorption spectroscopy.

Chapter 8 "Application of Gas Chromatography in Criminalistics" takes on the challenge of analysing trace evidence that can be easily volatized without decomposition through gas chromatography coupled with techniques like mass spectrometry. This section covers the analysis of various forensic evidence, including alcohol, organic compounds, drugs, explosives, ignitable materials, fingerprints, inks, paints, and toxins.

Chapter 9 "HPLC and HP-TLC" focuses on the crucial task of separating components in mixed crime scene samples. HPLC and HP-TLC are explored for their effectiveness in investigating poisoning cases and cases requiring component separation and trace impurity detection.

Chapter 10 "Forensic Aspects of Various Hyphenated Techniques" unveils the application of hyphenated analytical techniques, combining chromatographic and spectroscopic methods for analysing questioned samples such as paint, blood, saliva, explosives, and drugs.

Chapter 11 "Microscopic Techniques and Their Application in Forensics" delves into microscopic techniques like SEM, TEM, and AFM, enabling the scrutiny of minute morphological and structural details in trace samples.

Chapter 12 "EDX and X-Ray for Forensic Samples" reconnoitre the quantitative examination of elements in gunshot residue (GSR), paint, soil, and toxins are explored using EDX and X-ray techniques in forensic science in this chapter.

Chapter 13 "Nanotechnology in Forensic Science" The final chapter provides a comprehensive overview of nanotechnology's applications in forensic science and crime detection. It highlights nanotechnology's role in enhancing accuracy, precision, speed, and suitability in inquiries.

Collectively, these chapters strive to offer a comprehensive perspective on the diverse terrain of progress in analytical techniques for forensic sample analysis. They commemorate the achievements accomplished thus far, all the while recognizing the obstacles that await. As we embark on this expedition into the domain of enhanced analytical techniques, we extend an invitation to readers to uncover the potential of these advanced analytical techniques to bring about substantial transformations in how we tackle and overcome intricate identification hurdles.

Dr. Priyanka Chhabra
Prof. (Dr.) Divya Bajpai Tripathy

1

Introduction to Analytical Techniques for Forensic Analysis

Megha Walia[1]*, Bhoopesh Kumar Sharma[1] and Faray Jamal[2]

[1]*Department of Forensic Science, SGT University Gurugram, Haryana, India*
[2]*Central Forensic Science Laboratory, Bhopal, Madhya Pradesh, India*

Abstract
Forensic analysis is the application of scientific techniques to investigate and solve crimes or other legal issues. Analytical techniques play a crucial role in forensic analysis as they provide valuable information that can be used as evidence in court. Globally, the forensic sciences are utilized to settle disputes of the civil court, employ criminal laws, govern the created rules fairly, and safeguard public health. Forensic Science or Criminalistics is the application of science to law enforcement. Forensic scientists rely on instrumental examination of trace quantities of substances such as pharmaceuticals, toxicological specimens, fibers, glass, GSR, and soil etc. Individualization of evidence is facilitated by variances in manufacturing chemical composition, allowing for a high degree of differentiation even with minute pieces. The purpose of this chapter is to emphasize the qualitative and quantitative analytical techniques, such as IR Spectroscopy, UV-Visible Spectroscopy, AAS, NMR, Chromatography, Microscopic techniques, EDX, XRD, and nanotechnology, employed in criminalistics for the examination of vital and soupcon evidences that are procured from various scene regions.

Keywords: Analytical techniques, instrumentation, spectroscopy, NMR, chromatography, microscopic techniques, EDX, XRD

**Corresponding author*: megha_fosc@sgtuniversity.org

Priyanka Chhabra, Divya Bajpai Tripathy, Anjali Gupta, Rajeev Kumar, Kajol Bhati and Shruti Shukla (eds.) Advances in Analytical Techniques for Forensic Investigation, (1–34) © 2024 Scrivener Publishing LLC

1.1 Introduction

The evolution and development of Forensic Science is not something that has occurred in the recent past but has its root situated back to ancient Roman and Greek societies. As most of the English words are adopted and utilized in English, the term "forensic" is no exception and thus has its roots to the Latin language, wherein it refers to 'of the forum' where in ancient time law courts with discussion were held [1]. An area of study known as "forensic science" is one in which scientific principles are utilized in the course of a criminal investigation for the purpose of conducting an evaluation of the evidence that has been gathered over the course of the inquiry [2]. Forensic sciences use several disciplines, including the basic sciences-physics, chemistry, mathematics, and biology, along with law (both civil and criminal), engineering, dentistry, geology, microbiology, biotechnology to name a few and incorporate them to analyze the physical evidence [1]. In other words, forensic science applies scientific knowledge to the definition and execution of the law [3]. In fact, Forensic Discipline is acknowledged in and of itself as a science that draws from a variety of other fields. The amalgamation of all the sciences with the sole responsibility to assist the criminal justice system is the appropriate definition of Forensic Science. Forensic science is a realm that has indefinite possibilities [1].

The team that consists of people participating in the examination and investigation of crime scenes incorporate medics, police, and forensic professionals who are accountable for the collection of evidence. Laboratory-based forensic scientists/experts are more familiar with the many analytical procedures utilized for their analysis [2].

As a three-part structure, Forensic Science consists of

- Collection: Associated with Inquiry of Facts (Science);
- Examination: Associated with Generation of Results;
- Presentation: Associated with the Court of Law [3]

1.1.1 Forensic Analysis

Analysis of any crime scene requires the person to be competent in the domain of physical and biological sciences, including other sectors of technology and law enforcement. Forensic experts examine and analyze fingerprint ridges, fabrics, glass, and residues from gunshot, assess medications and poisons, investigate possibilities of forgeries, and inspect residues for any possible incendiary and explosive crimes [4]. Human body fluids such as blood, urine, seminal fluid, and saliva play a major role in the investigation of crimes like murder and rape [5]. Since forensics is primarily a scientific discipline, an extensive array of analytical methods is employed to examine evidence collected at the site of the crime. There is a plethora of information stored in this evidence; it just needs the right eye for identification. This motivation has fueled the development of forensic science, where information is gained via the analysis of numerous types of evidence to help the legal system in piecing together the past [2].

According to forensic community-recognized criteria, the result that is generated after thorough examination should be statistically correct and should always have high probability in reaching a fair and just decision. No categorical judgements are permitted unless the samples being compared have entirely distinct physicochemical profiles that are regarded as having a confidence level of one hundred percent [6–8].

Therefore, interpreting data as categorical while ignoring the "fuzziness of limits" may result in forensic malpractice.

Most known to occur during an investigation are biological, physical, and chemical evidence. Typically, these samples are prepared prior to examination utilizing analytical procedures to guarantee optimal analysis [2].

Application of analytical chemistry in forensic is one of the most helpful and initiating fields of research, with widespread usage in areas such as the examination of illicit and illegal narcotics in diverse matrices, the analysis of food adulteration, the analysis of adulteration of fuels and car chassis, and the analysis of frauds in works of arson [1].

They are two types of forensic analytical methods:

1. Destructive methods: This entails the destruction of the evidence and the loss of evidence integrity. Chromatographic procedures are examples.
2. Non-Destructive methods: This procedure preserves the integrity of the evidence because it does not entail the destruction of the evidence. Examples include microscopy and spectroscopy [9].

1.1.2 Introduction to Instrumentation in Forensic Science

In criminal and civil investigations, forensic science involves the use of sophisticated scientific methods. This right eye with the correct instrumental technique can not only just recognize, but detect and even segregate the articles found at the crime scene to forensically relevant material.

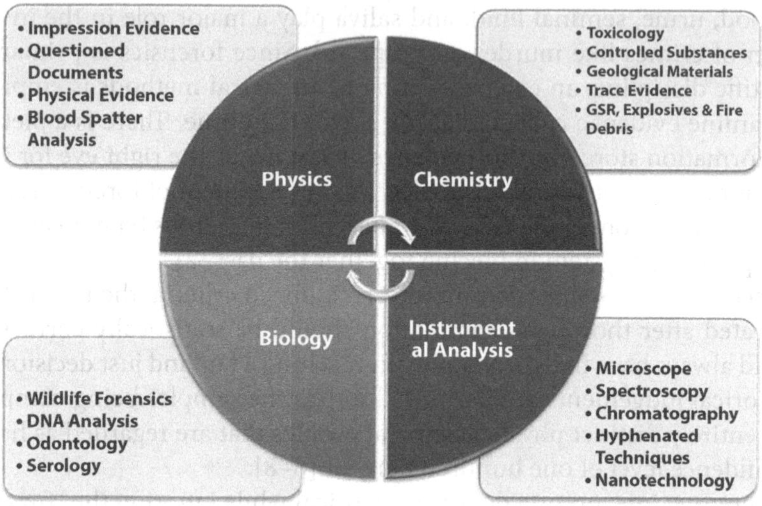

Figure 1.1 Types of evidence analyzed with various instrumental analysis.

This relevant material has stored incriminating stories regarding the event, the identity of the origin (who, what, with) and of the incident (how, when, why, where) that generated it [10]. The likelihood ratio method was given special study by Biosa *et al.*, who provided clarity on the interpretation of analytical data in the forensic context. The data has been classified into two categories using penalized logistic regression and the computation of likelihood ratios. Using data on alcohol biomarkers, the approach was utilized to categorize individuals who often consume alcoholic beverages [11]. Figure 1.1 depicts the physical, chemical, and biological evidence that can be analyzed by various instrumental techniques.

The numerous approaches to evidence analysis are going to be broken down into their essential components and outlined in this chapter [6–8].

1.1.2.1 Validation of Instrument

As never before, the legitimacy and credibility of forensic expert testimony, as well as its capacity to distinguish between defense and prosecution positions, are being challenged as well as questioned [12, 13].

Therefore, it is inevitable that the scientific basis of forensics would be questioned; thus, it is essential to shift the attention to the integrity of the investigation procedure. Thus prior to the deployment of any new forensic procedure, certain efforts must be performed to confirm the efficiency of the suggested method for its planned use i.e., every new procedure must be verified/validated. Analytical procedures have evolved greatly with time, from extremely subjective evaluations of data with limited information to objective evaluation using chromatographic and spectroscopic signals with detailed information [8]. To completely comprehend the efficiency of an instrument, experts must be conversant with the general features of investigative assays. This includes the limit of detection (LOD), the signal-to-noise ratio (S/N), the limit of quantification (LOQ), accuracy, precision, interference, and resilience. Due to the significance of such factors for defining evaluates, they are crucial mechanisms of validation of method. Numerous investigative equipment alter a specific characteristic of an analyte into an electrical indicator. Numerous factors, including arbitrary electrical transmissions, varying chemical concentrations innate to the sensor, which leads to undesired signals which might hinder the response of the target. Such irregular impulses are referred to as noise. The finest machinery enhances S/N by enhancing analyte signal, reducing noise, or both. A high S/N ratio reduces LOQ and LOD. These limits are often derived by gauging successive dilutions of an evidence in the matrix of interest and selecting the lowest concentration where readings fulfil S/N and other requirements in forensic toxicology [14].

1.1.2.2 Instrumentation for Organic Evidence

For the purpose of determining the presence of organic compounds like alcohols, alkenes, amino acids, carboxylic acids, aldehydes, ketones, esters, and phenols, among other things, organic analytical methods are utilized. The investigation reveals both the kind (the qualitative outcome) and the degree of something (quantitative result). Chromatography, UV-visible Spectrophotometry, GCMS, LCMS, Infrared Spectrophotometry, & Mass Spectrometry are some of the several analytical methods that are utilized in the process of analyzing organic substances [3].

1.1.2.3 Instrumentation for Inorganic Evidence

For the purpose of determining the presence of inorganic elements like C, B, P, K, Ca, Zn, S, Ba, Pb, V, Mo etc. in the unknown substances, inorganic analytical methods are utilized. The investigation reveals both the kind (the qualitative outcome) and the degree of something (quantitative result).

XRD, AES, AAS and NAA are few techniques that come under the category of the analytical methods that are utilized in the process of analyzing inorganic substances [3].

1.1.2.4 Instrumentation for Biological Evidence

Illicit and illegal substances, such as ethanol, benzodiazepines, MDMA, cocaine, LSD, barbiturates etc., used to be investigated evidences for a very long time, particularly in biological samples (blood, urine, viscera, and hair) derived from living and deceased humans. Research on legal or illegal substances in biological specimens, *in vivo* and post mortem, is in high demand because of the widespread drug usage that contributes to major public health problems across the world and disproportionately affects young people. During the Middle Ages, Europe saw an increase in the number of cases of poisoning caused by opium, arsenic, and hydrocyanic acid. At the same time period, Paracelsus, saw that the dose at which a drug is consumed determines whether it is a poison or not [1].

Arsenic was initially recovered from a variety of post-mortem biological samples in 1814 by Mathieu Joseph Bonaventure Orfila, who is also known as the Father of Toxicology. This study was the first to be systematized & classify poisons. He was the first person to propose that a poison must first be absorbed into the body or enter the bloodstream to have its harmful effects.

Jean Servais Stas came up with the first successful investigative method for removing alkaloids present in biological materials in the year 1851. Friedrich Julius Otto, segregated pure alkaloids, substantially changed the extraction method years later. This type of analysis is now often referred to as the StasOtto Method, and it continues to be one of the essential methods used in the drug extraction process [15].

When operating with biological samples, especially urine, having a full understanding of the metabolism of chemicals is essential for building diagnostic techniques. Wagmann *et al.* conducted research on *in vitro* methods to study the metabolites of several new psychoactive substances (NPS). Their findings highlighted the feasibility of zebrafish larvae for explaining the toxicokinetic of NPS, particularly in situations where studies on humans are impractical due to ethical considerations [16]. Putz *et al.* then carried out an extensive *in vivo* metabolic investigation centered on trenbolone; a drug commonly abused for the purpose of enhancing athletic performance [17]. The authors discovered new possible metabolites using Hydrogen Isotope Ratio Mass Spectrometry in conjunction with Liquid Chromatography. For the purpose of determining whether the detected trenbolone metabolites truly contribute anything of use to the standard doping control procedures, more research will be conducted. Since the credibility of forensic science has taken a significant hit in recent years as a result of a number of inefficient forensic pathologies

(Trager, 2018), thus it is vital to guarantee the examination of evidence by means of trustworthy analytical techniques [18]. After a procedure involving the creation of sodium hydroxide and hydride, the examination of hair is carried out using atomic absorption spectroscopy. This approach would make it possible to detect the inelastic light dispersion that occurs as a result of molecular vibration modes when the sample in question is exposed to a source of monochromatic light e.g., laser. In conjunction with the diameter of the hair shaft, the synchrotron radiation beam had a size of either 1 or 4 mm. It is still not quite clear the number of times hair shafts were counted in addition to the number of particles discovered. In accordance with the research arsenic has been discovered on just 1–2/100 hair shafts [19, 20].

This chapter discusses the philosophy behind contemporary technology as well as its most recent advancements in relation to the investigation of harmful substances found in biological fluids and tissues.

1.1.2.5 Instrumentation for Chemical Evidences

Recently, synthetic cannabinoids, compounds derived from fentanyl and cathinone, and other novel psychoactive drugs have been thrust into the mainstream of forensic analytical chemistry [1]. These chemicals are more commonly referred to by their acronym, NPS. The class of substances known as NPS, that are intended to simulate the effects of illegal recreational drugs that are already on the market, are the subject of a significant amount of research attention. The ever-increasing prevalence of NPS presents forensic laboratories with several difficult analytical hurdles [8]. In this context, it is of the utmost importance to do research, create new analytical methods, and conduct validation tests on those methods in order to meet the substantial demand posed by contemporary society for the clarification of forensic cases [1]. For instance, Cal *et al.* devised a bioanalytical procedure for the analysis of oral fluid and validated by using HPLC-MS that requires nominal evidence treatment prior to analysis [21]. On the other hand, Salerno *et al.* analyzed real "street" samples seized by GC-FTIR. Both approaches were successful in unequivocally determining the NPS that were being studied [22]. A collaborative research effort aimed at the synthesis and characterization of various NPS was presented by Bulska *et al.* with the intention of making the job of law enforcement authorities easier. The non-routine analytical methodology that was proposed to couple chromatography with combined XRD, and then mass spectrometry was used to identify the produced compounds. Also, NMR investigation was carried out in order to verify the compounds hypothesized chemical structures [23].

1.1.2.6 Instrumentation for Physical Evidences

Few qualified experts worldwide begin the task of documenting the type of bullets used and identifying the qualitative variations in GSR's chemical composition. Niewoehner [24] and Broiek Mucha *et al.* [25, 26] attempted a separate procedure for examination of GSR using SEM-EDX and interpreted results based upon chemical methods. It aids to identify the group of bullets that were utilized based on the GSR research. Analytical techniques are developed such as Inductively Coupled Plasma Mass Spectrometry (ICPMS) that offer more discriminating results than SEM EDX and are all being used to investigate the composition of primary residues [27]. Nevertheless, given that knowledge of both their morphology and the major important elements continues to be a useful tool for GSR examination. SEM-EDX is the GSR analytical approach that is more accurate [28].

1.2 Analytical Techniques for Evidence Analysis

These analytical techniques, along with others, are used to analyze different types of evidence, such as drugs, fibers, gunshot residues, and biological fluids, among others. The results of these analyses can provide important information that can be used in legal proceedings [10]. The subsequent section will encompass spectroscopy, chromatography, microscopy, and other emerging techniques that are frequently utilized in Forensic Science.

1.2.1 Spectroscopy

Spectroscopy is a technique that involves the measurement of the interaction between light and matter. It provides valuable information about the structure, composition, and dynamics of materials. There are many types of spectroscopy techniques, each of which uses a different region of the electromagnetic spectrum, from radio waves to gamma rays. The electromagnetic radiation (EMR) as represented in Figure 1.2 is the assorted scale of energy in the form of waves; they are arranged in the increasing and decreasing manner of their wavelengths and photon energies. The green color of leaves is result of the absorption and reflection of radiation from the electromagnetic spectrum.

When light strikes the surface of the leaf, it absorbs all the light except green color, thus only reflecting green light. The entire domain of spectroscopy is based on this interaction of light with the sample of our choice

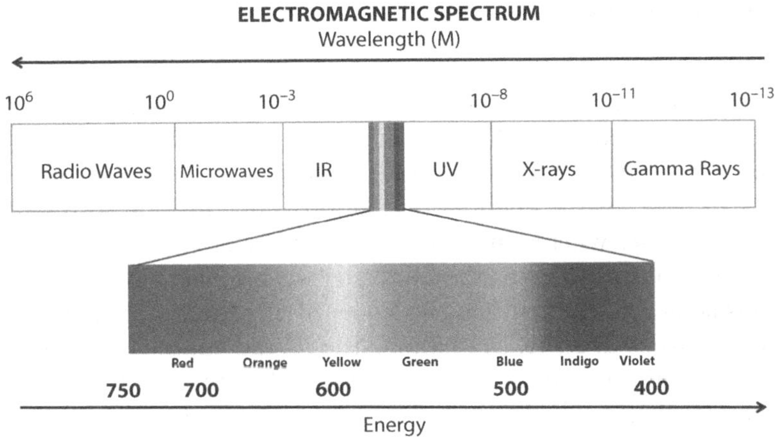

Figure 1.2 Electromagnetic spectrum.

to understand nature. EMR is composed of packets and bundles of energy called photons. The presence of photons imparts dual nature to the EMR; it behaves and propagates in the form of waves or particles. The waves move along in a perpendicular manner to each other. Thus, spectroscopy is the study of the electromagnetic spectrum and how dispersion of light occurs into various constituents and finally how matter behaves on interaction with light. Analytically speaking, every element or compound has a specific way it behaves when varying intensities of light are bombarded on it [10]. The output of the analysis is an electromagnetic spectrograph that quantifies the wavelength of the light that is emitted by the substance, in the form of graphs. The graph comprises lines that are unique to the specific element that emitted it, thus aiding the scientist in reaching a positive conclusion. Additionally, spectroscopy measures the amount of light absorbed by the substance, thereby deciphering the concentration of the element.

When heat is applied to a substance, it diffuses out light at a particular wavelength. Spectroscopy utilizes this chemical attribute for determining the characteristic element that is there in the sample. Spectroscopy is and can be utilized to identify numerous types of evidence that are recovered from the location of crime. Drugs, Fibers, Ink, Glass, Paint, Explosives, Trace elements and can additionally be used to identify contaminants that are found in the diverse material that is at our disposal for analysis [3].

The following section will shed some light on various classical and contemporary approaches in spectroscopy, namely; IR Spectroscopy, UV-Visible Spectroscopy, MS, AAS, AES and NMR.

1.2.1.1 *Infrared Spectroscopy*

There are two principal regions that aid in characterization of unknown substances; namely Ultraviolet-Visible and Infrared Region. Infrared (IR) region in comparison to the Ultraviolet (UV) region has lower energy-lower frequency but a higher wavelength. In case of UV-Visible spectroscopy, the analyte absorbs the energy of radiation and transition to the higher orbital takes place whereas in case of IR Spectroscopy there is not enough energy to be absorbed, thus the bonds between atoms vibrate. Thus, the output is achieved by identifying and quantifying the vibrational frequencies of the atoms upon IR irradiation. The IR radiation has a range from 700 nm to 1 mm. When the energy is absorbed by the bonds, they vibrate in a manner that is like that of a spring, they can rock, twist, stretch and bending in the direction of choice. The frequency, direction and manner of vibration are specific to each compound and thus aid in identification. To impart sensitivity to the technique it is ideally coupled with Fourier Transform which develops the final spectrogram post analysis, where Michelson Interferometers are used for the purpose of calibration. This is based on the principle of interference (constructive & destructive) radiation that is emitted by the evidence under evaluation. The technique is preferred as it is non-destructive in nature and is compatible for biological sample, counterfeited products, gun-shot residue, and explosives. Near-IR Spectroscopy has the same principle as of IR but it utilizes the near IR radiation that ranges between 0.7 mm and 1.4 mm for the analysis of evidence. The technique is quite popular for its ease and non-destructive approach. The energy in the radiation is less thus when the compound absorbs, the spectra achieved has a series of overlapping bonds; which aids in identifying elements that have high light scattering tendencies and strong absorption [10].

IR spectroscopy is commonly used in the analysis of organic molecules, such as polymers and biomolecules. It is also used in the analysis of inorganic materials, such as minerals and ceramics. However, IR spectroscopy has limitations, such as its inability to detect elements lighter than carbon and its sensitivity to sample preparation [29–31].

1.2.1.2 *UV-Visible Spectroscopy*

Ultraviolet Spectroscopy (UV) quantifies the wavelength of a beam and determines the proportion of various components that are present in an analyte [3]. It is a technique that uses the absorption or reflection of ultraviolet and visible light by a sample to determine its composition.

The absorption of light causes electrons in the sample to transition from the ground state to an excited state, and the energy of the absorbed light is equal to the energy difference between the two states. The absorption spectrum of a sample is a plot of the amount of light absorbed versus the wavelength of the light [10].

The technique that quantifies the absorption that occurs in the UV-Vis range; with the UV section being 190 nm to 350nm on the contrary to the visible region that extends from 350 nm to 800 nm. The primary postulate behind the working of UV Visible spectroscopy are the electronic transitions that take place in bonding and antibonding orbitals. These transitions occur in unsaturated compounds. The amount of light they absorb is measured through Beer-Lambert law, depending upon the concentration of sample and path length of light traveling within the sample. It is also suitable for analyzing myriad compounds. The governing principle of the technique is the excitation of electrons from ground level to a higher energy level after absorbing the desired intensity of transmitted light. The sample when bombarded with a light that has a high energy source, the electrons absorb energy and transition to a higher energy level. Conversely, over time the absorbed energy is lost and comes back to the previous state by releasing light of specific wavelength. Each element emits a light that is highly specific and unique thus aiding in elemental analysis and identification [10]. The output that is achieved through UV Spectroscopy is compared with the graphs in the database as part of the quantitative analysis to yield fruitful outputs. The technique is suitable for detecting drugs in blood, saliva and urine samples analyze the components of food additives, paint, dyes, petroleum products and can also be used to monitor air and water quality [3, 9, 31]. Such products are qualitatively and quantitatively analyzed through Spectroscopy making it the most ubiquitous tool. However, UV-Vis spectroscopy has limitations, such as its inability to distinguish between compounds with similar absorption spectra and its sensitivity to sample concentration [32, 33].

1.2.1.3 Nuclear Magnetic Resonance Spectroscopy (NMR)

NMR is an intriguing investigating tool that ascertains the structure of any chemical substance or molecule. The analysis through NMR takes into account nuclei spin and its magnetic moment under the influence of the peripheral magnetic field. The nucleus of an atom contains protons and neutrons that account for the arbitrary orientation spin. Thus, nuclei are considered as tiny magnets having random orientation that cancel out by each other. Under the influence of an external magnetic field, spin of all nuclei tends to be in or opposite direction of external magnetic field. Under the influence of radio frequency from an external source, the nuclei absorb specific energy and will move to a higher energy level from the ground energy level (also switches its orientation in opposite direction in respect to the orientation present under the influence of external magnetic field only). The wavelength and frequency at which this occurs is characteristic and unique to every compound. Upon removing the external source of radio frequency, the absorbed energy (specific to the compound) is released that is detected by the detector and nuclei come back to the ground state along with previous orientation. The detected energy is encoded in the form of peaks (as represented in Figure 1.3) that are characteristic to the compound.

Hydrogen is used in NMR as hydrogen has a single proton in the nucleus resulting in a better spectrum, Phosphorus is also an alternative for analysis of evidence. NMR is used for the examination of body fluids, toxins, drugs as well as for examining the post-mortem changes. Being extremely sensitive, NMR is used not only to elucidate the structure of compounds but can also be used to identify impurities thereby determining the quality making it an essential tool in the field of forensic.

NMR spectroscopy is commonly used in the analysis of organic molecules, such as proteins and carbohydrates. It is also used in the analysis of inorganic materials, such as minerals and catalysts. However, NMR spectroscopy has limitations, such as its sensitivity to sample purity and its inability to detect elements with low natural abundance [34, 35].

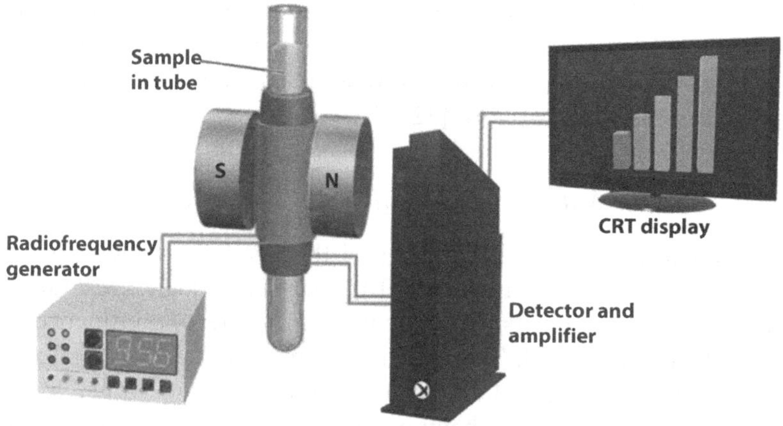

Figure 1.3 Diagrammatic representation of NMR.

1.2.1.4 Mass Spectrometer (MS)

Mass Spectroscopy when coupled with Gas Chromatography deciphers the m/z ratio of the molecule/s that is present in the evidence. The sample is loaded into the mass spectrometer; that will be turned into vapor and into ions (charged particles). These charged particles are then transferred through an electric and magnetic field. The distance it covers/travels will be directly proportional to the m/z ratio. The final output will be decoded by a detector. Each element has an extremely exclusive field; thus, MS is an indispensable tool for the precise examination of exhibits procured from various crime scenes [3, 9, 31]. MS analyses organic compounds by vaporizing them into gaseous form followed by segregating the ion as their mass/charge ratio (m/z).

Mass Spectrometer as represented in Figure 1.4 is made up of the following parts:

- An **ion source** where ionization takes place through electron impact, plasma desorption, fast atom bombardment, thermospray ionization, chemical ionization or through laser desorption;
- a **mass analyzer** where the ions get segregated through ion trap, magnetic sector, time of flight (TOF), or through a quadruple according to their mass to charge ratio; and
- a **detector** which can be faraday cups, photomultiplier tubes or scintillators that identifies the separated ions.

The mass spectrum is plotted wherein mass to charge ratio is plotted against their relative intensity. The highest intensity peak in the spectrum

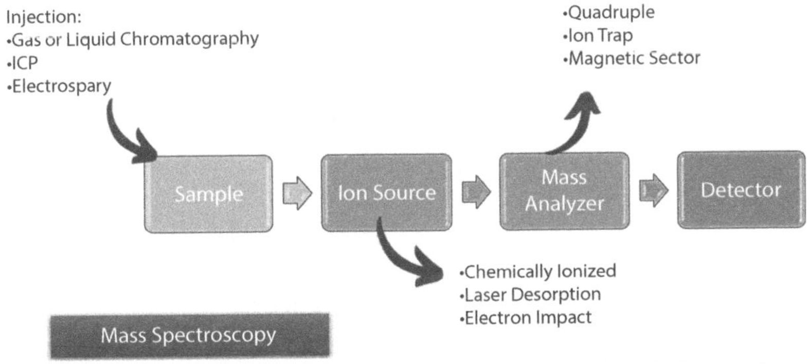

Figure 1.4 Flow chart representing the functioning of mass spectrometer.

is the point where the substance fragmented and ionized as per the molecular weight of the parent ion of the analyte. In order to increase efficiency; mass-spectroscopy is coupled with thin layer chromatography, gas or liquid chromatography to obtain more accurate analysis of forensic evidence.

The two properties of mass spectroscopy make it a suitable tool in analytical chemistry and is an ideal choice for Forensic Chemistry. Firstly, while transferring energy, if the source is monitored and is stable, the fragmentation of ions for the substance under evaluation can be reproducible. Lastly, the spectrum achieved post analysis is extremely specific to the substance and thus can be used for the purpose of identification.

The technique estimates the substance under examination both quantitatively and structurally. Both form of sample i.e., Solid and liquid can be examined through this technique [36]. 2.1.5 Atomic Absorption Spectroscopy (AAS) and Atomic Emission Spectroscopy (AES) Atomic Absorption Spectroscopy (AAS) quantifies the specific wavelength that is absorbed by atoms of substance under examination [3, 9, 31].

This type of spectroscopy considers the light absorbed and light emitted by atoms of analyte. These methods are quite effective when it comes to carrying out the elemental profiling of the analyte. AAS: As depicted in Figure 1.5, a typical atomic absorption spectrometer has four major components: the light source, the atomization system, the monochromator,

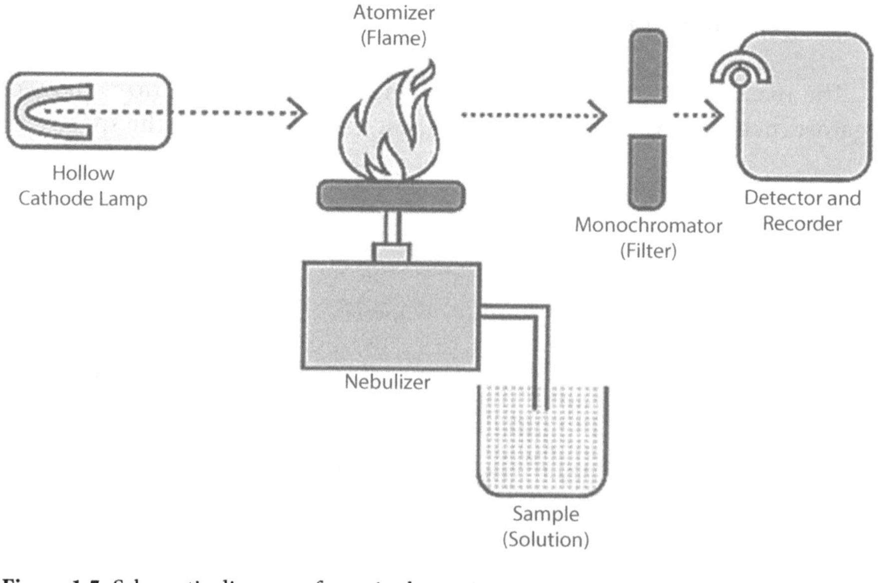

Figure 1.5 Schematic diagram of atomic absorption spectrometer.

and the detecting system. Liquid or solid samples are nebulized and subsequently atomized in either a flame or a graphite furnace. The unbound atoms are then illuminated by light, which is commonly emitted by a lamp with a hollow cathode, and experience electronic transitions from the ground state to excited electronic states by absorbing a light of certain wavelength that is characteristic to the atom [10].

As stated above, AAS depends on the element being sampled to absorb the radiation which is emanated by the source; it adheres to the Beer Lambert law. This law establishes a correlation between the quantity of radiation that is absorbed and the concentration of the element in the sample [37].

Between the sample and the detector, a monochromator is inserted to decrease background interference. The detector then translates the measured intensity of the light beam into absorption data. Therefore, it may be utilized for the purpose of carrying out the quantitative analysis of the element in the sample. Solid samples can be utilized for AAS analysis, although typically only in graphite furnaces with controlled electrical heating as opposed to a direct flame. Moreover, AAS is often exclusively employed to examine metal atoms. The primary reason is that these metals have single emission and absorption lines that are narrow, brilliant, and distinct [37]. The technique is suitable for deciphering various heavy-metal

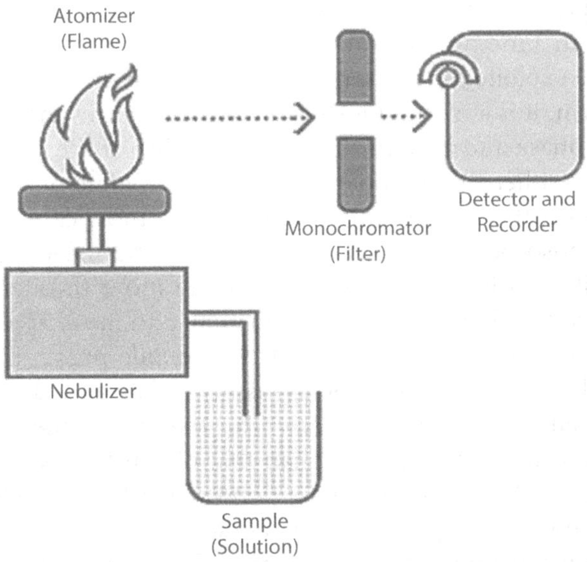

Figure 1.6 Schematic diagram of atomic emission spectrometer.

contaminants that are present in air, water, and soil samples. Paint and soil samples when analyzed using AAS can aid in identifying the location at which the crime took place [3, 9, 31].

AES: This method relies on the excitation of electrons to higher energy levels by the absorption of a certain wavelength at high temperatures. When excited species depart the high-temperature zone, they return to their ground states by emitting discrete wavelength packets of radiation. As depicted in Figure 1.6, these emissions travel via a monochromator or filter before being detected.

The excited levels have an extremely brief lifespan (10-8 s). This emission is specific to the element that can be found in the sample. As a result of the fact that the amount of radiation emitted is related to its concentration, quantitative analysis may also be done. This method can perform analyses on a wide variety of samples, including fibers, GSR, and combustible substances [10, 38, 39].

1.2.2 Chromatographic Techniques

Mikhail Tsvett, a Russian scientist, is credited with being the one who originally established chromatography in the year 1900. In the beginning, it was utilized for the purpose of separating the plant pigments found in a leaf. Chromatography is a technique that separates components of a mixture depending on the physical characteristics of those components. The basic principle of chromatography is based upon the fact that different components in a mixture have different physical and chemical properties, which can be exploited to separate them from each other. In its most fundamental form, it is a method for separating substances that makes use of a stationary phase and a mobile phase. The ability of the analytes to have an affinity for either the stationary phase or the mobile phase determines which direction the separation will proceed. In most cases, the analytes will become adsorbed on the stationary phase if they have a greater affinity towards it. This is because the analytes will move through the system at a slower speed. They have a greater tendency to move at a faster speed if they have a stronger affinity towards the mobile phase. Based on this fundamental concept, it is possible to readily isolate and identify the analytes contained inside any substance. The retention time of substances that move at a slow rate is greater than that of substances that move at a quicker rate, which has a shorter retention time [10]. In the chromatography technique known as paper chromatography, a trace quantity of a liquid combination is positioned close to the base of a sheet of paper. In the process of paper chromatography, the RF value is determined as the distance travelled by the substance divided by the distance travelled by the solvent. Chromatography is utilized in the arena of forensic science for the purpose of analyzing pigments found in fibers, testing for the presence of explosives or accelerants, and determining whether narcotics are present in bodily fluids or not. Paper chromatography has been superseded by more technologically advanced kinds of chromatography. The components of a mixture can be identified with the assistance of gas chromatography, which maps each spike to a distinct component of the mixture. The relative heights provide information about the proportional abundance of each component. In forensic laboratories, the chromatographic techniques of thin layer chromatography (TLC), gas chromatography (GC), and high-performance liquid chromatography (HPLC) are frequently utilized. In contrast to GC, the HPLC method may be carried out at ambient temperature. Therefore, HPLC can be utilized in the process of detecting the presence of combustible substances, such as explosives or accelerants [3, 9, 31].

1.2.2.1 Gas Chromatography (GC)

Gas chromatography is used to separate volatile compounds, which are compounds that can be easily vaporized. The sample is injected and vaporized by heating the column that is filled with a stationary phase. The mobile phase is an inert or noble gas like argon or helium which act as a carrier for a sample. Thus, this method involves transporting the analyte through the column in conjunction with the mobile phase (also known as carrier gas). At this point, the sample will be separated at various retention times depending on whether it has a stronger affinity for the stationary phase or the mobile phase. Even though this method offers a great deal of adaptability, it does have a few limitations. Because the sample must first be brought to the vapor state before it can be analyzed, this method cannot be used on substances that are thermally unstable. This is because such substances are more likely to undergo pyrolysis. It is feasible, however, to precisely segregate the components present in an analyte by making use of the required sample preparation processes and the use of protectants to maintain the authenticity of the sample. Some of the forensic samples that are extensively examined include illegal substances and the amount of alcohol in the blood. This method is also capable of detecting explosives and other flammable compounds, accelerants, and even pesticides and toxins. It is yet one of the fascinating types of chromatography that is frequently used in the arena of forensic all around the world [40, 41].

1.2.2.2 High Performance Liquid Chromatography (HPLC)

Liquid chromatography is used to separate non-volatile compounds, which are compounds that cannot be easily vaporized. The sample is dissolved in a liquid and passed through a column that is packed with a stationary phase and the mobile phase (in liquid state) in conjugation with prepared the sample is forced through the column at high pressure. In HPLC, the whole procedure is automated, and at the present time, several equipment come packaged along with autosamplers. The stationary phase (generally silica gel) can come in a variety of forms, such as normal phase, reverse phase, ion exchange, and size exclusion. The mobile phase of normal phase HPLC columns is less polar than the stationary phase. In columns that use the reverse phase separation technique, the stationary phase is nonpolar, while the mobile phase that is utilized is polar. Size exclusion columns employ acidic or basic columns and porous stationary phases. Ion exchange chromatography is used to separate charged compounds. The stationary phase is made up of charged groups, and the mobile phase is a solution of ions of opposite charge. The examination of each sample calls for the development of a unique protocol, which considers a variety of criteria, including the kind of column that will be utilized, the mobile phase, the pH of the mobile phase, the flow rate, the retention duration, and the pressure.

In HPLC, the detectors that are employed might also change depending on the type of material that is being examined. The ultraviolet/visible light detector, the fluorescence detector, the electrochemical detector, the conductivity detector, the evaporative light scattering detector, and the chiral detector are examples of commonly used detectors.

The HPLC technique is used to investigate illegal substances including opioids, pesticides, cannabis, alkaloids, plant toxins, and poisons [34, 42, 43].

1.2.2.3 High Performance Thin Layer Chromatography (HPTLC)

When it comes to the examination of forensic evidence, HPTLC is likely one of the chromatographic methods that is capable of the greatest degree of flexibility. In this method, an adsorbent or stationary phase-coated thin-layer chromatography or TLC plate is employed, and it is then incubated in a chamber that is saturated with the mobile phase. Before beginning the chromatographic development process, the material is also put very carefully onto the TLC plate. In this scenario, the length of time that the analytes contained in the sample have been traveling is considered when determining the retention period of the samples. This method is exceptionally helpful in the field of forensic science since it generates photographic evidence of the facts that can be effortlessly produced in court. In addition to this, every stage in this method is independent of the one that comes before it, which helps to keep any cumulative mistakes to a minimum. This method is typically used to evaluate samples such as illegal narcotics and poisons; however, it may also be used to identify samples of adulterants in food, counterfeit ink, and fabric, and even explosives. In addition, this method is widely used to examine materials. This method also provides outstanding automation, optimization, and detection capabilities while requiring only a little amount of sample preparation [34, 44].

1.2.3 Hyphenated Techniques

Hyphenated techniques refer to the combination of two or more analytical techniques in order to provide more comprehensive and accurate results than each individual technique could provide alone. These techniques have become increasingly popular in recent years, as they allow for a more complete understanding of complex systems and materials. Even if methods of chromatography are helpful for segregating the analytes and their detection is discovered through their retention time, it is not always feasible to estimate the chemical structure with complete accuracy. Because of this, these approaches are frequently combined with others that can shed light on the molecular structure. The most common hyphenated techniques involve coupling chromatography with spectroscopy, which can provide both separation and identification of analytes in a sample. GC, HPLC, and HPTLC are frequently combined or linked with other analytical instruments such as mass spectrometers (MS), FTIR, and nuclear magnetic resonance [45].

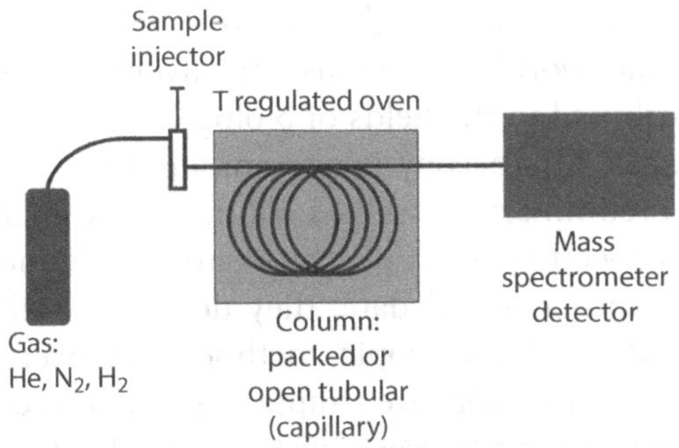

Figure 1.7 Diagrammatic representation of GC-MS.

In the GC-MS method, the material is first separated, as it would be in a standard GC analysis as represented in Figure 1.7.

After they have been isolated from one another, a specialized device is used to connect the 2 instruments. The analyte from the GC is then delivered to the MS via this device. Afterward, the MS sheds light on the composition of the molecule's structure. GC-MS is commonly used in forensic science, environmental analysis, and pharmaceutical analysis, among other fields [46]. In a manner analogous to this, when using LC-MS, once the chemicals have been separated using the chromatographic method, they are subjected to structural analysis by the MS. LC-MS is commonly used in drug discovery, proteomics, and metabolomics.

Fourier Transform Infrared Spectroscopy-Gas Chromatography (FTIR-GC): This technique combines the ability of FTIR to identify functional groups with the separation capabilities of GC. FTIR-GC is commonly used in the analysis of polymers, plastics, and other organic materials. High Performance Liquid Chromatography-Nuclear Magnetic Resonance Spectroscopy (HPLC-NMR): This technique combines the separation capabilities of HPLC with the structural information provided by NMR. HPLC-NMR is commonly used in the analysis of natural products, such as plant extracts.

Like FTIR and MS, HPTLC may also be used with other analytical techniques. The connection that ties the two together is an essential component of hyphenated strategies like these. Overall, hyphenated techniques provide powerful analytical tools that allow for the identification and quantification of complex mixtures. These techniques have become essential tools in many fields of forensic science, and their use is likely to continue to grow in the future [45–48].

1.2.4 Microscopic Techniques

The microscope is an instrument that has revolutionized the way we see and understand the world around us. Its invention and development have greatly contributed to the fields of biology, chemistry, medicine, and many other sciences. Microscopy is one among the most popular methods adopted for preliminary as well as confirmatory analyses of forensic evidence. Though spectroscopic and chromatographic methods can yield precise structural and chemical data, they do not actually represent the substance morphology. Microscopic methods get over this restriction and give objective findings that are simple to present in court rooms. The modern microscope, however, was developed in the 19th century. It was made possible using new technologies, such as better lenses and improved illumination sources. With these advancements, scientists were able to study microscopic structures in greater detail and with greater accuracy. The microscope is used in medicine to diagnose diseases, study cells and tissues, and develop new drugs and therapies. The microscope is also used in forensics to analyze evidence, such as hair, fibers, and bloodstains. This section emphasizes on optical, electron, and probe microscopes [10].

1.2.4.1 Optical Microscope

One of the most compliant and widely utilized instruments for visualizing forensic evidence encountered at crime scenes are Optical Microscopes. They can examine the samples by striking evidence with a proper light source that produces photons. The resulting photons then interact with the sample under examination, and a set of objective lenses gathers the light that is reflected and scattered as a result from the specimen [49].

The simple and compound microscopes are the two main categories of optical microscopes. Simple Microscope: It is a simple device that uses a convex and concave lens to magnify objects. Compound microscope: It is one of the most frequently used microscopes in laboratories. For higher magnification, this microscope utilizes numerous lenses and different light sources.

The magnification of a compound microscope (Figure 1.8) typically ranges from 40X to 2,000X. The compound microscope is made up of numerous objectives with a variety of magnifications and condenser lenses, while the simple microscope just has one lens. Compound microscopes are the most common type of optical microscope used in any forensic laboratory. An appropriate source of light, a condenser lens for the collection of light rays and then focusing light from the light source and impounding it on to the specimen, and a variety of objective lenses for gathering and

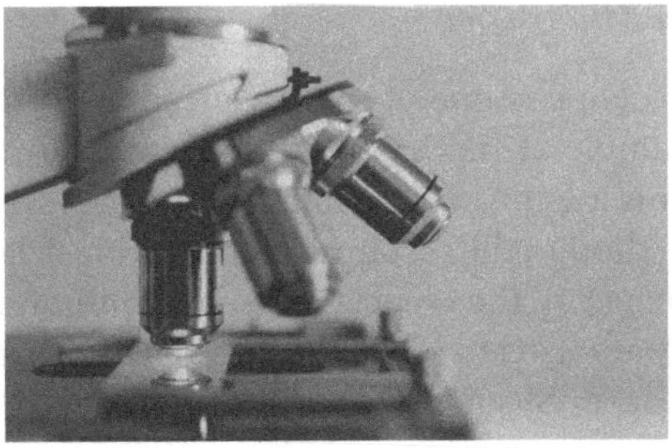

Figure 1.8 Compound microscope.

focusing light from the specimen are used to compensate for a compound microscope. The objective lens provides high magnification, while the eyepiece lens magnifies the image further and allows the observer to see the specimen in detail. For the investigation of various types of evidence, fluorescence microscopes, phase contrast microscopes, polarized microscopes, bright field microscopes, and stereo microscopes are microscopes used in often practices. Though these are the further modifications of typical optical microscopes.

In forensic science, a compound microscope is used in several applications, including:

1. Examination of trace evidence: A compound microscope is used to examine small particles of evidence, such as hair, fibers, and dust, which can be crucial in criminal investigations. The microscope allows forensic experts to study the morphology and characteristics of these particles, helping to identify their origin and potential relevance to the investigation.
2. Examination of fingerprints: A compound microscope is used to examine the ridge patterns of fingerprints, which can help to identify suspects or link a suspect to a crime scene.
3. Ballistic analysis: A compound microscope is used to examine bullets and cartridge cases in ballistic analysis. By studying the marks left on the bullet or cartridge, forensic experts can determine the type of firearm used and potentially link the firearm to the crime.
4. Miscellaneous analysis: Optical microscopes can also be used to examine materials like fibers, glass, paints, and even disputed documents up to an extent [50].

1.2.4.2 Electron Microscope

An Electron Microscope is one of the advanced and precise microscopes that can view a sample at higher resolution with substantial magnification. Electron beams are the critical source of image formation in electron microscopes. Even though the resulting picture is black and white, electron microscopes can magnify the objects up to two million times with appreciable quality. They are used to study the internal structure of cells, viruses, and other microscopic objects [51].

Scanning Electron Microscope (SEM), and Transmission Electron Microscope (TEM) are the two most prevalent kinds of electron microscopes. The Scanning Electron Microscope is used to examine the material's surface morphology while the Transmission Electron Microscope is used for material's internal structure analyses.

The scanning electron microscope (SEM) creates a three-dimensional image by moving an electron beam across the surface of a subject. In the SEM technique, the impact of incoming electrons on the sample generates the emission of backscattered and secondary electrons that characterize the surface morphology, while in the TEM approach, transmitted electrons are detected. Under Transmission Electron Microscope (TEM), an electron beam travels through a thin piece of a specimen under examination. Image of interior structure of the specimen is created as a result that is viewed on the computer screen or through the ocular unit.

SEM is well suited for conducting materials, so that the incident electrons may readily interact with the surface of the sample being examined. Therefore, the sample preparation for SEM requires coating with a metal, like gold. On the other hand, the samples used in TEM must be extremely thin for the electrons to easily pass through them. As per the type of evidence obtained from crime scenes, SEM has found more use in forensic science than TEM. These methods make it simple to photograph small samples and see their minute outer surface or interior surface characteristics. Several biological pieces of evidence, such as hairs, fibers, pollens, teeth, skin cells, and bone cells, are frequently analyzed in forensic materials with the aid of SEM and TEM. An image of pollen grains as examined through SEM is represented in Figure 1.9.

Beside this, electron microscopy has also been used to investigate a variety of anthropogenic and geological samples [51–53].

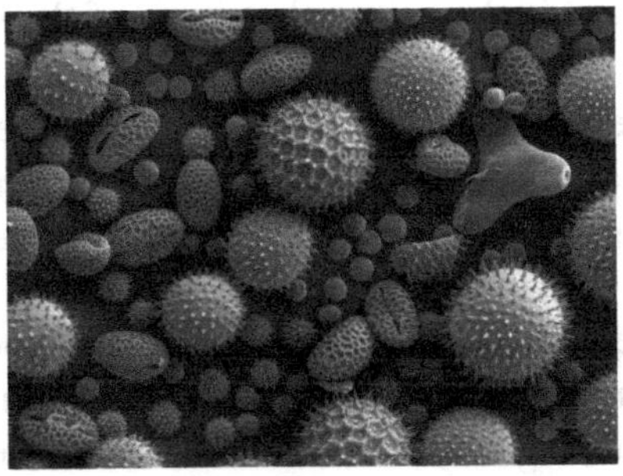

Figure 1.9 An image through SEM showing pollen grains.

1.2.4.3 Stereomicroscope

It is a type of microscope that provides a three-dimensional view of the object being observed. This is achieved by using two eyepieces and two separate objective lenses, which work together to create a stereo image. The specimen's surface reflects the light from a stereomicroscope, also known as a dissecting microscope. The light's reflection in a stereo microscope creates a 3D image and has a large working space that is beneficial for dissecting or creating a three-dimensional image of evidence to view the minute details. It is used to study larger specimens that cannot be viewed under a compound microscope. The stereomicroscope also makes surface features more evident [3, 9, 31].

The stereo microscope is widely used in various fields, including forensic science, due to its ability to provide a high level of detail and clarity.

In forensic science, the stereo microscope is used for a variety of purposes. One of its primary applications is in the examination of evidence collected from crime scenes, such as hairs, fibers, and other small particles. The stereo microscope allows forensic scientists to view these objects in three dimensions, which can reveal details that might not be visible with a traditional microscope. For example, the stereo microscope can be used to identify the color, texture, and shape of fibers, which can help link them to a suspect or a particular location.

Another important application of the stereo microscope in forensic science is in the analysis of tool marks. Tool marks are often left at the scene of a crime and can provide valuable evidence in identifying the perpetrator. The stereo microscope can be used to examine these marks in detail, allowing forensic scientists to determine the type of tool used and to compare it to tools found in the possession of suspects.

The stereo microscope is also used in forensic anthropology to examine bones and other skeletal remains. By examining these remains under a stereo microscope, forensic scientists can identify unique features that can help identify the individual, such as the shape of the skull or the presence of certain bone abnormalities. The paint chips, bug larvae, fake and genuine coins, gunshot residues, bullet striations, cartridge markings, currency notes, and other small pieces of evidence can be examined through a stereomicroscope. Image of two spent cartridges and fiber as viewed through stereomicroscope is shown in Figure 1.10.

In conclusion, the stereo microscope is a valuable tool in forensic science due to its ability to provide a detailed, three-dimensional view of objects. Its applications in examining evidence collected from crime scenes, analyzing

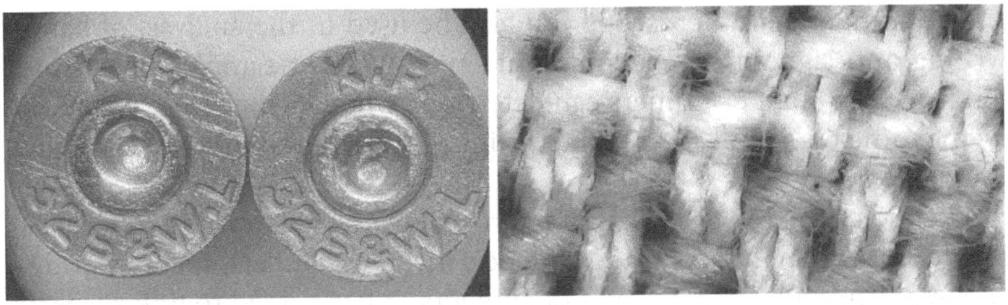

Figure 1.10 Images taken from stereo microscope.

tool marks, and examining skeletal remains make it an essential tool for forensic scientists in their investigations [10, 54, 55].

1.2.4.4 Comparison Microscope

A comparison microscope is a specialized tool used in forensic science for the side-by-side comparison of two separate specimens, usually bullets, fibers, or other trace evidence. The comparison microscope consists of two optical microscopes that are joined with the help of prisms and mirror to a single eyepiece. The microscope has two separate optical paths that allow the examiner to view each specimen simultaneously, making it easier to compare the two specimens.

Comparison of two samples can be done simultaneously under two objectives of comparison microscopes. The sample under examination is usually kept under left objective lens and the control or the known specimen under the right objective lens. The image is formed on the monitor or in the ocular unit that can compare the specimens under both the objective lenses [3, 9, 31]. One of the most significant applications of a comparison microscope in forensic science is the analysis of bullet fragments. When a firearm is discharged, the bullet may fragment upon impact with the target, leaving tiny pieces of metal behind. By comparing the markings left on a fragment to those left on a known bullet fired from the same gun, forensic scientists can determine whether the fragment came from that gun or a different one. This technique is known as ballistic fingerprinting and has been used to link suspects to crimes where firearms were used. Another application of a comparison microscope is in the analysis of fibers found at a crime scene. By comparing fibers found on a suspect or at the scene of the crime to fibers found on the victim or at the suspect's residence, forensic scientists can determine whether there is a link between the suspect and the crime scene.

The comparison microscope can also be used in the analysis of handwriting and signatures. By comparing two different samples of writing, forensic document examiners can determine whether they were produced by the same person or not. This technique is often used in cases involving fraud or forgery.

In conclusion, the comparison microscope is a valuable tool in forensic science for the analysis of trace evidence, including bullets, spent cartridge case markings, fibers, hairs, and documents. It has helped to link suspects to crimes and has been used to secure convictions in numerous criminal cases [10, 50, 56].

1.2.4.5 Energy Dispersive X-Ray Coupled Microscopy in Forensic Science

The Energy dispersive X-ray (EDX) spectroscopy has been found to be a very effective elemental mapping technique that can analyze the elemental composition of the material under examination. The sample is exposed to an electron beam which causes the generation of secondary electrons such as the backscattered electrons, auger electrons and others. These electrons are specific to a particular element in the sample under examination, making it simple to get both quantitative and qualitative information about that specific component. Thus, the distinctive X-ray emissions from the components are identified that characterize the analyte. When EDX is coupled with the electron microscope, then electron gun serves as the source for both the instruments. To efficiently gather scattered electrons, the EDX detector is often placed in the proximity of the sample. Si-lithium or silicon drift detectors are majorly used detectors for the purpose. The electron beam's accelerating voltage and the sample's thickness play a vital role in determining the elemental information as can also be seen in electron microscopy. In forensic science, EDX and SEM have frequently been used together to evaluate samples and to gather maximum information from the specimen that can further be compared with the control sample for presentation in the courtroom. This technique is often used to evaluate common forensic evidence, such as: biological material, explosives, contaminants, etc. Additionally, this method is used to evaluate pigments, glass, and gunshot residue [57, 58].

1.2.5 X-Ray Diffraction (XRD)

XRD is a method for assessing a material's crystallinity. Elastic or inelastic scattering occurs in XRD when X-rays, typically of greater energy, strike the atoms that are organized in a material. In inelastic scattering, the energy of the scattered rays is not the same as the energy of the incident rays whereas in elastic scattering, the scattered rays have the same energy as the incident electron. As a result, depending on the sample's crystal orientation, there may be constructive or destructive interference. Bragg's law, which considers the angle between the radiation and the crystal planes, the wavelength of the radiation, and the distance between the crystal planes, governs constructive interference. It is possible to learn more about the sample's crystallinity by using the Bragg equation. The angle between the incident ray and the crystallographic planes is typically fixed or varied throughout analysis. The X-ray sources are often created by exposing metals like copper, molybdenum, or iron to a high-voltage electron beam while they are in a vacuum. The samples can be examined as complete crystals or in pulverized form. The category of X-ray diffraction method can also be chosen based on the type of sample to be studied. This approach frequently employs charge coupled, solid state, or scintillation detectors. Drugs, minerals, and other metals crystalline structures have all been frequently examined using XRD. However, it has also been employed in forensic science to examine paints, pigments, bones, and even fibers [59–61].

1.2.6 Nanotechnology

The study of nanomaterials, or substances with a size in the nanoscale range, is known as nanotechnology. Nanomaterials possess improved optical, magnetic, and electrical properties as a result of their small size. They have a wide array of uses in a variety of applications because of their characteristics. Nanomaterials including nanoparticles, nanoshells, nanofibers, and nanotubes are frequently employed in a variety of fields. Nonetheless, these nanoparticles are routinely functionalized, meaning that a guest molecule or functional group is regularly added to their surface in order to change them. The inherent qualities of nanoparticles are further improved via functionalization [62].

The two most common techniques for generating nanomaterials are the bottom-up and the top-down techniques. In the first bottom-up approach, a precursor salt solution, and a catalyst or reducing agent are used to make nanomaterials. The bulk material is crushed to nanoparticles using a variety of mechanical and chemical processes in the top-down approach. These nanomaterials are characterized using a variety of spectroscopic, electron, and probe microscopic methods. To obtain elemental information, EDX is typically combined with electron microscopes. Nanomaterials have been extensively employed in forensic research to create sensors that can find explosives, gunshot residue, and other poisons and pesticides. Since they can easily attach to a fingerprint's ridges due to their nano size, they have also been utilized to identify latent fingerprints, enabling for more sensitive and selective fingerprint recognition with better contrast [63–66].

1.3 Conclusion

Forensic science may provide answers to crucial issues about any crime and be used in civil or criminal proceedings. Forensic analysis is essentially the study and application of analytical concepts to any legal issues. The importance of forensic science in the criminal justice system is crucial.

The examination and evaluation of different forensic evidence is crucial since it can be the foundation of any criminal inquiry or crime investigation. In addition to conducting criminal investigations, analyzing different types of evidence is necessary to put legislation and security measures into effect.

Almost all study domains employ a variety of analytical approaches to address issues, and technology is always opening new avenues for research. By using various tools and techniques, forensic investigators continue to identify harmful components of society including drug misuse. Over the years, a variety of analytical techniques have been used to analyze samples such as gunshot residue, illegal drugs, explosives, biological evidence, blood, semen, DNA material, saliva, pollen grains, fabrics, paints, diatoms, pigments, and questioned documents. This chapter has provided a quick overview of the numerous chemical and elemental analytical instruments used for the investigation of innumerable forensic evidence.

Chromatography techniques like HPLC, GC, HPTLC and TLC, spectroscopic techniques like UV-Vis, IR, NMR, Raman, AAS and AES have been utilized for preliminary and confirmatory analysis of evidence. Typically, a Mass Spectrometer is used in conjunction with these approaches to get structure-related information of the evidence. AAS is the most common approach to identify and evaluate metallic compounds. Investigators today investigate the microscopic features of various pieces of evidence that are gathered at crime scenes using a broad variety of analytical procedures and sophisticated equipment. The presence of substances like nicotine and cocaine in hair is identified by the HPLC, and the presence of alcohol and different trace elements is determined through the GC. AAS aids in the analysis of bodily fluids. The microscope is a powerful instrument that has greatly contributed to our understanding of the world around us. Its invention and development have led to many important discoveries in the fields of biology, chemistry, medicine, and many other sciences. Usually, optical and electron microscopic methods give a precise visual of the evidence. In addition to these conventional techniques, emerging analytical technologies, like as nanotechnology and lab-on-a-chip devices, hold great potential for analyzing a wide range of forensic evidence. Recent years have seen a significant advancement in forensic analysis that aids in crime scene reconstruction. Finally, the field of forensic analysis expands significantly through dealing large number of criminal cases.

Referencces

1. B. S. De Martinis, "Forensic analytical chemistry," *Brazilian J. Anal. Chem.*, vol. 5, no. 21, pp. 6–7, 2018.
2. C. Aitken, A. Nordgaard, F. Taroni, and A. Biedermann, "Commentary: Likelihood ratio as weight of forensic evidence: A closer look," *Front. Genet.*, vol. 9, 2018.
3. M. Manimala and K. D. Vijay, "A Review on Forensic Analytical Chemistry," *Pharmatutor*, vol. 5, no. 12, p. 12, 2017.
4. M. Sharma, "Analytical Instrument in Trace Evidence Analysis used in Forensic Sciences," *J. Forensic Sci. Crim. Investig.*, vol. 5, no. 4, 2017.
5. S. Kamanna, J. Henry, N. H. Voelcker, A. Linacre, and K. Paul Kirkbride, "A mass spectrometry-based forensic toolbox for imaging and detecting biological fluid evidence in finger marks and fingernail scrapings," *Int. J. Legal Med.*, vol. 131, pp. 1413–1422, 2017.
6. A. Martyna, D. Ramos, G. Zadora, and C. Aitken, *Statistical analysis in forensic science: evidential value of multivariate physicochemical data.* John Wiley & Sons, 2013.
7. C. C. G. Aitken *et al.*, "ENFSI guideline for evaluative reporting in forensic science," 2015.
8. P. O. and G. Z. Alberto Salomone, "New Approaches in Forensic Analytical Chemistry," *Front. Chem.*, vol. 9, p. 224, 2021.
9. J. A. Siegel and K. Mirakovits, *Forensic science: the basics.* CRC Press, 2015.
10. J. Brier and L.D. jayanti, *Handbook Of Analytical Techniques For Forensic Samples*, vol. 21, no. 1. 2020.
11. G. Biosa, D. Giurghita, E. Alladio, M. Vincenti, and T. Neocleous, "Evaluation of Forensic Data Using Logistic Regression-Based Classification Methods and an R Shiny Implementation." *Front. Chem.*, vol. 8. 2020.
12. K. Pyrek, "Forensic Science Under Siege: The Challenges of Forensic Laboratories and the Medico-Legal Death Investigation System/Kelly M. Pyrek." Amsterdam, 2007.
13. J. Fraser and R. Williams, "The contemporary landscape of forensic science," in *Handbook of Forensic Science*, Willan, pp. 1–20, 2013.

14. M. L. Smith *et al.*, "Modern instrumental methods in forensic toxicology," *J. Anal. Toxicol.*, vol. 31, no. 5, pp. 237– 253, 2007.
15. B. Levine and S. Kerrigan, *Principles of forensic toxicology*, vol. 2. Springer, 1999.
16. L. Wagmann *et al.*, "How to Study the Metabolism of New Psychoactive Substances for the Purpose of ToxicologicalScreenings—A Follow-Up Study Comparing Pooled Human Liver S9, HepaRG Cells, and Zebrafish Larvae." *Front. Chem.*, vol. 8. 2020.
17. M. Putz, T. Piper, and M. Thevis, "Identification of Trenbolone Metabolites Using Hydrogen Isotope Ratio Mass Spectrometry and Liquid Chromatography/High Accuracy/High Resolution Mass Spectrometry for Doping Control Analysis." *Front. Chem.*, vol. 8. 2020.
18. R. Trager, "Forensics in crisis," *Chem. World.*, 2018.
19. J. Kawai, "Forensic analysis of the Wakayama arsenic murder case," in *Forensic Analysis-From Death to Justice*, IntechOpen, 2016.
20. A. T. Navare, J. G. Mayoral, M. Nouzova, F. G. Noriega, and F. M. Fernández, "Rapid direct analysis in real time (DART) mass spectrometric detection of juvenile hormone III and its terpene precursors," *Anal. Bioanal. Chem.*, vol. 398, pp. 3005–3013, 2010.
21. L. Calò, L. Anzillotti, C. Maccari, R. Cecchi, and R. Andreoli, "Validation of a Bioanalytical Method for the Determination of Synthetic and Natural Cannabinoids (New Psychoactive Substances) in Oral Fluid Samples by Means of HPLC-MS/MS." *Front. Chem.*, vol. 8. 2020.
22. T. M. G. Salerno, P. Donato, G. Frison, L. Zamengo, and L. Mondello, "Gas Chromatography—Fourier Transform Infrared Spectroscopy for Unambiguous Determination of Illicit Drugs: A Proof of Concept." *Front. Chem.*, vol. 8. 2020.
23. E. Bulska *et al.*, "Comprehensive Protocol for the Identification and Characterization of New Psychoactive Substances in the Service of Law Enforcement Agencies." *Front. Chem.*, vol. 8. 2020.
24. L. Niewoehner, "Chemometric Analysis of GSR data–first results," in *ENFSI Firearms Working Group Meeting, Metropolitan Laboratory, The Forensic Science Service, London, UK*, vol. 29, 1998.
25. Z. Brozek-Mucha and G. Zadora, "Frequency of occurrence of certain chemical classes of GSR from various ammunition types," *Z Zagadnien Nauk Sadowych*, vol. 46, pp. 281–287, 2001.
26. Z. Brozek-Mucha and A. Jankowicz, "Evaluation of the possibility of differentiation between various types of ammunition by means of GSR examination with SEM–EDX method." *Forensic Sci. Int.*, vol. 123, no. 1, pp. 39–47, 2001.
27. R. D. Koons, "Analysis of gunshot primer residue collection swabs by inductively coupled plasma-mass spectrometry." *J. Forensic Sci.*, vol. 43, no. 4, pp. 748–754, 1998.
28. B. L. Gulson, J. C. Eames, and J. D. Davis, "Evaluation of exhibits from a murder case using the lead isotope method and scanning electron microscopy." *J. Forensic Sci.*, vol. 47, no. 5, pp. 1015–1021, 2002.

29. S. Bell and Y. Xu, "Infrared spectroscopy| Industrial applications," in *Encyclopedia of Analytical Science*, Elsevier, pp. 124–133, 2018.
30. M. El-Azazy, "Introductory Chapter: Infrared Spectroscopy - A Synopsis of the Fundamentals and Applications," M. El-Azazy, Ed. Rijeka: IntechOpen, p. Ch. 1, 2018.
31. A. V Ewing and S. G. Kazarian, "Infrared spectroscopy and spectroscopic imaging in forensic science," *Analyst*, vol. 142, no. 2, pp. 257–272, 2017.
32. J. A. Räty, K.-E. Peiponen, and T. Asakura, *UV-visible reflection spectroscopy of liquids*, vol. 92. Springer Science & Business Media, 2004.
33. F. A. Settle, "Chemical instrumentation, evolution of instrumentation for uv-visible spectrophotometry," *J. Chem. Educ.*, 1986.
34. C. M. Hussain, D. Rawtani, G. Pandey, and M. Tharmavaram, *Handbook of Analytical Techniques for Forensic Samples: Current and Emerging Developments*. Elsevier, 2020.
35. M. V. S. Elipe, "LC-NMR and other hyphenated NMR techniques: Overview and applications," 2011.
36. E.De Hoffmann and V. Stroobant, *Mass spectrometry: Principles and applications*. John Wiley & Sons, 2007.
37. S. P. Singhal, "Atomic absorption spectroscopy in forensic chemistry," *Can. Soc. Forensic Sci. J.*, vol. 7, no. 1, pp. 7– 17, 1974.
38. G. M. Hieftje, "Atomic Emission Spectroscopy—It Lasts and Lasts and Lasts," *J. Chem. Educ.*, vol. 77, no. 5, p. 577, 2000.
39. G. L. Moore, *Introduction to inductively coupled plasma atomic emission spectrometry*. Elsevier, 2012.
40. J. Swinley and P. de Coning, *A practical guide to gas analysis by gas chromatography*. Elsevier, 2019.
41. L. M. Blumberg, "Theory of gas chromatography," in *Gas chromatography*, Elsevier, pp. 19–97, 2021.
42. M. K. Ghosh, *HPLC methods on drug analysis*. Springer Science & Business Media, 2012.
43. S. Ahuja and M. Dong, *Handbook of pharmaceutical analysis by HPLC*. Elsevier, 2005.
44. P. S. Variyar, S. Chatterjee, and A. Sharma, "Fundamentals and theory of HPTLC-based separation," *High performance thin-layer Chromatogr.*, pp. 27–39, 2011.
45. S. Gocan, "10 Hyphenated Techniques," *Adv. Chromatogr. Vol. 47*, vol. 47, p. 353, 2009.
46. O. D. Sparkman, Z. Penton, and F. G. Kitson, *Gas chromatography and mass spectrometry: A practical guide*. Academic press, 2011.
47. M. J. Bogusz, "Hyphenated liquid chromatographic techniques in forensic toxicology.," *J. Chromatogr. B. Biomed. Sci. Appl.*, vol. 733, no. 1–2, pp. 65–91, 1999.
48. C. G. Awuchi, H. Twinomuhwezi, and C. G. Awuchi, "Hyphenated techniques," in *Analytical Techniques in Biosciences*, Elsevier, pp. 125–145, 2022.

49. R. Haynes, *Optical microscopy of materials*. Springer Science & Business Media, 2013.
50. S. Saadat, G. Pandey, and M. Tharmavaram, "Microscopy for forensic investigations," *Technol. Forensic Sci. Sampling, Anal. Data Regul.*, pp. 101–127, 2020.
51. S. Amelinckx, D. Van Dyck, J. Van Landuyt, and G. van Tendeloo, *Electron microscopy: Principles and fundamentals*. John Wiley & Sons, 2008.
52. J. I. Goldstein *et al.*, "The SEM and its modes of operation," *Scanning Electron Microsc. X-ray Microanal. Third Ed.*, pp. 21–60, 2003.
53. B. Fultz and J. M. Howe, *Transmission electron microscopy and diffractometry of materials*. Springer Science & Business Media, 2012.
54. L. C. da Silva Nunes and P. A. M. dos Santos, "An application of stereoscopy and image processing in forensics: Recovering obliterated firearms serial number," in *5th Iberoamerican Meeting on Optics and 8th Latin American Meeting on Optics, Lasers, and Their Applications*, vol. 5622, pp. 208–212, 2004.
55. P. Sharma, P. Aneja, S. K. Choudhary, and S. Mathur, "Forensic Applications of Stereo Microscope," in *Forensic Microscopy*, CRC Press, pp. 156–181, 2022.
56. A. Chansiri, J. Boonpanya, G. Eksintkun, and S. Noimanee, "A study of toolmark casting by using polymer for comparison microscope analysis in applied biomedical forensic," in *2016 9th Biomedical Engineering International Conference (BMEiCON)*, pp. 1–3, 2016.
57. V.-D. Hodoroaba, "Energy-dispersive X-ray spectroscopy (EDS)," in *Characterization of Nanoparticles*, Elsevier, pp. 397–417, 2020.
58. G. Zadora and Z. Brożek-Mucha, "SEM–EDX—a useful tool for forensic examinations," *Mater. Chem. Phys.*, vol. 81, no. 2–3, pp. 345–348, 2003.
59. L. Brügemann and E. K. E. Gerndt, "Detectors for X-ray diffraction and scattering: A user's overview," *Nucl. Instruments Methods Phys. Res. Sect. A Accel. Spectrometers, Detect. Assoc. Equip.*, vol. 531, no. 1–2, pp. 292–301, 2004.
60. M. Kotrlý, "Using X-ray diffraction in forensic science," *Zeitschrift für Krist. Mater.*, vol. 222, no. 3–4, pp. 193–198, 2007.
61. A. Bishnoi, S. Kumar, and N. Joshi, "Wide-angle X-ray diffraction (WXRD): technique for characterization of nanomaterials and polymer nanocomposites," in *Microscopy methods in nanomaterials characterization*, Elsevier, pp. 313–337, 2017.
62. G. Pandey, D. Rawtani, and Y. K. Agrawal, "Future aspects of halloysite nanotubes in forensic investigations," *J. Nanomedicine Res.*, vol. 6, no. 2, p. 2, 2017.
63. M. Tharmavaram, G. Pandey, and D. Rawtani, "Surface modified halloysite nanotubes: A flexible interface for biological, environmental and catalytic applications," *Adv. Colloid Interface Sci.*, vol. 261, pp. 82–101, 2018.
64. D. Rawtani, M. Tharmavaram, G. Pandey, and C. M. Hussain, "Functionalized nanomaterial for forensic sample analysis," *TrAC Trends Anal. Chem.*, vol. 120, p. 115661, 2019.

65. M. R. KV, V. K. K, P. D. Ghode, and B. E, "Review On Recent Analytical Techniques Used in Forensic Sciences," *Am. J.PharmTech Res.*, vol. 10, no. 2, pp. 164–173, 2020.
66. B. J. Jones, "Microscopy in forensic sciences," in *Springer Handbook of Microscopy*, Springer, pp. 1507–1524, 2019.

2

Forensic Sample Collection and Preparation

Anuj Sharma[1], Poonam Kumari[2], Abhishek R. Rai[2], Varad Nagar[2], Vaibhav Sharma[2], Archana Gautam[3], Tina Sharma[3], Rajeev Kumar[4] and Mahipal Singh Sankhla[3,5]*

[1]Department of Forensic Science, School of Science, ITM University, Gwalior, Madhya Pradesh, India
[2]Department of Forensic Science, Vivekananda Global University, Jaipur, Rajasthan, India
[3]Department of Forensic Science, (UIAHS) Chandigarh University, Mohali, Punjab, India
[4]Department of Forensic Science, SBMS, Galgotias University, Greater Noida, U.P., India
[5]University Centre for Research and Development, (UCRD), Chandigarh University, Mohali, Punjab, India

Abstract

The collection of the sample and its preparation for forensic purposes depends upon the type of sample matrix and the analytes which are taken into consideration, whether the sample is wet or dry. It becomes challenging for Investigator officers to use a standardized method for sample preparation and collection due to the complexity and variety of sample matrix. While making the standardized method for the collection of samples such as fiber, toxic substances, biological fluid, etc. it should be taken into consideration that the integrity of the sample should be maintained, for that chain of custody needs to be maintained till the sample is presented in a court of law. Proper care should be done so that the rate of error while collecting the sample gets minimized. Before the sample is collected it should make sure that the sample analyzed is relevant and the nature and integrity of the sample are maintained. This chapter covers the different method used for collection and their preparation for use in forensic science.

**Corresponding author*: mahi4n6@gmail.com

Priyanka Chhabra, Divya Bajpai Tripathy, Anjali Gupta, Rajeev Kumar, Kajol Bhati and Shruti Shukla (eds.) Advances in Analytical Techniques for Forensic Investigation, (35–68) © 2024 Scrivener Publishing LLC

Keywords: Forensic science, collection, preparation, sample matrix

2.1 Introduction

The collection and selection of samples provide several unique difficulties [1]. The kind and quality of the sample(s) provided to the laboratory have a major role in determining the relevance of any finding. As a result, many pre-analytical factors should be taken into account during sample collection to ensure that there are enough samples of sufficient quality and quantity. Gather cups, bottles, pipes, syringes, needles, cotton, lemons, spoons, silver paper, and any other suspicious household goods since, in some cases, the evidence found at the scene may be the most helpful to forensic investigators. Blood, plasma or serum, urine, hair, nails, exhaled air, oral fluid, and gastric content are the samples that must be obtained *in vivo*. These samples ought to be collected during hospital admission, before the start of treatment [2, 3]. A common origin for the suspect, the evidence, or the crime scene must be determined. The standard is put through the same tests as the sample that was taken at the scene. As a result, the likelihood that the samples are of a common origin is established. The sample's features are next examined. The samples that share an identifiable trait are grouped according to those traits. Class distinctions alone, however, are insufficient to distinguish the offender from a large pool of suspects. As a result, for the inquiry to be successful, individual qualities are identified, examined, and contrasted. When reconstructing what might have happened, the physical evidence found at the crime scene and its surroundings are crucial [4]. For the destruction of the crime scene, the change in climate or environment is responsible.

For the reconstruction of a crime scene, every stage in crime scene processing is crucial from the crime scene to the court. The reconstruction should be in synergy with all major domains such as science, policing, and law that all create a complex system in forensic science [5]. During the reconstruction, it involves many stakeholders from different domains, and information from multiple sources such as witness testimony, digital and physical record, and evidence from the crime scene is included and helps in reconstruction [6].

Physical evidence includes any item that is tangible and was uncovered at the crime scene. Chemical and biological data are likewise considered to be physical proof [7, 8]. Physical evidence can be broken down into numerous forms, including ballistic division, questioned documents, traces, impressions, and digital evidence [9]. Physical evidence is used to support or refute facts. These details are used to reconstruct the crime scene, and as a result, the perpetrator, the suspect, and the victim are recognized and distinguished. Different sorts of evidence are gathered, including standard, control, and the questioned sample, to support the facts [10].

2.2 Collection and Preservation of Evidence at the Crime Scene

A successful criminal investigation and following legal actions depend on the careful and important process of gathering and preserving evidence at a crime scene. To ensure the integrity of the investigation process and make it possible for justice to be served, it is crucial to properly collect and secure various forms of evidence. The identification, documentation, and security of various sorts of evidence, which might include tangible, digital, and documentary evidence, are crucial tasks for crime scene investigators, law enforcement agents, and forensic specialists. For each of these categories to remain authentic and admissible in a court of law, certain strategies must be used to overcome specific obstacles [11].

2.2.1 Physical Evidence

Physical evidence includes a diverse range of tangible items and materials uncovered at a crime scene that may offer priceless information about the type of crime, the identities of those responsible, and the general chronology of events. Crime scene investigators methodically gather, record, and preserve this type of evidence, which ranges from the minute to the significant, to support criminal investigations [12].

2.2.2 Biological Evidences

Blood, saliva, semen, and other biological samples gathered during a crime scene investigation can potentially include a wealth of genetic and non-genetic data. Through the use of common biochemical and immunological chromatographic assays, the examination of gathered biological evidence can reveal details about the make-up of biological fluids. The determination of a DNA profile to identify the donor, however, is the biggest and most crucial purpose of forensic analysis. Although frequently employed in serology-based, forensic genetics, techniques have many drawbacks, including sample consumption, non-parallel processing, and different degrees of selectivity and sensitivity. The several kinds of kits that forensic management uses vary considerably [13]. Whatever the format, having the right sample containers, making sure they are properly marked, and maintaining a chain of custody are essential for the collection to go well and produce a positive toxicological result. Wide-bore pipettes or disposable hypodermic syringes with the appropriate needle gauges and lengths can be used to collect biological fluids. Different samples should be kept in separate containers, and plastic (particularly polypropylene) with screw caps is most often helpful because it does not break, especially when frozen. Samples should be quickly collected if volatile xenobiotics (such as solvent abuse or anesthesia gas intoxication) are to be analyzed [14]. There are various ways for collecting oral liquid, however it is important to keep in mind that the sample may be diluted by the buffer, preservative, or other chemicals contained in the devices. Sweat is only helpful for qualitative analysis; it should be collected over the course of at least one week (without preservatives); it is non-invasive; however, it is difficult to collect and takes some time to create an acceptable volume for analysis. The collection from the appropriate chamber is desirable, a preservative is not necessary, and the sampling location should be stated on the label [15]. Qualitative/screening analysis can be useful because there are enormous volumes available. To fill a 10 mL plastic jar with a screw cap, collect all the fluids that are available (about 2–5 mL in adults and 1 mL in neonates); this liquid is crucial for the analysis of certain psychotropic substances (such as ethanol) and biochemistry. Bile collection in a 10 mL plastic screw-top jar with all of the available bile (and no preservative) is especially helpful in situations when life has been prolonged beyond the prior dosing and when urine is not present [16, 17]. Urine is always obtained for screening because it often contains higher amounts of the parent xenobiotic and its metabolites than other samples and because it can be very valuable if collected up to 96 hours after intoxication. Urine is always collected for screening and is collected in 30 mL or as much as is possible for a plastic screw-top container [17].

The procedure of sample preparation is crucial for the efficient measurement of analytes from a variety of materials when creating biological evidence. This will be crucial for analyzing their bioactivity, toxicity, and safety. As a result, the appropriate sample preparation technique should be quick, easy, and produce the highest analyte recovery while causing little to no matrix interference. Even in methanolic solutions, monitoring the residual enzymatic activity is strongly advised since some enzymes, such as hydrolases and phosphatases may still be active. Galactosyltransferase, alkaline phosphatase, and urease substrates can be monitored for urine samples to gain insight into the samples' residual enzymatic activity. The most frequent techniques are urine and blood samples put a lot of focus on sample storage at low temperatures, preferably at 80°C right after collection. This is due to inadequate metabolic suppression [18]. The results for labile metabolites should, however, be taken with considerable caution because this may not guarantee precise amounts of all metabolites. 500 mL of urine was added to 500 mL of ultrapure water containing 1 percent (v/v) formic acid after it had been defrosted at 4°C. After that, 1 mL of ethyl acetate was added, and everything was well mixed by overhead shaking for an hour. One gram of sodium sulfate was then added, manually shaken for one minute, and then allowed to crystallize for 20 minutes [18]. The samples were centrifuged at 3000g for 3 min, and after that, 320 L of the organic phase was transferred to an injection vial and dried to dryness in a water bath at 40°C using a constant stream of nitrogen. When the residue was mixed with 120 liters of ultrapure water that also contained 0.4 percent (v/v) formic acid, a dilution factor of 1 was achieved. The residue was first vortexed in 40 liters of methanol that contained the formic acid solution. At 4 °C, serum samples were quickly vortexed after which 50 L was transferred to a fresh polypropylene tube. This was mixed with 100 L of cold acetonitrile that contained 1 percent (v/v) formic acid, vortexed, and then left to stand for an hour at 4 °C [9].

It is still essential to improve the pre-analytical and analytical techniques used to assess EVs in blood samples. With the physical energy involved in blood collection, platelet activation is a possibility; to reduce this activation, it is advised to use a butterfly system with needles that seem to be 21 gauge or bigger. To further reduce the impacts of pressure and fibroblast contamination, it is advisable to discard the first few milliliters of blood storage and distribution. However, additional research is needed to find the most effective venipuncture approach for EV isolation. Additionally, hemolyzed samples must not be used, and if they are, the results from the analysis must be used carefully [19]. The selection of anticoagulants (such as EDTA, heparin, and citrate) for plasma collection is still up for debate. A series of tiny hollow microneedles were introduced into the epidermis after the pH level of the heart surface was evaluated. This allowed for continuous glucose monitoring and blood glucose assessment by measuring glucose in the ISF. The detection of glandular secretions is done from various kinds of biochemical sensors, skin-like sensors are crucial because they can be used to monitor secretions in real-time on skin or gland surfaces and accomplish non-invasive medical detection [20].

2.2.3 Trace Evidences

Trace evidence collection and preservation is a rigorous and important procedure that is crucial to criminal investigations. This painstaking process entails painstakingly locating, cataloguing, and safeguarding tiny shards of items that might provide crucial insights into the specifics of a crime. These minute pieces, including fibers, hair, glass shards, paint chips, and gunshot residue, have the power to provide important details about the crime scene, the participants, and the events that took place. Investigators must first pinpoint possible trace evidence sources within the context of the crime scene [21]. For instance, in burglary investigations, they could search through broken windows for paint chips or trapped fibers that might reveal information about the entryway. One cannot stress the significance of detailed documentation; each item of trace evidence must be meticulously documented, including its position, nature, and context. Making use of resources like photographs, sketching, and thorough notes guarantees an accurate portrayal of the facts [22].

Personal protective equipment (PPE) is a crucial safety measure when gathering evidence. Investigators are shielded from any dangers and cross-contamination that might jeopardize the reliability of the evidence by wearing gloves, masks, and coveralls. The prevention of cross-contamination is maintained while data are gathered from diverse sources. To avoid blending evidence, different regions or objects should be handled individually, and gloves or equipment should be changed. Different trace evidence kinds need specialized gathering methods. To gather fibers and hair, for instance, tweezers, tape lifts, and micro-vacuum systems are used. Forceps are used to carefully gather glass shards, which are then put in safe containers to stop them from shattering [18]. Clean tools are used to gently scrape or lift paint chips, and adhesive stubs or wipes are used to blot people's hands and clothing of gunshot residue. Each technique for gathering evidence is designed to maintain the integrity of the data. The proper packing is necessary for preservation as well. To prevent contamination and preserve its condition, trace evidence is stored inside sterile, airtight containers. Depending on the type of evidence, a certain type of packaging, such as envelopes, plastic containers, or glass vials, is used. It is crucial to have a clear chain of custody. The evidence's route is methodically tracked by labelling every container with detailed information, including item description, location, date, and the collector's identification. When the evidence is taken to the lab and subsequently presented in court, precise record-keeping is essential. To avoid deterioration or contamination, the conditions of the evidence must be maintained during transportation and storage.

To ensure the preservation of the evidence, a safe, climate-controlled location is selected. The chain of custody is meticulously upheld throughout this procedure, recording each transfer and interaction with the evidence [23, 24].

2.2.4 Impression Evidence

Identification, documentation, and preservation of markings or patterns left at a crime scene are all steps in the painstaking process of gathering and preserving impression evidence. These impressions, which include tyre tracks, bite marks, tool marks and footprints, have the ability to reveal important details about the parties involved and the order in which the events took place [25]. The integrity of impression evidence is guaranteed throughout the investigation and judicial procedures by following this step-by-step approach. First, impression evidence is located and recorded [26]. Recognizing possible sources of imprints, such as footprints close to points of entrance or tyre markings on surfaces, is necessary to accomplish this. It is essential to record their position, look, and context, which may be done through photographs, sketching, and detailed notes. The foundation for proper portrayal is this thorough documentation. Wearing personal protective equipment (PPE) is crucial when dealing with impression evidence. To protect the safety of the investigator and to avoid contaminating the evidence, gloves and shoe coverings are used. Avoiding cross-contamination is crucial [27]. Each collection is kept distinct in order to prevent the blending of evidence from various sources or regions. Tools and gloves are adjusted properly to avoid any accidental mixing. Specialized gathering methods are required for various sorts of impression evidence. Footprints and tyre tracks can be lifted with adhesive lifters onto flexible sheets or cast using dental stone or plaster to form a mold [28]. On the other hand, pictures with supporting scale references are the ideal way to record tool marks. In rare circumstances, the complete item with the mark may be gathered. In order to preserve impression evidence, packaging is essential. Large tyre tracks and tool-marked surfaces are examples of items that need to be preserved in their natural condition since they cannot be directly retrieved. Evidence preservation strategies include burying tyre tracks to protect them from environmental deterioration. It is impossible to exaggerate the value of labelling. It is essential to mark gathered goods and related materials correctly. It contains crucial details such as an explanation of the impression, its location, date, and the collector's name [29].

Latent prints – The choice of whether to examine a piece of evidence for latent fingerprints at the crime scene or package it and send it to the lab depends primarily on the surface in question. If the surface is porous, the laboratory is better suited to processing it chemically. The article should be formatted and submitted as an appropriate result. However, if the surface is flat, fingerprint powder will stick to the oils and perspiration that were left behind by the pores in the friction ridges of the fingers; this procedure is simple to carry out at the crime scene. Packaging for evidence that will be processed in a laboratory should minimize friction on the print-bearing surface. It is advised against merely putting the item in a plastic bag because this could cause friction. It is essential to immobilize the item in a way that enables transfer while handling this form of evidence [30]. Now with the advancement in research, fingerprint can be developed even if they exposed to liquid [31]. Even these fingerprints are developed by nanoparticles [32–34] and magnetic Nanoparticles [35].

Post-mortem fingerprints: To positively identify the deceased, the investigator must first thoroughly dry the cadaver's fingers and palms. After that, they are directly imprinted with normal fingerprint ink and an ink roller or pad. The fingerprint Spoon II (a curved metal plate with a slot for a fingerprint card) is next used to press the separate fingers, and it is then 16 released. A large cylindrical object, such as a beaker or bottle, trapped in plain bond paper secured by elastic bands, over the palms of the cadaver is rolled over the palms after they have been similarly linked to obtaining the impressions [36].

2.2.5 Explosives

Quick collection of conventional explosive particles is necessary because the majority of solid explosives of interest have low vapor pressures. The swab method of sample collection is the method of choice everywhere. For removing traces of explosive residue from surfaces, the most often used swipe materials are made of TeflonTM-coated fiberglass, Nomex®, an aromatic polyamide (also known as an aramid), and cotton fabric (Muslin). A woven cotton cloth called muslin is frequently used for sampling and collecting trace explosives [37]. Numerous stations also use fiberglass covered with polytetrafluoroethylene (PTFE) and Nomex®. For the swipe to be effective at gathering explosive particles, it must meet the following criteria: It must be able to tolerate high temperatures (up to 200°C), be able to adequately collect explosive particles while being selective enough to pass over other compounds, be unaffected by multiple swab sampling, and be competitively priced if it is used to introduce the sample into the IMS [38, 39]. To design swipe materials that meet these objectives, a full understanding of the processes involved is required. It is necessary to have a thorough grasp of the processes involved in order to design swiping materials that satisfy these requirements. A vacuum suction-impact collecting device was used to gather the wipe samples; it was originally designed to do so for uranium particles on a carbon impaction plate [40]. A flow rate of around 2.0 L/min is achieved using vacuum pumping to move the wipe sample's particles, and impaction is employed to collect them onto the carrier (carbon disc). While explosives should be handled and stored with extreme caution, they are stable in a room. Once the residue is in the laboratory, it must be divided for the synthesis of organic and inorganic extracts [41].

Electric detonators taken from IEDs, which are used to detonate powerful bombs, are gathered. Compared to debris that is gathered from other locations of the blasting site, post-blast debris that is collected from the blast area's center exhibits more favorable results [42]. The crater mark left by an explosion is a sign that devices were employed and can provide numerical data on the explosive that was used for the blast in the case of high explosive filler, which produces a lot of pieces and smaller-sized pieces than low explosive filler [43].

Cotton swabs are used on 'witness plates' positioned close to a controlled explosion to simulate the absorption of residues on prospective witnesses. This data is then analyzed using a UV detector and HPLC. According to the results, EGDN, NG, PETN, RDX, and TNT were present. In order to determine whether 2,4-dinitrotoluene (DNT) was present on the fingerprint, the authors also developed a novel method using surface-enhanced Raman scattering (SERS) from a cotton swab coated with AgNPs. Swabs were also used to demonstrate how to spot TNT on objects including soil samples, bare hands before and after washing, and materials like metal, plastic, cardboard, carpet fabric, wood, and surfaces wrapped with adhesive tape. The examination was carried out using three various immunochemical tests. A NIR-Hyperspectral system with a spectrometer (Headwall photonics model 1002A-00371) was employed for the measurement of explosive residues on handprints, courtesy of FOSS (FOSS A/S, Denmark). With a spectral resolution of 7 nm and a total of 142 bands recorded for each spectrum, the NIR wavelength range covered the region from 1000 to 1700 nm. With a line of 320 pixels, the spectrometer was modified for line mapping [44].

2.2.6 Hair and Fibers

Normally, one can remove individual hairs with their fingers or tweezers; however, vacuum sweepers can also be used for this purpose. The paper that contains the hair is then folded in the "druggist fold" and placed inside of an envelope that is properly labeled with identity information and sealed. The center of the paper should contain the piece of proof. The paper should be folded twice lengthwise in non-parallel folds so the flaps overlap. Fold over the end by tucking the smaller inside the larger. The resulting packet should be put inside a regular envelope and sealed [45]. The sample region should first be brushed to remove any loose hairs following accepted norms. These loose hairs should be packaged separately. The root should then be added to the standards after that. Samples of head hair should be collected from the crown, neck, sides, and front of the head, among other areas. Collect 12 hairs at a minimum. Cutting the hair as close as feasible to the skin or scalp is a less popular technique for achieving standards. The best method for gathering fibers as evidence is to pick them up with your hands or tweezers. Another method for gathering fibers is to use a vacuum sweeper with an in-line canister attachment on the hose [46]. A filter that needs to be replaced after each user must be included in the canister. Tape is a third technique to pick up this kind of thing. Using tape to gather this kind of evidence is the third technique. The advantage of not contaminating the samples is that you can pick up the evidence with your fingers, tweezers, or tape. Packaging – Vacuum sweepings should be put in distinct containers and labeled according to their origin. Small amounts or single fibers should be placed in a paper that has been folded in the "druggist fold," which is then sealed in a paper envelope with identification information [47].

Hair is a sample taken from outside the body and is susceptible to contamination from such sources. Before continuing with the study, the analyst must choose whether to take a measure to try to remove external contamination.

Some researchers have used straightforward solvent rinse methods, whereas others have employed many phases involving solvents, water, and detergents. To assess the extent of removal of external drug contamination before analyzing the material, it may be appropriate to keep these wash solutions so they can be tested for the drug. Methanol, acetone, sodium dodecyl sulfate, dichloromethane, and other organic solvents are some of the hair-washing techniques used in decontamination processes. The speed and effectiveness of hair analysis have been increased by certain recently discovered procedures, such as ultrasonic- and microwave-assisted extraction [48]. Three miniature techniques—hollow-fiber liquid-phase microextraction, headspace solid-phase microextraction, and microextraction by packed sorbent—significantly reduce the quantity of organic solvents utilized and the amount of harmful waste produced during the cleanup processes.

2.2.7 Documentary Evidence

To maintain the validity and authenticity of legal, investigative, or historical topics, documentation must be gathered and preserved. To guarantee that the integrity of the evidence is maintained, the procedure requires a thorough and precise approach. The categories of documented evidence that must be gathered must be clearly identified from the start. This entails carefully evaluating how each document relates to the situation or objective at hand. Obtaining the proper authorization and making sure all legal and regulatory requirements are satisfied are equally important. This can entail getting the required subpoenas, warrants, or permission from the necessary parties [49].

The next step is to create a well-organized strategy that outlines the parameters, goals, and techniques for gathering and maintaining the evidence. The roles and duties of the people engaged in the gathering, preservation, and custody of the evidence should also be made explicit in this strategy [50]. A key component of the procedure is thorough documentation. All papers destined for collection should be listed in detail, with all relevant metadata, including dates, sources, locations, and custodians, being meticulously recorded. The value of the evidence in the context it was designed for is enhanced by this contextual information [51].

In the actual collecting phase, a variety of items are gathered, including written documents as well as electronic data, audio recordings, and films. Maintaining the admissibility and reliability of electronic evidence requires the use of forensically sound techniques. Using archival-quality materials and keeping a regulated atmosphere assist stop degradation for tangible documents. Physical and electronic evidence require different preservation techniques [52]. To prevent degradation, physical documents require a safe, climate-controlled environment. Their durability is ensured by acid-free storage options. The creation of forensic pictures of storage devices and the use of write-protected media are required for electronic evidence to prevent any unintended adjustments. Encryption adds an additional degree of security, particularly for sensitive electronic documents. The chain of custody must be meticulously maintained. This calls for a thorough record of all transactions and changes in ownership. It is important to correctly document the names, dates, and signatures of everyone who interacts with the evidence [53].

Storage that is strategically secure is essential. To protect against environmental influences, physical documents need to be stored in safe and regulated environments. Electronic evidence requires secure servers with tight access restrictions for storage. Regular backups protect against technological issues that might cause data loss. Strict access restrictions are part of security measures to prevent unauthorized access to both physical and electronic evidence. Access restrictions and encryption together improve the security of critical electronic documents. The process of organizing and cataloguing evidence entails creating a thorough system for indexing and classifying the items gathered. Effective cataloguing is built on metadata, which includes information on the type of document, the date, its importance, and linkages to other pieces of evidence [54].

2.2.8 Digital Evidences

A crucial stage in electronic device-related investigations is the gathering and storage of digital evidence. Digital evidence is vulnerable to being altered or destroyed, which emphasizes how important it is to protect its integrity from the start. In the first phase, prospective digital evidence that is relevant to the inquiry must be carefully identified. This includes a variety of technological gadgets that each contain important data, including laptops, cellphones, hard discs, and USB drives. In order to prevent manipulation or destruction, it is crucial to secure the evidence that has been detected [55].

To reduce the potential of remote interference, this calls for turning off devices, unplugging them from the internet, and putting them in a Faraday bag. The collecting and storing of digital evidence is an essential step in investigations involving computer devices. Because digital evidence may be manipulated or deleted, it is crucial to maintain its integrity from the beginning [56]. Prospective digital evidence that is pertinent to the investigation must be carefully recognized in the initial step. This covers a range of technology devices, such as computers, telephones, hard discs, and USB drives, that each carry crucial data. The evidence that has been found must be secured in order to avoid tampering or destruction. This suggests shutting off gadgets, disconnecting them from the internet, and placing them in a Faraday bag to lessen the possibility of remote influence. However, this procedure is complex and necessitates adherence to rigid guidelines [57].

A fundamental requirement is to rely on authorized employees for the gathering and processing of evidence. To maintain accountability and transparency, every activity involving the evidence should be thoroughly documented. The selection of tools and methods for data extraction demands considerable thought. It is essential to use specialized tools designed for digital forensics since they guarantee accuracy and preserve data integrity. It is essential to tenaciously keep the evidence intact [58]. This involves preserving the whole evidential process, from the initial collection to the final presentation, in addition to retaining the extracted data. Digital evidence must be physically stored in a secure location that is protected from hacking or unauthorized access. Following these procedures maintains the chain of custody and the value of the evidence. It is strongly advised for people working on investigations involving digital evidence to get advice from qualified digital forensic experts. Their knowledge guarantees adherence to best practices, reducing the possibility of fraud or corruption [59].

2.3 Legal Considerations

In every legal situation, paying close attention to legal issues is essential to guaranteeing the fairness, integrity, and legality of proceedings. The foundation of the entire system of justice is made up of legal considerations, which include a variety of norms, regulations, and moral standards that direct the behavior of all parties. judicial concerns are crucial in determining the path of judicial processes, affecting outcomes, and preserving public confidence in the legal system. These issues range from protecting constitutional rights to respecting due process. Upholding justice and the rule of law requires a thorough awareness of and unwavering commitment to these legal issues, whether in litigation, commercial disputes, investigations, or any other area of law. This essay explores the complex world of legal considerations, demonstrating their importance and influence on numerous areas of the legal system [60].

2.4 Chain of Custody

The historical history of a piece of evidence from the time it is gathered at a crime scene to the time it is presented in court is known as the "chain of custody" in forensic science. It entails keeping track of how evidence is used, moved, handled, and stored in order to guarantee its reliability, credibility, and legal admissibility [61, 62].

2.4.1 Importance and Significance of Chain of Custody in Forensic Science

1. Preservation of Evidence Integrity: Ensuring a safe and uninterrupted chain of custody is important for preserving the integrity of the evidence. The reliability and accuracy of the evidence can be jeopardized by improper management, contamination, or unauthorized access.
2. Credibility in Court: The credibility of the evidence in court is improved by a well-documented chain of custody. It eliminates concerns about tampering or manipulation by giving

confidence that the evidence provided is identical to that which was gathered at the crime scene.

3. Admissibility: For evidence to be admitted in court, a proper chain of custody must be maintained. In order to avoid the presentation of incorrect or misleading information, courts frequently demand verification that the evidence has been handled and preserved properly.
4. Authentication: The chain of custody records serve to establish the reliability of the evidence and to demonstrate its provenance, preventing its replacement, alteration, or fabrication.
5. Protection from Legal Disputes: Accurate chain of custody records offer a strong defense against claims made by adversaries who could contest the truthfulness or dependability of the evidence. The handling of the material exhibits a high degree of professionalism and openness [63, 64].

2.5 Admissibility in Court

The evaluation of evidence for its admissibility in court involves determining its appropriateness and relevance for a trial or legal action. Specific requirements must be satisfied in order for evidence to be considered credible, fair, and suitable. Not all evidence is immediately accepted. Depending on the jurisdiction and the sort of evidence at question, these criteria may change. Relevance and materiality are factors that affect whether or not evidence is admissible; the evidence must have a direct bearing on the case and its resolution. Considerations regarding hearsay or privileged information, the expertise of individuals presenting the evidence, authentication to confirm its veracity, and other factors all play a part. What is admissible is influenced by the idea of a secure chain of custody, character evidence restrictions, precautions against undue bias, and the rules controlling expert testimony. In the end, judges uphold the need to uphold fairness and dependability in the courtroom by making determinations on the admissibility of evidence in accordance with accepted legal principles and processes. This procedure makes sure that only relevant, reliable, and objective evidence informs legal judgements.

2.6 Forensic Laboratory Analysis

Examination and analysis methods: Forensic science plays an essential role in criminal investigations, providing crucial insights through evaluating and analyzing physical evidence. A variety of strategies are used to reveal the intricate details underlying crimes, victims, and perpetrators [65]. It highlights primary inspection and analysis procedures in forensic science, suggesting how fingerprints, DNA profiling, toxicology, and other modalities aid in the resolution of legal mysteries [66].

2.7 DNA Analysis

DNA analysis is a fundamental component of modern forensic examination that promotes investigations at diverse crime sites. Here's an example of its application, including the types of crime scenes and devices employed [67]. DNA analysis is used to identify people, link suspects to crime scenes, and establish familial links. DNA is extracted from biological samples such as blood, hair, saliva, or body tissues [68].

2.7.1 Types of Crime Scenes Where an Expert Can Find DNA

Homicide Scene: The bloodstains and biological samples of a murder victim are obtained from the crime scene. DNA analysis contributes in the identification of prospective culprits and the confirmation of victims' identities [69].

Sexual Assault Case: DNA can be extracted from bodily fluids or skin cells found on victims or at crime scenes. The comparison of the DNA profile to databases aids in the identification of criminals [70].

Burglary or Theft: DNA left behind by perpetrators on objects like as gloves or tools can be used to connect them to the crime scene. Hair and fibers can also be analyzed as traces of evidence [71].

Hit-and-Run Incident: DNA collected from biological material on a vehicle involved can aid in the identification of victims or witnesses, as well as potentially linking the car to the scene [72].

2.7.2 Techniques Used

PCR (Polymerase Chain Reaction): PCR amplifies DNA segments, producing enough material for analysis. PCR reactions are carried out using thermal cyclers [73].

Gel Electrophoresis: This method isolates DNA fragments based on their size. UV light is used to visualize the generated DNA bands [74].

DNA Sequencers: This method Decoders decode DNA sequences and provide precise genetic information for comparison [75].

Capillary Electrophoresis: Modern DNA analysis employs capillary electrophoresis for high-resolution separation of DNA fragments, enhancing accuracy [76].

2.8 Fingerprint Analysis

The examination and analysis of fingerprints in forensic science is a multistep process that involves the following.

2.8.1 Collection

Fingerprints can be collected from a variety of surfaces, including skin, glass, metal, and plastic. The method of collection will vary depending on the surface and the condition of the fingerprint [77].

Roll impressions: This is the most common method of collecting fingerprints. The person's fingers are rolled onto a piece of paper or cardstock [78].

Flat impressions: This method is used to collect fingerprints from smooth surfaces, such as glass or metal. The person's fingers are pressed onto the surface [79].

Landmark impressions: This method is used to collect fingerprints from curved surfaces, such as the inside of a drinking glass. The person's fingers are pressed onto the surface and then rolled slightly.

2.8.2 Development

Once the fingerprints have been collected, they need to be developed so that they can be seen more clearly. This can be done using a variety of methods, such as powder dusting, iodine fuming, or cyanoacrylate fuming. Once fingerprints have been collected, they need to be developed so that they can be seen more clearly [80].

Powder dusting: This method involves dusting the fingerprint with a fine powder, such as black powder or fingerprint powder. The powder adheres to the sweat and oil left by the fingers, making the ridges visible [81].

Iodine fuming: This method involves exposing the fingerprint to iodine vapors. The iodine vapors react with the sweat and oil left by the fingers, making the ridges visible [82].

Cyanoacrylate fuming: This method involves exposing the fingerprint to cyanoacrylate vapors. The cyanoacrylate vapors react with the moisture in the fingerprint, creating a plastic film that makes the ridges visible [83].

2.8.3 Lifting

Once the fingerprints have been developed, they need to be lifted so that they can be transported to the laboratory for analysis. This can be done using a variety of methods, such as tape lifting or lifting film. Once the fingerprints have been developed, they need to be lifted so that they can be transported to the laboratory for analysis [84].

Tape lifting: This method involves lifting the fingerprint using a piece of tape.

Lifting film: This method involves lifting the fingerprint using a piece of lifting film.

2.8.4 Analysis

In the laboratory, fingerprint examiners will analyze the fingerprints using a variety of techniques, including microscopy, comparison, and classification [85].

Microscopy: This technique involves examining the fingerprints using a microscope. This allows the fingerprint examiner to see the ridges and minutiae in great detail [86].

Classification: This technique involves classifying the fingerprint into one of the following patterns: arches, loops, whorls, or composites [87].

Comparison: The fingerprint examiner will compare the unknown fingerprint to a database of known fingerprints. This comparison is done using a variety of factors, including the pattern of the ridges, the number and type of minutiae, and the overall quality of the print [88].

2.8.5 Evaluation

The fingerprint examiner will evaluate the results of the analysis and make a determination as to whether or not the fingerprints match.

Verification: The fingerprint examiner's findings will be verified by another fingerprint examiner. The examination and analysis of fingerprints is a complex and specialized process that requires a high level of training and expertise. Fingerprint examiners play an important role in forensic science by helping to identify suspects and solve crimes [89].

2.9 Ballistic Analysis

Forensic ballistics is the scientific examination of firearms, ammunition, and gunshot residue (GSR) for the purpose of reconstructing a crime scene or identifying a suspect [90]. Forensic ballistics is a complex and specialized field, and ballistics experts must have a thorough knowledge of firearms, ammunition, and GSR. They must also be able to use a variety of scientific equipment and techniques to examine and analyze this evidence. Ballistics evidence can be a valuable tool for law enforcement in reconstructing crime scenes and identifying suspects.

2.9.1 Visual Examination

Ballistics experts carefully examine the physical characteristics of bullets, cartridges, and GSR to identify their class characteristics (e.g., caliber, type of firearm, and manufacturer) and individual characteristics (e.g., unique markings left by the firearm's rifling) [91].

Comparison microscopy: Ballistics experts use comparison microscopes to compare the individual characteristics of bullets and cartridges to known exemplars from a suspect's firearm. This can be used to identify the firearm that was used to fire a particular bullet or cartridge [92].

2.9.2 Gunshot Residue Analysis

Ballistics experts can also analyze GSR to determine the distance from which a gun was fired, the type of firearm that was used, and whether the shooter was wearing gloves [93].

2.9.3 Trajectory Analysis

Ballistics experts can use the trajectory of a bullet to determine the shooter's position relative to the victim. This can be done by examining the angle of impact of the bullet and the distance between the bullet's entry and exit wounds [94].

Here are some specific examples of how forensic ballistics can be used in criminal investigations:

To identify the firearm that was used to fire a particular bullet or cartridge. This can be done by comparing the individual characteristics of the bullet or cartridge to known exemplars from a suspect's firearm [95]. To determine the distance from which a gun was fired. This can be done by analyzing the amount of GSR that is deposited on a surface or by examining the trajectory of the bullet [96]. To determine the shooter's position relative to the victim. This can be done by analyzing the angle of impact of the bullet and the distance between the bullet's entry and exit wounds [97].

Forensic ballistics is a valuable tool for law enforcement in investigating crimes involving firearms. By examining and analyzing ballistic evidence, ballistics experts can help to identify the firearm that was used, the shooter's position, and the distance from which the gun was fired. This information can be crucial in solving crimes and bringing criminals to justice.

2.10 Toxicology Analysis

Forensic toxicology is the field of science that deals with the detection, identification, and quantification of drugs and other toxins in biological samples. Forensic toxicologists use a variety of methods to analyze biological samples [98].

2.10.1 Spectroscopy

Spectroscopy is a technique that uses electromagnetic radiation to identify and quantify substances. Common types of spectroscopies used in forensic toxicology include ultraviolet-visible (UV-Vis) spectroscopy, infrared (IR) spectroscopy, and Raman spectroscopy [99].

2.10.2 Chromatography

Chromatography is a technique that separates mixtures of substances into their individual components. Common types of chromatography used in forensic toxicology include gas chromatography (GC) and liquid chromatography (LC) [100].

2.10.3 Immunoassays

Immunoassays are techniques that use antibodies to detect and quantify specific substances. Immunoassays are often used to detect drugs in biological samples [101].

2.10.4 Mass Spectrometry

Mass spectrometry is a technique that uses electric and magnetic fields to separate ions according to their mass-to-charge ratio. Mass spectrometry is often used to identify and quantify drugs and other toxins in biological samples [102].

The specific methods used in forensic toxicology will vary depending on the type of sample being analyzed and the substances being sought. For example, GC is often used to analyze drugs in blood samples, while LC is often used to analyze drugs in urine samples. Immunoassays are often used to detect drugs in hair samples, while mass spectrometry is often used to identify and quantify drugs and other toxins in tissue samples.

2.11 Quality Control Measures

Quality control measures in forensic science are critical processes and procedures put in place to ensure the accuracy, reliability, and validity of the scientific analyses and findings conducted during the investigation and analysis of evidence. These measures are crucial to maintain the integrity of forensic evidence and to ensure that the results are both scientifically sound and defensible in a court of law [103].

2.11.1 Validation of Methods

Before a forensic method is used in casework, it undergoes rigorous validation to ensure its accuracy, sensitivity, specificity, and reliability. This involves testing the method using known samples and establishing its limitations [104].

2.11.2 Calibration

Instruments used in forensic analysis must be calibrated regularly to ensure accurate measurements. This involves comparing the instrument's readings to known standards and making adjustments if necessary [105].

2.11.3 Quality Assurance Programs

Laboratories implement quality assurance programs to ensure that all aspects of their operations, from evidence collection to analysis and reporting, meet established standards. This includes regular audits and reviews of procedures [106].

2.11.4 Documentation and Record Keeping

Detailed records are maintained at every step of the analysis process, including notes on procedures, observations, calculations, and any deviations from standard protocols. Evidence Preservation is the proper storage and preservation of evidence are crucial to prevent contamination, degradation, or loss over time [107].

2.11.5 Documentation and Reporting of Evidences

Documentation and reporting of evidence in forensic science involves comprehensive and accurate record-keeping of all procedures, observations, and findings during the analysis process. This meticulous documentation ensures the transparency, traceability, and reliability of the investigation [108]. It encompasses detailed notes on evidence collection, preservation, and analysis methods, as well as any deviations from standard protocols. The final report summarizes the results, interpretations, and conclusions, serving as a critical communication tool for conveying scientific findings to legal proceedings [109]. Precise documentation and reporting uphold the integrity of forensic analysis, enabling transparency, reproducibility, and the just administration of the law.

2.12 Challenges and Emerging Technologies

Challenges in evidence collection: Challenges in evidence collection encompass issues related to maintaining the integrity and credibility of collected materials [110]. 0d. Additionally, variations in collection techniques due to different personnel, lack of standardized procedures, and difficulties in preserving fragile or transient evidence such as trace materials or biological fluids can hinder accurate analysis and interpretation [111]. Striking a balance between thoroughness, speed, and maintaining the original state of evidence while considering legal and ethical constraints remains a continuous challenge [112].

2.12.1 Contamination

Contamination in forensic science refers to the unintended introduction of foreign substances or materials into evidence, which can compromise the integrity and reliability of analyses and conclusions [113].

2.12.2 Microbial Contamination

Bacteria, fungi, and other microorganisms can grow on evidence if it's not properly stored or handled, altering its characteristics and potentially impacting analysis results [113].

2.12.3 Packaging and Storage Contamination

Inadequate packaging or storage conditions can lead to contamination from external sources, potentially degrading the evidence over time [114].

2.12.4 Preservation Difficulties

Preservation difficulties in forensic science arise due to various factors that can compromise the integrity and reliability of collected evidence over time. Biological evidence, such as DNA, may degrade if not stored under proper temperature and humidity conditions. Decomposition, contamination, and evaporation can affect volatile substances and fluids [115]. Physical evidence like firearms or tool marks might be susceptible to corrosion or environmental wear. Additionally, digital evidence faces challenges in maintaining its authenticity and preventing data loss or corruption [116]. Balancing the need to preserve evidence for extended periods, adhering to legal requirements, and accounting for the potential impacts of storage conditions remains a complex challenge in forensic science [117].

2.13 Handling Digital Evidence

Handling digital evidence in forensic science involves specialized procedures to collect, preserve, and analyze electronic information from various devices and digital platforms [103]. As technology advances, the challenges and complexities of digital evidence increase. Properly handling this evidence requires stringent adherence to established protocols to ensure its authenticity, integrity, and admissibility in legal proceedings. Digital evidence can include data from computers, mobile devices, cloud services, social media, and more [118]. Collecting digital evidence demands a forensically sound approach, often involving creating forensic images of storage media to prevent changes or corruption of the original data. Chain of custody must be meticulously maintained to track who accessed the evidence and when. Preservation involves safeguarding against accidental data alteration, intentional tampering, or data degradation [119]. State-of-the-art tools and techniques are used to recover deleted or encrypted files, analyze metadata, and reconstruct timelines of digital activities. Adapting to the evolving landscape of technology is crucial, as new encryption methods, communication platforms, and data storage mechanisms continuously emerge [120]. Professionals in digital forensics must stay updated with advancements and legal standards while upholding the highest ethical standards to ensure that digital evidence remains a reliable and effective component of modern forensic investigations.

2.14 Emerging Technologies

Emerging technologies are revolutionizing the landscape of forensic science, enhancing investigative capabilities and improving the accuracy of analyses. One significant advancement is the utilization of advanced DNA sequencing techniques, enabling the extraction of more detailed genetic information from even degraded samples [121]. Digital forensics tools have also seen remarkable growth, allowing experts to extract, analyze, and interpret evidence from digital devices, networks, and online platforms. Artificial Intelligence (AI) and machine learning algorithms are playing an increasingly crucial role in automating tasks like facial recognition, pattern recognition in fingerprints, and even predicting crime hotspots based on historical data patterns [122]. High-resolution imaging technologies, such as 3D scanning and photogrammetry, aid in the detailed documentation of crime scenes and the subsequent analysis of physical evidence like footwear impressions or tool marks. Nanotechnology applications offer improved visualization of latent prints and trace evidence, while isotopic analysis assists in determining geographical origins of materials [123]. Furthermore, block chain technology is being explored to maintain an unalterable chain of custody for digital evidence. While these technologies hold immense promise in bolstering forensic capabilities, their integration must be approached thoughtfully, ensuring legal compliance, addressing potential biases, and maintaining the highest standards of accuracy and ethics [124].

2.15 Advances in DNA Analysis

Advancements in DNA analysis have propelled forensic science to new heights, transforming the way investigations are conducted and evidence is interpreted [125]. One notable breakthrough is the advent of rapid DNA analysis, allowing for swift on-site identification of individuals. This is particularly valuable in cases of missing persons, disaster victim identification, and eliminating suspects during initial investigations. Additionally, next-generation sequencing (NGS) technologies have revolutionized DNA profiling by enabling the analysis of multiple loci simultaneously, enhancing the discrimination power and accuracy of identifications [126]. NGS can even recover DNA from highly degraded or mixed samples, expanding the potential pool of evidence that can be analyzed. Furthermore, miniaturization and automation of DNA analysis processes have streamlined workflows, reduced sample consumption, and accelerated results. Forensic laboratories now possess the capacity to process larger caseloads efficiently, addressing the longstanding issue of backlogs [127]. The development of probabilistic genotyping software allows analysts to handle complex mixtures and low-template DNA samples more effectively, providing more robust and objective interpretations of results. Despite these advancements, ethical and legal considerations, along with potential biases in DNA databases, must be carefully managed. The expansion of DNA databases raises concerns about privacy and misuse of genetic information. As DNA analysis continues to evolve, ensuring its responsible and equitable implementation will be paramount to fully realizing its potential in forensic science [128].

2.16 AI and Machine Learning in Forensic Analysis

Advancements in AI and machine learning are reshaping forensic science by revolutionizing the way evidence is analyzed, patterns are recognized, and investigations are conducted. In the realm of forensic analysis, AI-powered algorithms are streamlining tasks such as fingerprint and facial recognition, reducing human error and speeding up identification processes [129]. Machine learning techniques are enhancing the accuracy of DNA analysis by identifying complex patterns in genetic data that might not be apparent to human analysts. Additionally, AI-driven tools are assisting in the analysis of digital evidence, enabling rapid extraction and interpretation of information from various sources like social media, emails, and encrypted data [130]. Machine learning models can predict crime patterns based on historical data, aiding law enforcement agencies in resource allocation and preventive measures. These technologies are also valuable in analyzing large datasets, identifying correlations between seemingly unrelated pieces of evidence, and uncovering hidden trends that might aid investigations [131].

2.17 Cyber Forensics Techniques

Emerging technologies are fundamentally reshaping the landscape of cyber forensics, enabling more efficient and effective responses to digital crimes. Advanced data analytics and machine learning algorithms are being harnessed to rapidly process and analyze massive volumes of digital evidence, aiding in the identification of malicious activities and patterns indicative of cyberattacks [132]. Blockchain technology is revolutionizing the field by providing tamper-proof, transparent, and traceable records, enhancing the credibility of digital evidence and maintaining the integrity of the chain of custody. The advent of quantum computing, although in its nascent stages, has the potential to significantly impact cyber forensics by potentially breaking current encryption methods and prompting the development of quantum-resistant cryptographic techniques [133]. Furthermore, advancements in memory forensics allow investigators to extract valuable information directly from a computer's memory, providing insights into sophisticated attacks that attempt to evade traditional detection methods. Challenges, however, persist, such as ensuring the ethical use of AI in cyber investigations, addressing the dynamic nature of digital evidence, and maintaining up-to-date knowledge in this rapidly evolving field [134]. In the face of an ever-expanding digital threat landscape, these emerging technologies hold immense promise for cyber forensics, bolstering cyber defense strategies, and aiding in the pursuit of cybercriminals [135].

2.18 Conclusion

In conclusion, modern forensic investigations rely heavily on the meticulous handling, gathering, and preservation of physical, documentary, and digital evidence. The wide range of evidence types necessitates a thorough understanding of each one's distinctive qualities and the procedures required for protecting them. It is crucial to uphold the integrity and reliability of gathered evidence that the legal framework governing the admissibility of evidence in court, including the chain of custody and standards of admissibility, is followed. The investigative process' mainstay, forensic laboratory analysis uses specialized methods for looking over and analyzing evidence. These techniques, which range from the intricate analysis of DNA to the minute details of fingerprint and ballistic analysis, offer priceless insights that can solve challenging criminal puzzles. The accuracy and dependability of the analytical results are ensured by strict quality control procedures, enhancing the credibility of forensic findings. A just legal process is supported by the thorough documentation and reporting of evidence-based findings, which further facilitates open communication with legal stakeholders.

Despite this, gathering evidence is still difficult due to concerns about contamination, problems with preservation, and the complex management of digital evidence. The answers to these problems also advance with technology. Emerging technologies have the potential to revolutionize the field and improve investigative abilities. Examples include sophisticated DNA analysis methods, the use of AI and machine learning in forensic analysis, and the dynamic field of cyber forensics.

The ongoing development of forensic methods and technologies in this dynamic environment emphasizes the increasing significance of interdisciplinary cooperation among law enforcement, legal experts, and scientists. To take advantage of new opportunities, address problems, and ultimately serve justice through thorough, evidence-based investigations, there must be seamless synergy between these domains. As we look to the future, the fusion of experience and innovation promises a new era in forensic science, one that consistently pushes the limits of our knowledge and capabilities in the quest for justice and truth.

References

1. Negrusz, A. and G. Cooper, *Clarke's analytical forensic toxicology*. 2013: Pharmaceutical press.
2. Dinis-Oliveira, R.J., *et al.*, *Collection of biological samples in forensic toxicology*. 2010. **20**(7): p. 363-414.
3. Dinis-Oliveira, R.J., T.J.T.m. Magalhães, and methods, *Forensic toxicology in drug-facilitated sexual assault*. 2013. **23**(7): p. 471-478.

4. Rawtani, D., *et al.*, *Functionalized nanomaterial for forensic sample analysis.* 2019. **120**: p. 115661.
5. Morgan, R.M. and P.A.J.P.i.P.G. Bull, *The philosophy, nature and practice of forensic sediment analysis.* 2007. **31**(1): p. 43-58.
6. Morgan, R.M., *et al.*, *Crime reconstruction and the role of trace materials from crime scene to court.* 2020. **2**(1): p. e1364.
7. James, S.H. and J.J. Nordby, *Forensic science: an introduction to scientific and investigative techniques.* 2002: CRC press.
8. Saferstein, R., *Forensic Science Handbook, Volume 1.* 2002: Prentice Hall Englewood Cliffs, NJ.
9. Dash, H.R. and K.J.H.o.D.P. Vajpayee, *Collection, Preservation, and Transportation of Biological Evidences.* 2020: p. 1-16.
10. Rao, P.K., *et al.*, *Physical Evidence and Their Handling.* 2020: p. 55-78.
11. Lee, H.C. and E.M. Pagliaro, Forensic evidence and crime scene investigation. *J. Forensic Investig.*, 2013. **1**(2): p. 1-5.
12. Kirk, P.L. and P.L. Kirk, *Crime investigation: physical evidence and the police laboratory.* 1953.
13. Lee, H.C. and C.J.C.m.j. Ladd, *Preservation and collection of biological evidence.* 2001. **42**(3): p. 225-228.
14. Jones, C.E.J.A.C.L.R., *Evidence destroyed, innocence lost: The preservation of biological evidence under innocence protection statutes.* 2005. **42**: p. 1239.
15. Lee, H.C., *et al.*, *Forensic applications of DNA typing: part 2: collection and preservation of DNA evidence.* 1998. **19**(1): p. 10-18.
16. Ballou, S.M., *et al.*, *The biological evidence preservation handbook: best practices for evidence handlers.* 2013.
17. Cunningham, H.M., *et al.*, *Effective Long-term Preservation of Biological Evidence.* 2014.
18. Lee, H.C., *et al.*, *Collection and Preservation of Physical Evidence, in Forensic DNA Applications.* 2023, CRC Press. p. 203-224.
19. Bathrick, A.S., *et al.*, *Long-Term Preservation of Biological Evidence with Commercial Off-the-Shelf Preservatives.* 2017. **67**(4): p. 519-535.
20. Badeaux, D.J.T.T.A.L., *The DNA's over there... right next to the jelly: The problems with the preservation of evidence in Texas.* 2009. **11**: p. 333.
21. Schwartz, T.R., D.S. Rothenberg, and B.L.J.H.o.T.E.A. Clark, *Trace evidence recognition, collection, and preservation.* 2020: p. 1-31.
22. Touroo, R. and A.J.V.F.P. Fitch, Volume 1, *Crime scene findings and the identification, collection, and preservation of evidence.* 2018: p. 9-25.
23. Touroo, R. and A.J.V.P. Fitch, *Identification, collection, and preservation of veterinary forensic evidence: on scene and during the postmortem examination.* 2016. **53**(5): p. 880-887.
24. McGillivray, B.J.A. and e. nursing, *The role of Victorian emergency nurses in the collection and preservation of forensic evidence: a review of the literature.* 2005. **13**(2): p. 95-100.
25. Bodziak, W.J.J.F.L.E.B., *Shoe and tire impression evidence.* 1984. **53**: p. 2.

26. Bodziak, W.J., *Footwear impression evidence: detection, recovery and examination*. 2017: CRC Press.
27. Charron, J., *et al.*, *Interpol Review Paper of Marks and Impression Evidence 2019-2022*. 2023. **6**: p. 100308.
28. Watkins, D. and K. Brown, *Impression and Pattern Evidence, in Handbook of Forensic Photography*. 2022, CRC Press. p. 122-138.
29. LeMay, J., S. Adams, and A.J.J.o.F.I. Stephen, *Validation of vinyl static cling film for the collection and preservation of dust impressions*. 2011. **6**(4): p. 317-332.
30. Sanders, N.J.J.o.f.i., *Recovery of fingerprint evidence from post-blast device materials*. 2011. **61**(3): p. 281.
31. Aseri, V., *et al.*, *A comparative study on scanned fingerprint after applying lubricants and without scanned fingerprint on porous surface;(white paper)*. 2022. **69**: p. 1515-1531.
32. Verma, R.K., *et al.*, *Zinc oxide (ZnO) nanoparticles: Synthesis properties and their forensic applications in latent fingerprints development*. 2022. **69**: p. 36-41.
33. Awasthi, K.K., *et al.*, *Friction Ridge Analysis: Applications of Nanoparticles for Latent Fingerprint Development*. 2023, Springer.
34. Lohar, S., *et al.*, *Comparative study of development of latent fingerprint by using cost effective waste materials*. 2022. **68**: p. 848-853.
35. Sharma, A., *et al.*, *Latent Fingerprint Development from Magnetic Nanoparticles, in Friction Ridge Analysis: Applications of Nanoparticles for Latent Fingerprint Development*. 2023, Springer. p. 39-46.
36. Lee, H.C. and E.M.J.J.o.F.I. Pagliaro, *Forensic evidence and crime scene investigation*. 2013. **1**(2): p. 1-5.
37. RÖßLER, R., *et al.*, *A snapshot of an early Permian ecosystem preserved by explosive volcanism: new results from the Chemnitz Petrified Forest, Germany*. 2012. **27**(11): p. 814-834.
38. Sisco, E., *et al.*, *Quantifying the stability of trace explosives under different environmental conditions using electrospray ionization mass spectrometry*. 2017. **165**: p. 10-17.
39. Lee, H.C., T. Palmbach, and M.T. Miller, *Henry Lee's crime scene handbook*. 2001: Academic Press.
40. Thurman, J.T., *Practical bomb scene investigation*. 2017: CRC Press.
41. Kennedy, J. and P. Kennedy, *Fire, Arson and Explosion Investigation*. 1977: Investigations Institute Chicago, IL.
42. SACHTLEBEN, D.J.J.F.I.o.E., *Vehicle-Borne Improvised Explosive Devices*. 2011: p. 405.
43. Korajlić, N., A. Dautbegović, and D. Muharremi, *Notion, Classification and Procedures on Collection, Preservation and Transportation of Traces Caused by Explosion*. 2009.

44. Hayden, W.E., *Evidence spoliation issues affecting the fire and explosion investigator: Developing a guideline for the fire and explosion investigator to avoid and defend against evidence spoliation claims.* 2004: Touro College.
45. Robertson, J., C. Roux, and K.G. Wiggins, *Forensic examination of fibres.* 2017: CRC press.
46. SPRINGER, F.J.F.e.o.f., *5.2 Collection of Fibre Evidence from Crime Scenes.* 1999: p. 101.
47. Buzzini, P. and J.C.-C.J.F.e.m.F.s.t.c. Yu, *General principles and techniques of trace evidence collection.* 2017: p. 75-98.
48. Ahola, M., *et al., On the scent of an animal skin: new evidence on Corded Ware mortuary practices in Northern Europe.* 2018. **92**(361): p. 118-131.
49. Nichols, B., *Introduction to documentary.* 2017: Indiana University Press.
50. Platt, J.J.T.S.R., *Evidence and proof in documentary research: 1 Some specific problems of documentary research.* 1981. **29**(1): p. 31-52.
51. Ahmed, J.U.J.I.J.o.M. and S. *Sciences, Documentary research method: New dimensions.* 2010. **4**(1): p. 1-14.
52. Grazioli, S. and S.L.J.I.J.o.E.C. Jarvenpaa, *Consumer and business deception on the Internet: Content analysis of documentary evidence.* 2003. **7**(4): p. 93-118.
53. Battipaglia, G., *et al., Five centuries of Central European temperature extremes reconstructed from tree-ring density and documentary evidence.* 2010. **72**(3): p. 182-191.
54. Burgdorf, A.-M.J.C.o.t.P., *A global inventory of quantitative documentary evidence related to climate since the 15th century.* 2022. **18**(6): p. 1407-1428.
55. Granja, F.M. and G.D.R. Rafael. *Preservation of digital evidence: application in criminal investigation. In 2015 Science and Information Conference* (SAI). 2015. IEEE.
56. Munkhondya, H., A. Ikuesan, and H. Venter. *Digital forensic readiness approach for potential evidence preservation in software-defined networks. in ICCWS 2019 14th International Conference on Cyber Warfare and Security: ICCWS.* 2019.
57. Kumar, S., *et al., An enhanced digital forensic investigation framework for XSS attack.* 2022. **25**(4): p. 1009-1018.
58. Danielsson, J. and I. Tjostheim. *The need for a structured approach to digital forensic readiness. in IADIS International Conference e-commerce.* 2004.
59. Sonmez, Y.U. and A.J.I.J.o.I.S.S. Varol, *Review of evidence collection and protection phases in digital forensics process.* 2017. **6**(4): p. 39-45.
60. Saferstein, R., *Criminalistics: An introduction to forensic science.* 2004.
61. Evans, M.M. and P.A.J.A.j. Stagner, *Maintaining the chain of custody evidence handling in forensic cases.* 2003. **78**(4): p. 563-569.
62. Giannelli, P.C., *Chain of custody.* 1996.
63. Damascena, N.P., *et al., Recommendations for procedures related to the evidence chain of custody in forensic anthropology in Brazil.* 2022. **7**(4): p. 609-622.

64. Cosic, J., Z.J.C.t. Cosic, and application, *Chain of custody and life cycle of digital evidence*. 2012. **3**(2).
65. Douglas, J.E., *et al.*, *Crime classification manual: A standard system for investigating and classifying violent crime*. 2013: John Wiley & Sons.
66. Basu, S., *The history of forensic science in India*. 2021: Routledge.
67. San Pietro, D., *et al.*, *Is forensic science in danger of extinction?* 2019. **59**(2): p. 199-202.
68. Butler, J.M., *Forensic DNA typing: biology, technology, and genetics of STR markers*. 2005: Elsevier.
69. Oosthuizen, T. and L.M.J.F.S.I.G. Howes, *The development of forensic DNA analysis: New debates on the issue of fundamental human rights*. 2022. **56**: p. 102606.
70. Aparna, R. and R.S.J.F.s.i. Iyer, *Tears and eyewear in forensic investigation—A review*. 2020. **306**: p. 110055.
71. Suppajariyawat, P.J.S.S.A., *TRACE EVIDENCE: A ROLE AND IMPACT ON FORENSIC SCIENCE AND THE CRIMINAL JUSTICE SYSTEM*. 2021. **7**(3): p. 50-66.
72. Amankwaa, A.O. and C.J.W.I.R.F.S. McCartney, *The effectiveness of the current use of forensic DNA in criminal investigations in England and Wales*. 2021. **3**(6): p. e1414.
73. Lorenz, T.C.J.J., *Polymerase chain reaction: basic protocol plus troubleshooting and optimization strategies*. 2012(63): p. e3998.
74. Lee, P.Y., *et al.*, *Agarose gel electrophoresis for the separation of DNA fragments*. 2012(62): p. e3923.
75. Liu, L., *et al.*, *Comparison of next-generation sequencing systems*. 2012. **2012**.
76. Kaushik, S., V.J.F.D.T.P. Sahajpal, Applications, and Advancements, *Capillary Electrophoresis Issues in Forensic DNA Typing*. 2020: p. 223-238.
77. Su, B.J.A. and b. chemistry, *Recent progress on fingerprint visualization and analysis by imaging ridge residue components*. 2016. **408**: p. 2781-2791.
78. Friesen, J.B.J.J.o.C.E., *Forensic chemistry: The revelation of latent fingerprints*. 2015. **92**(3): p. 497-504.
79. Kumar, P., *et al.*, *Effects of latent fingerprint development reagents on subsequent forensic DNA typing: A review*. 2015. **32**: p. 64-69.
80. Sari, S.A.J.A.J.o.C., *Comparison between latent fingerprint identification using black powder and cyanoacrylate glue*. 2018. **30**(12): p. 2615-2620.
81. Qiu, Z., *et al.*, *A general powder dusting method for latent fingerprint development based on AIEgens*. 2018. **61**: p. 966-970.
82. Hu, Z., *et al.*, *A highly stable ScNb2VO9: Eu3+ phosphor with wide band excitation for visualization of latent fingerprints based on the powder dusting method*. 2023. **165**: p. 112300.
83. Wilshire, B.J.E., *Advances in fingerprint detection*. 1996. **20**(1): p. 12-15.
84. King, R.S., P.M. Hallett, and D.J.F.s.i. Foster, *Seeing into the infrared: A novel IR fluorescent fingerprint powder*. 2015. **249**: p. e21-e26.

85. Cole, S.A.J.B., *Individual and collective identification in contemporary forensics*. 2020. **15**(3): p. 350-375.
86. Garrett, B. and G.J.J.o.E.L.S. Mitchell, How jurors evaluate fingerprint evidence: The relative importance of match language, method information, and error acknowledgment. 2013. **10**(3): p. 484-511.
87. Win, K.N., *et al.*, *Fingerprint classification and identification algorithms for criminal investigation: A survey*. 2020. **110**: p. 758-771.
88. Lee, S.M., H.J. Kim, and Y.P.J.P.A. Jang, *Chemometric classification of morphologically similar Umbelliferae medicinal herbs by DART-TOF-MS fingerprint*. 2012. **23**(5): p. 508-512.
89. Isensee, F., *et al.*, *nnU-Net: a self-configuring method for deep learning-based biomedical image segmentation*. 2021. **18**(2): p. 203-211.
90. Chang, K.H., *et al.*, *Gunshot residue analysis and its evidential values: a review*. 2013. **45**(1): p. 3-23.
91. Haag, M.G. and L.C. Haag, *Shooting incident reconstruction*. 2020: Academic press.
92. White, P., *Crime scene to court: the essentials of forensic science*. 2010: Royal society of chemistry.
93. Birkett, J., *et al.*, *Understanding ballistics a primer for courts*. 2021: The royal society.
94. Zeichner, A.J.A. and B. Chemistry, *Recent developments in methods of chemical analysis in investigations of firearm-related events*. 2003. **376**: p. 1178-1191.
95. Smith, J.A.J.J.o.f.s., *Beretta barrel fired bullet validation study*. 2021. **66**(2): p. 547-556.
96. Hueske, E.E.J.T.F.L.H.P. and Practice, *Firearms and toolmarks*. 2011: p. 227-264.
97. Wallace, J.S., *Chemical analysis of firearms, ammunition, and gunshot residue*. 2018: Crc Press.
98. Ojanperä, I., *et al.*, *Current use of high-resolution mass spectrometry in drug screening relevant to clinical and forensic toxicology and doping control*. 2012. **403**: p. 1203-1220.
99. Steuer, A.E., L. Brockbals, and T.J.F.i.C. Kraemer, *Metabolomic strategies in biomarker research–new approach for indirect identification of drug consumption and sample manipulation in clinical and forensic toxicology?* 2019. **7**: p. 319.
100. Merone, G., *et al.*, *Fast LC–MS/MS screening method for the evaluation of drugs, illicit drugs, and other compounds in biological matrices*. 2022. **5**: p. 100105.
101. Usui, K., *et al.*, *Application of modified QuEChERS method to liver samples for forensic toxicological analysis*. 2014. **32**: p. 139-147.
102. Usman, M., *et al.*, *Forensic toxicological analysis of hair: A review*. 2019. **9**(1): p. 1-12.
103. Arshad, H., A.B. Jantan, and O.I.J.J.o.I.P.S. Abiodun, *Digital Forensics: Review of Issues in Scientific Validation of Digital Evidence*. 2018. **14**(2).

104. Budowle, B., *et al.*, *Criteria for validation of methods in microbial forensics.* 2008. **74**(18): p. 5599-5607.
105. Vidaki, A. and M.J.F.S.I.G. Kayser, *Recent progress, methods and perspectives in forensic epigenetics.* 2018. **37**: p. 180-195.
106. Muharam, I. and C.J.H.o.D.P. Paintner, *Validating Forensic DNA Workflows 50.* 2022: p. 1087.
107. Wheate, R.M. and A.J.I.C.o.E. Jamieson, *A tale of two approaches-the NAS report and the Law Commission consultation paper on forensic science.* 2010. **7**(2).
108. Zephro, L., A.J.F.a. Galloway, and t.U.S.j. system, *Report writing and case documentation in forensic anthropology.* 2019: p. 89-108.
109. Daluz, H.M., *Fingerprint analysis laboratory workbook.* 2018: CRC Press.
110. Stoyanova, M., *et al.*, *A survey on the internet of things (IoT) forensics: challenges, approaches, and open issues.* 2020. **22**(2): p. 1191-1221.
111. Cruzes, D.S., *et al.*, *Case studies synthesis: a thematic, cross-case, and narrative synthesis worked example.* 2015. **20**: p. 1634-1665.
112. Cowie, H., *et al.*, *Measuring workplace bullying.* 2002. **7**(1): p. 33-51.
113. Gruber, J., C.J. Hargreaves, and F.C.J.F.S.I.D.I. *Freiling, Contamination of digital evidence: Understanding an underexposed risk.* 2023. **44**: p. 301501.
114. Palmiere, C., *et al.*, *Bacterial translocation and sample contamination in postmortem microbiological analyses.* 2016. **61**(2): p. 367-374.
115. Rao, P.K., *et al.*, *Biological evidence and their handling.* 2020: p. 35-53.
116. Watterson, J., V. Blackmore, and D.J.F.E. Bagby, *Considerations for the Analysis of Forensic Samples Following Extended Exposure to the Environment.* 2006. **15**(4).
117. Girma, G.J.E.A.J.o.B.S., G. Microbiology, *Microbial bioremediation of some heavy metals in soils: an updated review.* 2015. **7**(1): p. 29-45.
118. Guarino, A. *Digital forensics as a big data challenge. in ISSE 2013 Securing Electronic Business Processes: Highlights of the Information Security Solutions Europe 2013 Conference.* 2013. Springer.
119. Granja, F.M., G.D.R.J.I.J.o.E.S. Rafael, and D. Forensics, *The preservation of digital evidence and its admissibility in the court.* 2017. **9**(1): p. 1-18.
120. Bakardjiev, D.K.J.J., *Officer body-worn cameras-capturing objective evidence with quality technology and focused policies.* 2015. **56**: p. 79.
121. Rees, H.C., *et al.*, *The detection of aquatic animal species using environmental DNA–a review of eDNA as a survey tool in ecology.* 2014. **51**(5): p. 1450-1459.
122. Mich, L.J.H.o.e.-T., *Artificial intelligence and machine learning.* 2020: p. 1-21.
123. Zappi, A., *et al.*, *Extracting information and enhancing the quality of separation data: a review on chemometrics-assisted analysis of volatile, soluble and colloidal samples.* 2023. **11**(1): p. 45.
124. Pyrek, K., *Forensic science under siege: The challenges of forensic laboratories and the medico-legal investigation system.* 2010: Elsevier.

125. Julian, R.D., *et al.*, *What is the value of forensic science? An overview of the effectiveness of forensic science in the Australian criminal justice system project.* 2011. **43**(4): p. 217-229.
126. McKiernan, H. and P.B. Danielson, *Molecular diagnostic applications in forensic science, in Molecular diagnostics.* 2017, Elsevier. p. 371-394.
127. Dowd, E., *Backlogged or Logjammed? An Analysis of the Patterns that Surround the Rape Kit Backlog Across Jurisdictions.* 2020.
128. Sabatello, M., *et al.*, *Structural racism in the COVID-19 pandemic: Moving forward.* 2021. **21**(3): p. 56-74.
129. Gupta, B., P. Agarwal, and D.J.I.-M.s.J.o.P.R. Devalia, *TRACKING MISSING PERSONS USING FACIAL RECOGNITION.* 2023. **10**(1).
130. Dunsin, D., *et al.*, *A Comprehensive Analysis of the Role of Artificial Intelligence and Machine Learning in Modern Digital Forensics and Incident Response.* 2023.
131. Tachizawa, E.M., M.J. Alvarez-Gil, and M.J.J.S.C.M.A.I.J. Montes-Sancho, *How "smart cities" will change supply chain management.* 2015. **20**(3): p. 237-248.
132. Samtani, S., *et al.*, *Cybersecurity as an industry: A cyber threat intelligence perspective.* 2020: p. 135-154.
133. Grimes, R.A., *Cryptography apocalypse: preparing for the day when quantum computing breaks today's crypto.* 2019: John Wiley & Sons.
134. Naik, A., *et al.*, *From Portfolio Optimization to Quantum Blockchain and Security: A Systematic Review of Quantum Computing in Finance.* 2023.
135. Bashirpour Bonab, A., *et al.*, *Quantum Technologies for Smart Cities: A Comprehensive Review and Analysis.* 2022.

3

Vibrational Spectroscopy in Forensic Sample Analysis

Harjeet Singh[1], Noble George[1,2], Deepti Attitiniti[2] and Shivani R. Pandya[1,2*]

[1]*Centre of Research for Development, Parul University, Vadodara (Gujarat), India*
[2]*Dept. of Forensic Science, PIAS, Parul University, Vadodara (Gujarat), India*

Abstract

Vibrational spectroscopy (VS) has undergone significant improvements over the past several decades, given its non-destructivity, selectivity, efficiency and portability, notably in the field of forensics, compared to other scientific techniques. Raman Spectroscopy (RS) and Infrared spectroscopy (IRS) conjugated with chemometrics has emerged as a viable technique for the investigation of forensic evidence in light of these advancements. Body fluids are rarely observed at crime scenes in their pure form, in such cases VS with mapping can identify the biological fluids even in heterogeneous condition contaminated with sand, grit or dirt. This approach may be used to distinguish between the organic and inorganic components in ballistic studies. Additionally, they play a significant role in resolving vehicular accident scenarios by examining trace evidence like paints. They are quite helpful in detecting the narcotics even at low concentration whenever it comes to the substance of abuse situations. However, improved VS methods would be generated as the need for extracting in-depth and versatile information out of primary evidences is inevitable. Furthermore, these methods have already shown their utility in forensics and will continue to do so for many years to come. This section of the book discusses the significance of VS towards the distinction and identification of diverse crime scene evidence beyond other conventional approaches.

***Keywords*:** Vibrational spectroscopy, chemometrics, infrared spectroscopy, raman spectroscopy, non-invasive, forensic evidences

**Corresponding author*: shivpan02@gmail.com; mailgsbtm@gmail.com

Priyanka Chhabra, Divya Bajpai Tripathy, Anjali Gupta, Rajeev Kumar, Kajol Bhati and Shruti Shukla (eds.) Advances in Analytical Techniques for Forensic Investigation, (69–92) © 2024 Scrivener Publishing LLC

3.1 Fundamentals of Vibrational Spectroscopy (VS)

It is a non-invasive identification technique that examines a chemical's vibrational energy. Each chemical bond in a molecule possesses its own vibrational energy leading to have a unique fingerprint as a result of this unique vibrational energy, the output indicating the peak strengths at various vibrations. This fingerprint is useful for determining chemical structure, identifying and characterizing compounds ultimately identifying contaminants. This is accomplished by comparing the test fingerprints to known compound fingerprints.

A very wide variety of sample types are studied using vibrational spectroscopy, which can be used for anything from a quick identification test to a comprehensive, entire spectrum, qualitative and quantitative examination. Over an expansive assortment of thermal readings and physical status, samples can be analyzed in bulk or in tiny quantities. Also vibrational spectroscopy offers a wide range of possibilities and having the capability to solve a variety of significant and difficult analytical issues.

3.2 General Forms of Vibrational Spectroscopy

Current vibrational spectroscopy comprises a diverse set of techniques centered on two substantially separate manifestations; (i) infrared absorbing and (ii) Raman scattering [1]. Because they combine a number of advantages, the spectroscopic technologies such as infrared and Raman have already risen in popularity in forensic applications [2–4]. Both Raman and mid-IR spectroscopy offer distinctive fundamental vibrations that are widely utilized to decide and identify molecular architecture, and are equally complementary to one another, and both are frequently required to fully quantify a molecule's vibrational energies (Figure 3.1).

Although certain vibrations may be brisk in both RS and IR spectroscopy, both of them result from separate procedures and principles. Imprecisely, RS excels at symmetric vibrations of non-polar groups, whereas IRS thrives at asymmetric polar group vibrations. The exploration of association of radiation with molecular vibrations is a component of both IR and RS, although they vary in the way in which photon energy is conveyed to the molecule via influencing its vibrational state. Without an analyst who is conversant with the fundamentals of spectral interpretation, the full potential of IRS and RS cannot be fulfilled.

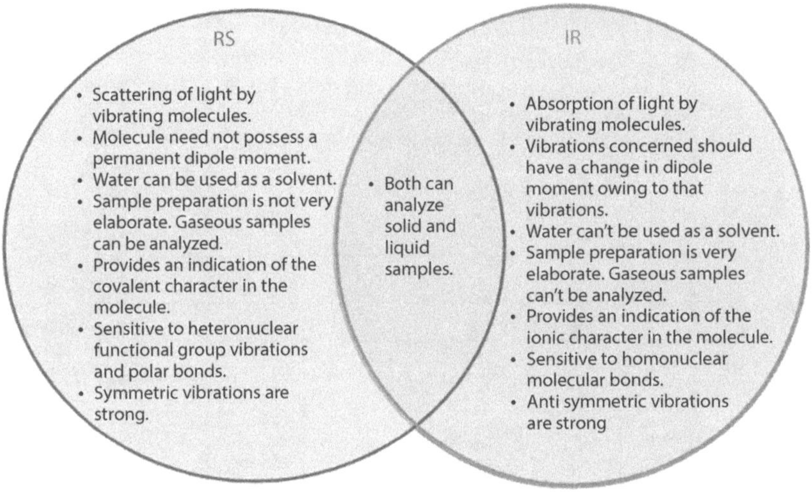

Figure 3.1 General comparison between Raman and IR spectroscopy.

3.2.1 Raman Spectroscopy: Science of Elastic and Inelastic Scattering of Photons

The elastic and inelastic scattering of radiant energy is the essential concept underpinning RS (Figure 3.2) [5]. Radiation can be absorbed, reflected, or dispersed when it strikes a sample [6]. Elastic or Rayleigh scattering is the situation that takes place when the energies of the photons produced by scattering and the radiant energy are identical [7, 8]. Inelastic or Raman scattering, on the other hand, is an occurrence in which the power of the incoming rays will be more or less than the power of photons produced by dispersion [7, 8]. This scattering is further categorized into stokes and anti-stokes resulting from the power that photons carry after getting scattered [8]. As a result, Raman scattering yields information on molecule vibrational structures that will serve as a molecular footprint. Furthermore, "Surface Enhanced Raman Spectroscopy" (SERS) is a variation of 'Raman' that modifies and increases the basic approach's susceptibility and differentiation [9, 10].

RS is a potent method that creates significant spectrum variation between samples and substrates that causes disruptions to allow for visual separation. A categorization confidence value of 70% was generated by the Support Vector Machines Discriminant Analysis (SVMDA) approach, indicating that all physiological fluids were correctly identified and none of the substrates causing disturbance was identified as one of the 5 biological fluids. False positive results are prevented by combining chemometrics and

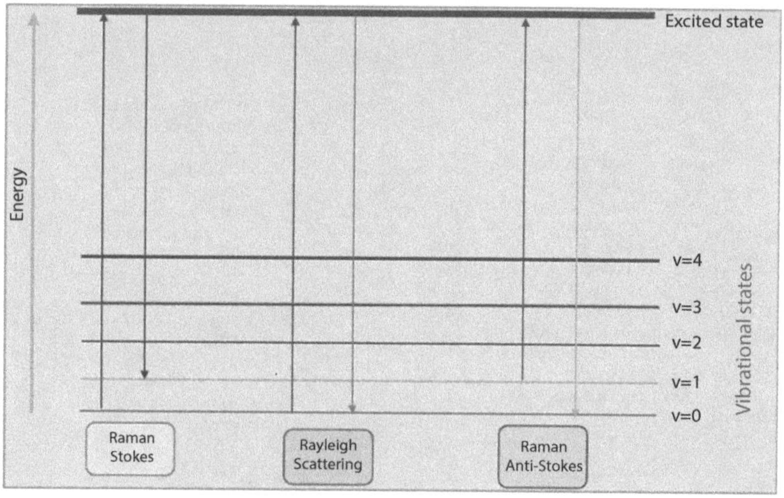

Figure 3.2 Graphical representation of the principal of Raman Spectroscopy. (Image was reused with permission) [11].

Raman spectroscopy for the identification and segregation of biological fluids [11, 12]. Despite being dependent on the spectroscopic characteristics of the substrates, physiologic fluids' spectral fingerprints may be extracted using RS and the Hypothetical Addition Multivariate Analysis with Numerical Differentiation (HAMAND) program. The program searches for inputs to the band of an unidentified chemical using the standard spectrum of the target analyte [11, 12], because the target's input can be seen independently after using HAMAND on the data. Additionally, it does not rely on any substrate characterization in the question; rather, it searches for the elements of a target feature that has been defined. Likewise, HAMAND evaluates the amount of biological fluids in a smear without the necessity of additional complicated equipment and provides quick findings.

3.2.2 IR Spectroscopy: Technique Based on Interaction of Infrared Radiation with Matter

Dispersive IR spectroscopy has certain flaws, which led to the development of Fourier Transform Infrared Spectroscopy (FT-IR), a technique that measures all wavelengths collectively, as opposed to individually. The interferometer is a straightforward optical apparatus that produces a distinctive response for each IR frequency that is "recorded" and produces spectra. The beam splitter absorbs IR light and separates it all into two optical streams. Two beams interfere with one another to form the interferometer, which produces the interferogram as a signal. The observed signal cannot be directly analyzed in order to produce identification, but it may be determined by using a mathematical method known as "Fourier Transformation" to decode the component frequencies. It could be done using a computer that displays the spectrum data for evaluation [13].

The fundamental idea behind the FT-IR involves specimen exposure with infrared light to capture the vibrations of the subject particles' molecular bonds [14]. FT-IR has two regions, namely, functional group (which represents functional groups of given samples or compounds) and fingerprint region (which provides unique details about the given compound). The major advantages of FT-IR are speed, sensitivity, mechanical simplicity, and internal calibration of samples. Due to its non-destructive nature, it has become a promising tool for analysis of evidence found at scenes. FTIR is useful for analyzing a range of evidences like biofluids, chemical and physical evidence like hair, paints, documents and even gunshot residues. Invariably it has become an accepted diagnostic tool for biomarkers identification [13].

ATR-FT-IR, which holds for "Attenuated Total Reflectance Fourier Transform Infrared," was developed as a result of advances in the area of spectroscopic percussion. It has been used in a multitude of biological research and is capable of probing numerous levels of assimilated species at a solid or liquid interface. It has gained attention for its diagnostic capabilities following discrimination of health from diseased samples [14]. Another variation, FTIR-PAS stands for 'Fourier Transform Infrared Photoacoustic Spectroscopy', which deals with depth of spectral analysis and thermal properties and to differentiate between optical and opaque substances [15]. Because of the enhanced speed and sensitivity of Fourier transform infrared (FT-IR) spectroscopy, the implementation of IR to forensic investigation became more prominent [16].

3.2.3 Chemometrics: Data Driven Science to Extract Chemical Information

Chemometrics is an articulation that uses statistical and mathematical approaches to build the most efficient experimental setups and to get knowledge from intricate analytical data. Moreover, Raman and IR spectra offer characteristics that resemble fingerprints of materials, leading to very complicated spectra. Therefore, to analyze, measure, or categorize vibrational spectroscopic data, multivariate statistical techniques are necessary [17]. Depending on the circumstances at hand and the information required, several chemometric approaches can be used in forensic investigation.

The most popular unsupervised approach is principal component analysis (PCA), which is used in particular to extract the relevant details from a dataset in a confined area based on the variance of the data. It is crucial to stress that PCA is an exploration method rather than a classification method [4, 18]. The assessment of the FT-IR data appears to require the use of multivariate statistical approaches (MSA) in order to enable feature extraction, accurate evaluation and identification of produced spectra [17]. Another supervised pattern recognition technique is Linear Discriminant Analysis (LDA). The criteria in LDA are a maximum discrimination among the specified classes, whereas PCA chooses a direction that maintains maximal structure in a lower dimension [19, 20]. Combining PCA with LDA is particularly beneficial since it increases classification efficiency by automatically choosing the most important characteristics to include in the classification model.

3.3 The Deployment of Vibrational Spectroscopy in Forensics and Criminal Investigations

As crime rates and methods of operation evolve, innovative, quick, and precise analytical methodologies are necessary in the forensic domain [11, 21]. Even though there are commonalities, never two different murder scenes are identical. The backdrop in which a felony is committed may fluctuate depending on the circumstances. This has an impact on the sorts of proof found in criminal investigations. As a reason, identifying, differentiating and evaluating such buried proofs would be a tough and time-consuming task for an analyst [11, 21–24]. Techniques must be quantifiable and even have corresponding statistical certainty in order to remove the effect of an investigator and allow for the objective determination of the likelihood of error. In order to boost output, it could have been better for procedures to be automated and commercial. As discussed earlier, in forensic investigations, RS and IR spectroscopy are increasingly gaining attention as they are quick, effective, precise and conclusive [1]. RS is a multidimensional, viable, touchless and non-destructive validation technique for analyzing forensic evidences [11, 25]. It rely upon inelastic dispersion of laser beam by vibration of molecules [1, 11], therefore, could differentiate chemicals following the dispersion phenomenon. In light of the enhanced speed and sensitivity of Fourier transform infrared (FT-IR) spectroscopy, the deployment of the mentioned spectroscopy to forensic investigation grew more common with its development [16]. Both the techniques are useful in their own way and some of the chemical and biological compounds are discussed in the approaching sections which can be analyzed maneuvering RS and FT-IRS.

3.3.1 Biological Fluids

Biological fluids recovered at a criminal investigation site potentially act as a conduit, linking the scene and the victim or charged. As an outcome, forensic investigation of such bodily fluids is critical in determining if a criminal or victim exists [26, 27]. A scientific investigator's preferred gadget should be one that may be used at a crime scene to identify all bodily fluid samples found without tampering with or corrupting the evidence. Comparing spectroscopic approaches to conventional chemical tests, there are a number of benefits making them meritorious. As noted earlier, spectroscopic techniques are quick, focused, and most importantly, noninvasive. Some of the relevant biological fluids which are established evidences are addressed in detail below.

i. Blood

Blood is an important body fluid for the clinical and diagnostic disciplines as well as for thorough forensic analysis. The benefactions from Hb predominate the average spectrum of peripheral blood. The heme group's strong peak at the wavelengths 753 cm^{-1}, 1372 cm^{-1}, 1577 cm^{-1} and 1620 cm^{-1}, phyrin and pyrrole rings could be seen. Phenylalanine, on the other hand, guarantees that blood seems to have a greater extent at 1002 cm^{-1} while a broad amide III indication at 1245 cm^{-1} [28]. Many individuals are experimenting with serum samples in order to apply them as a source of identification. Researchers can now identify (i) age; (ii) race and (iii) gender of an 'unidentified blood' shade by using RS. Blood serves as a connecting tissue in both human beings and animals. Identification of these samples belonging to human or animal is therefore crucial. RS have the capability to discriminate human and animal on the basis of respective 'fingerprint regions' of animal and human blood. Therefore, RS is useful in identifying the source of blood.

A blood sample's provenance may be ascertained using RS in combination with chemometrics, as demonstrated by Gregory *et al.* [28]. Visible variations were discovered when the absorption spectra from the bloodstream and a variety of other animals were examined [28]. McLaughlin *et al.*

in their study has successfully categorized ten unidentified samples as either human or animal during the blind assessment. Ten distinct spectra from cattle blood were collected in total, which were also classified as animal (Figure 3.3). Therefore, it is possible to use this technology to identify the species of origin of a blood sample that produces without any incorrect findings [28]. It has also been proven that the gender can be distinguished

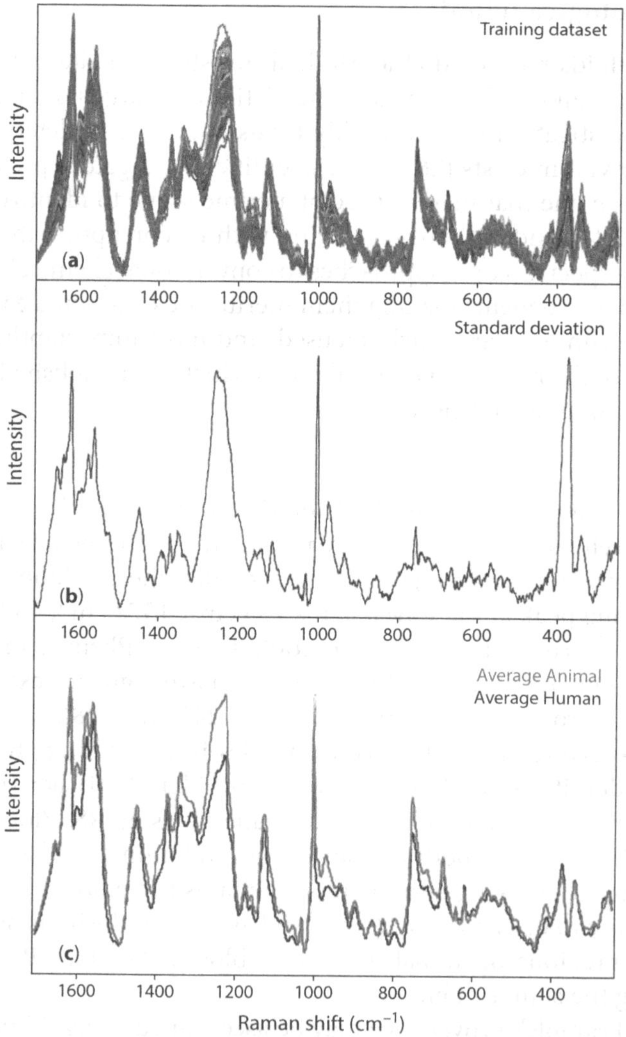

Figure 3.3 (a) Comparative Raman spectra of all 11 species (b) Standard deviation of 11 species' precompiled Raman spectra and (c) the average of all the animal (n = 100) and humans (n = 10) spectra. (The spectral graph has been reproduced with authorization) [28].

from the procured blood sample by RS. As that male and female blood differs biochemically, RS can be used to confirm the gender of blood donors. Coagulation factors are twice as abundant in the plasma of women as in those of males [12].

The levels of globulin, cholesterol, alkaline phosphatase as well as hematocrit are different between men and women. Gender variations in lipoprotein, the main dietary fat-carrying molecule in human blood that could be identified biochemically, are present [12]. RS research on blood for gender determination came to the conclusion that there are only slight variations in the 930 to 975 cm^{-1}, 1210 to 1230 cm^{-1}, and 1560 to 1580 cm^{-1} peaks. The accuracy of sex distinction produced by combining an algorithm with an artificial neural network was nearly 98% [12, 29].

Usually body fluids in their pure form, are rarely detected at crime scenes. It is possible that the area has environmental contaminants or contaminants from other bodily fluids. Even in samples tainted with sand, grit, or soil, RS with chemometric mapping may identify blood. The ability to distinguish peripheral blood from menstrual blood is a crucial step in a sexual assault investigation. There weren't many tactics that could be used at the crime scene prior to RS. There are just a few peaks that differ in their relative intensities, but the spectra imprints of menstrual and peripheral blood are quite alike in structure. When contrasted to menstrual blood, the tryptophan peak in peripheral blood is more prominent at 744 cm^{-1}, whereas the peaks related to heme group is at 1125 cm^{-1} [30]. Following chemometrics combined with RS, 100% discrimination is possible and even vaginal fluids and menstrual blood can be distinguished [7, 30].

DNA analysis of a blood cannot reveal biological age, in contrast to race and gender. Therefore, particular care has been taken to ascertain the biological age of the blood specimen's donor. In a study on the impact of age of blood samples, Kyle *et al.* (2018) divided the contributors into 3 age categories: new-borns (< 1 year old), adolescents (11–13 years old), and the elderly (43–68 years old) [31]. RS and chemometrics were utilized to analyze the samples. The frequency is stronger at the surges at 320 cm^{-1}, 375 cm^{-1}, 1030 cm^{-1}, 1570 cm^{-1} and 1620 cm^{-1} when determining the donor's age group. The period after the deposition of a blood stain may be determined using 375 cm^{-1} stretching frequency, a recognized indicator for met-Hb [29]. The amplitudes of 375 cm^{-1} in adult, neonatal, and teenage donors were noticeably varied. Implicating that this rise might indeed be utilized to establish the correspondent's biological age and time frame of blood-spatter accumulation. The magnitude of the peak at 375 cm^{-1} varied according to the age groups. The spectra exhibited excellent contributor differentiation based on chronological age despite the influence of factors like food, health, etc. on the donors [31]. E. Mistek *et al.* (2016) employed dried blood traces and RS for the first time to differentiate between races [32]. The findings suggested that RS might be used to distinguish between races in peripheral blood. Blood content quantitatively differs by race, and RS, which is supported by chemometrics, was able to identify these differences [32].

ii. Semen

Semen is a bodily fluid conjured up of both cellular and noncellular substances. The cellular part predominantly contains WBCs, epithelial cells, and sperm cells. While the non-cellular component contains the seminal plasma, which feeds the sperm cells. Semen is a crucial piece of proof in accusations of sexual assault. In the past, researchers used the existence of sperm cells to verify the presence of semen. The lack of sperm cells within semen led to the development of the disorder known as azoospermia. By employing RS along with chemometrics the examination of seminal fluid provide details of the presence of semen in the total fluid [33]. Choline produced the first discernible signal during the observation of the surge at 715 cm^{-1}, while fructose along with tyrosine accounts for significant crest at 830 cm^{-1} [29, 33]. Additionally, they noticed an increase in lactate, tyrosine, but also tryptophan at 850 cm^{-1}. A significant notch was produced at 958 cm^{-1} by spermine phosphate hexahydrate and citrate [29, 33]. RS hence proved that sperm cells are not necessary for studying semen and hence the condition of azoospermia was neglected while examining the semen samples.

iii. Oral Fluid

It is transparent fluid contains water, that can be retrieved using non-invasive approaches, and. The salivary production from the glands, oral microorganisms and cells from the mouth make up the majority of the oral fluid. Currently, it is used to screen for substance abuse instead of blood and urine. It has recently been discovered that the content of illicit drug chemicals is markedly larger in oral fluid than in blood, and they are easily detectable at lower quantities [25]. False positive readings are a downside of the traditional assays used for oral fluid monitoring. While SERS allows the identification of substances at microgram amounts in oral fluid [25]. The amino acids predominate in saliva's Raman spectrum. In saliva, phenylalanine exhibits large peaks at 1003 cm^{-1} and 1444 cm^{-1}, while tyrosine has a faint signal at 853 cm^{-1} [25]. Spectra of dehydrated saliva remnants were used to distinguish between smokers and non-smokers. An algorithm accurately predicted outcomes by differentiating certain spectral areas between the two groups. In light of this, a proposal has been introduced that modified RS can be used in criminal justice [34].

iv. Vaginal Secretions

It is a blend of leucocytes, delaminated cell components, vaginal mucosal releases and peptides from the genital tract [35, 36]. The vaginal fluid approach exploits immunological investigations (basically based on female hormones). As mentioned in the above sections, RS had 100% discrimination towards blood, employing potent chemo-metrics and RS [37].

Ideally, forensic methods for bodily fluid studies might be modelled after Raman and IR spectroscopy. Both are ideal for investigating crime scenes because of their non-invasive, quick, and conclusive characteristics [35, 38]. Also the sophisticated approaches like SERS, help to circumvent susceptibility and sample size restrictions [39]. Investigators can evaluate complicated spectrum data sets and retrieve data using descriptive stats and chemometrics, leading to more precise and comprehensive conclusions [27].

3.3.2 Ballistics

i. Gun Shot Residues

Through identifying whether discovered ballistic proof came from a certain firearm, forensics experts try to connect offenders to specific shooting instances. This method relies on tool mark analysis, which evaluates striations on fired bullets or cartridge casings as being exclusive to a particular weapon [40, 41]. Unfortunately, tool mark evaluations rely on the expertise of the examiner, which invites bias and examiner discrepancies. For said purpose of reconstructing firing incidents, the latest events in analytical technology have increased the utility of gunshot residue (GSR) [41].

GSR is made up of the burned and somewhat unburnt remnants of the firing of firearms. Usually the analysis of gunshot residues is done through XRD and SEM-EDX [40]. Although these techniques are highly reliable, they cannot detect organic GSR particles. VS is capable of coupling the analytical information with a single GSR particulate, minimizing the probability of mislead convictions significantly in contrast to bulk GSR studies [42]. Contrary to that, Raman is used to detect both organic and inorganic GSR particles [3]. The major advantage of utilizing RS is, it can distinguish the body fluids, ink, sand and other contaminants from GSR particles, confirming its screening capability [43]. It establishes a chemical and statistical linkage between the accused and the crime scene and has the potential to be quick, sensitive, portable, solvent-free and precise for GSR identification [44]. The Raman method has emerged as a key tool for analyzing the organic components, especially in lead-free ammunition, and is notably helpful for identifying various metal anions in GSR particulates, such as Ba and Pb [41, 43]. Eventually the traditional and non-toxic GSR particulates could easily be distinguished. This method offers microscopic viewing of the GSR particles along with chemical data. GSR from various gun-and-ammunition configurations could easily be distinguished using ATR-FT-IR spectroscopy. Goudsmits *et al.* (2015), insightful study on ATR-FT-IR spectra produced by a "dark-colored GSR" having its Raman signature masked by fluorescence. Spatially Offset Raman Spectroscopy (SORS) prevents Raman scattering and fluorescence from canisters and enables consumers to get a Raman spectrum of the components [44].

ii. Explosives

Incendiaries are very powerful, delicate and hazardous materials employed in both civilian and military settings as well as in terrorist acts. Given the wide range of explosive compounds which come from army, industrial and improvised channels and can be discovered intact, concealed in canisters, the exploration of incendiary devices can be very difficult and intricate. IRS and RS are the well-established methods for the examination of explosives. Even more, handheld devices have been introduced to the crime scenes for the detection and analysis of explosive compounds [45].

Explosive compounds create a distinctive infrared spectrum, which makes IRS beneficial for identifying the main constituents in mass bombs, similar to what numerous forms of forensic evidence do [46]. The basic vibrational and rotational shifts of all the explosives usually found in the mid-IR region, making IRS a rather honed for explosive detection [47]. Nevertheless, it is still challenging to find these energetic components required to make explosive devices, and they continue to pose the biggest hazard to army and ordinary workers [48]. Plastic explosives have been satisfactorily subjected to ATR-FT-IR both in bulk and following extraction [49]. Visually looking for particles in fingerprints and detecting the FTIR spectra of the particles are the integrated functions of ATR-FTIR spectromicroscopy. With the use of the above feature, it is feasible to determine from a suspect's fingerprints solely if they have dealt explosive [50, 51]. For the investigation of explosives at the crime scenes, recent advancements in portable FT-IR apparatus seems to be promising. IR has the capability to be employed for remote explosives monitoring. In an investigation, many explosive substances were identified using FT-IR spectroscopy and monitored at a five-meter distance [52, 53].

Due to their quick collection periods, lower error rates and non-invasive nature, vibrational spectroscopic methods seem appealing for the investigation of explosives [54, 55]. Low sensitivity issues can prevent RS and IRS from finding widespread use in practice. RS is constrained by this limitation, whereas SERS can get around it. SORS is restricted to non-metallic canisters [56]. However, it is very helpful for precise chemical analysis of materials in sealed canisters that are inaccessible by traditional RS techniques [52, 57].

3.3.3 Document and Ink Evidences

Document examination plays a crucial role in forensics, for the examination and comparison of handwritings, ink analysis, printing processes, papers and even currency notes as well as the characteristics of documents. Knowing the legitimacy of the document and establishing a relationship between the culprit and a crime scene are two of the main benefits of ink analysis [58]. While analyzing the ink, the fact to consider is that there is a tiny chemical interaction that takes place between the ink and the paper [59]. In order to detect that, the vibrational techniques became a promising tool for analysis of inks. Both FT-IR and RS help us to determine the chemical and elemental composition of the ink. FT-IR is used for differentiating the inks and toners based on intensity and peaks related to different components of the dyes, which gives information regarding their pigments and particular functional groups [60]. The spectrum also provides 'molecular fingerprints' of the ink samples [1]. ATR-IR spectra help to know about the type of materials used on paper, various binding agents and minerals, while RS deals with the course and shape of the curve that corresponds to florescence intensity and is capable of determining both chemical and elemental composition and its structure [61]. Notably, Raman spectral analyses have even succeeded in distinguishing the inks from the same manufacturer at different times [62] and even able to determine the order of handwritten strokes, being non-invasive in nature [63]. Extended Raman Spectroscopy techniques *i.e.* Micro-Raman spectroscopy is showing promising non-invasive method for determination of the origin of the ink of counterfeit currencies [64].

3.3.4 Trace Evidences

At a crime scene, often tiny physical evidence such as fiber, hair, etc. are left behind and even they could transfer from one place to another. According to 'Locard's principle of exchange', "when two objects come in contact with each other, there will always be an exchange of material". The most commonly found trace evidences at the crime scenes are hair, paint chips, soils, fibers, glass and tapes. These evidences play a significant role and help to find the culprit for the crime scene. But the handling and analysis of trace evidence requires the utmost care and specialized techniques. Some of the major trace evidences are discussed in the succeeding sections in light of RS and IRS.

i. Hair Evidence

The most prevalent scientific proof discovered at scenes is hair, which could be found anywhere in the environment. As growth is continuous, there is constant loss and replacement of hair strands as they get transferred during the act of crime and it plays a vital role in investigations. Care should be taken while inspecting the hair specimen and the features of the body area, color, length and breakage must be considered. Currently, the most common method for hair analysis is microscopic examination. However, with advancements in technology, spectroscopic methods have gained a lot of attention, and can dramatically enhance the data obtained from them. Both FT-IR and Raman Spectroscopy have been used to identify the "melanin granules" in hairs. Foggia *et al.* studied bleaching of hair samples by ATR-FT-IR [65], and found it useful for the identification and visualization of the stretching and vibrations of lipids in cortex and cuticle regions. Boll *et al.* has worked on differentiation of dyed and non-dyed hairs and its classification using statistical approach from the results of ATR-FT-IR analysis [66]. FT-IR helps to know the layer of hair by absorbing at different intensities containing particular functional groups [67]. This information is highly reliable for comparing the questioned sample with the standard hair samples [4]. ATR-FT-IR along with chemometric analysis can differentiate the origin of hair i.e. between human, felines and canines which is non-invasive, rapid and reliable [68].

ii. Fiber Evidences

Fiber is one of the most common pieces of evidence usually found in cases like homicide and sexual assaults. These fibers are ubiquitous and could be found in fingernails, hair, clothes etc. These may be natural or synthetic fibers that could help in developing a link between a crime scenes to a suspect. To evaluate the worth of fiber proof, manufacturing, chemical and physical qualities are needed. The forensic examiner generally uses textile and fiber proof while analyzing fibers. Textile fibers of different origin, dyed using various pigments could also be differentiated and identified using Raman imaging and multivariate techniques (Figure 3.4) [69].

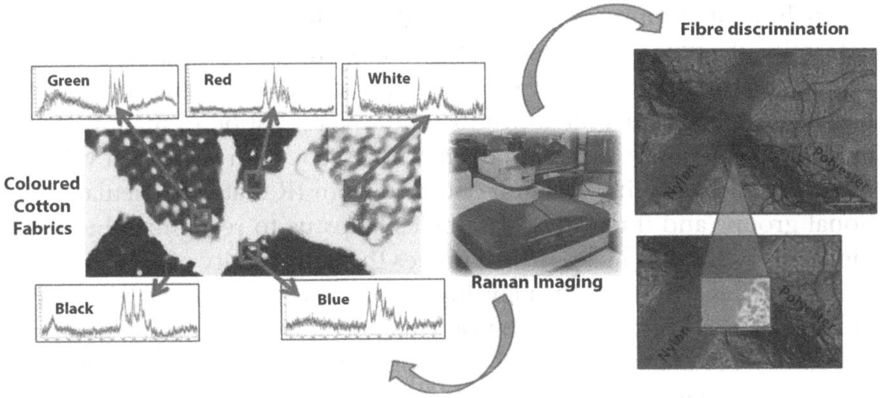

Figure 3.4 Graphical representation of differentiation of colored textile fibers through Raman imaging (Image is used with authorization) [69].

The foremost method for analyzing natural and synthetic fiber evidence is microscopy, though for further specificity of fiber type IR is very useful [70]. RS is used for the determinations and differentiation of fibers of various ages, which are exhibiting acceptable results while compiled with chemometrics i.e. multivariate analysis and hence forensic expert will get to know the origin and deposition time of the evidence at scene of crime [71]. In contrast to previous methods, RS and IRS have been utilized to discriminate between the two types of polymers. Variants of FT-IR i.e. reflectance-FT-IR (r-FT-IR), FT-IR-microspectrometer with ATR mode (mATR-FT-IR) and ATR-FTIR studies between the amide-based fibers wool, silk and polyamides were carried out by Peet *et al.* [72]. All mentioned variants showing promising and accurate results with non-invasiveness, but among r-FT-IR, mATR-FT-IR and ATR-FT-IR, r-FT-IR is showing very accurate and acceptable results and hence useful for forensic evidence analysis [72].

iii. Paint Evidences

Numerous types of paper, wood, plastics, metals and other general covering substances are covered with paint. The three main components of paint are binder, solvent and pigment [5, 73]. The paint chips are usually found in hit and run cases and on vehicles and buildings. As Locard's principle says, interaction between two things results in the transfer of material. This transfer of material provides valuable information about the suspect and the crime scene. Rather than light microscopy, IR and Raman spectroscopy obtain specific chemical information regarding binders, pigments and additives from paint sample [74].

Analysis of automotive paint through FT-IR helps forensic experts to determine the types of organic binders and resins, but the pigments are not detectable using the same [75]. However, Micro-Raman spectrophotometer (M-RS) enables the identification and differentiation of main pigment by comparing paint chip found from crime scene with suspected vehicle's paint. The chemical information obtained from IR that is particular functional groups and intensities of samples helps us to recognize the make, model and year of vehicles, which proves the authenticity of art [75].

M-RS plays a vital role in analyzing the paint, as it enables *in situ* analysis of paint without further preparation which avoids handling and contamination of trace material [76]. RS is not only applicable to organic samples, Gelder *et al.* has identified the presence of calcite and barium sulphate by identifying characteristic Raman band and additional information like binder can be extracted by combining IR spectroscopy [77]. Surface Enhanced Raman Spectrophotometry (SERS) aids in the identification of the chemicals, including fuchsin, crystal violet and other dyes, as well as the monitoring of crystal violet ageing [73, 78].

3.3.5 Controlled Substances

i. **Illicit Drugs**

Illicit drugs are those which are highly addictive and illegal substances. These are not prescribed by doctors and encountered by law enforcement agencies. This includes cocaine, marijuana, opioids, etc. prepared from naturally occurring substances or totally synthetic form for an instance, amphetamines, MDMA etc. [79]. Usually, illicit drug cases are examined by forensic science laboratories using X-ray, Mass, IR, Raman for their various analysis and are all validated by Scientific Working group of the Analysis of Seized Drugs (SWGDRUG) (Figure 3.5) [80]. Since from last few decades, RS and SERS techniques shows promising, rapid and accurate results for the determination of the quantification of novel psychoactive substances (NPS). In said context, Muhamadali *et al.* have conducted study on discrimination and quantification of methcathione and aminoindane derivative by combining Principal component analysis (PCA) along with RS and SERS [81]. Dong *et al.* have developed rapid direct detection method of Methamphetamine (MAMP) from urine using dynamic surface-enhances Raman spectroscopy (D-SERS) [82]. In addition to above, Han *et al.* developed portable kit for the sensitive and reliable Surface-enhanced Raman scattering (SERS) where kit includes two sealed reagent tube, standard SERS reagent and mini Raman device and

	Method	Discrimination	Substances	Identify (qualify)	Amount (quantify)	Destroy sample?	Lab	Point of care	Cost (USD)	Ease of use	Time required for results
Most discriminatory	Mass Spectrometry	★★★★★	Virtually any	Identify (qualify)	✓	Yes	✓		$5000 (used, older)–200.000+ (new, advanced models) Plus recurring costs (reagents, servicing)	Intermediate–advanced (depending on model)	Minutes
	Infrared spectrometry	★★★★★	Virtually any	✓	✓	No	✓	✓	$4000 (used, older)–100.000 (new, advanced models) Portable: 10,000–60,000 Plus recurring costs (licensing, servicing)	Basic–advanced (depending on model)	Second to minutes (Inc. Portable)
	Raman Spectroscopy	★★★★★	Virtually any	✓	✓	No	✓	✓	$5000 (used, older)–100.000 (new, advanced models) Portable: 10,000–60,000 Plus recurring costs (licensing, servicing)	Basic–advanced (depending on model)	Seconds to minutes (Inc. Portable)
	X-ray diffractometry	★★★★	Crystalline (solids)	✓	✓	No	✓		$50,000–250,000+ Plus recurring costs (reagents, servicing)	Advanced—expert	Minutes to hours

Figure 3.5 Tabular representation of most discriminatory methods for the identification and quantification of illicit drug. (Table is reused with authorization) [80].

can detect MDMA and Methacathione (MC) with the detection limit of 0.1 ppm [83]. Due to accuracy and rapidity now a days many scientists are focusing on developing effective methodology for the detection of various class of illicit drugs like cocaine, amphetamines, Banzodiazepams and other designer drugs [84–87]. Near Infrared Spectroscopy (NIR) followed by Chemometrics for the NPS screening has been validated and applied successfully for "in site" detection of illicit drugs at Rome [88]. ATR-FTIR and FT-Raman spectroscopy are applied for the detection and quantification of most important alkaloids in poppy milk [89].

3.4 Conclusions and Future Prospects

Contrary to other scientific disciplines, forensics occupies a special position owing to its significant and immediate influence on society. In order to effectively assess proof without taking into account bias, forensic procedures must have good approaches. Disruptive methods must also be resisted in order to safeguard the material for later study. In general, forensic techniques must be effective and trustworthy. Owing to both precise and noninvasive characters, VS techniques such as RS and IR in conjugation with chemometrics are indeed excellent resources for investigators. This guarantees that studies are impartial as well as preserves the material. Since most technical facilities are furnished either with an IR or RS, simultaneously, the approaches mentioned above are anticipated to have a significant influence on investigative processes by proving their viability. The search for something like a feasible alternative could find a solution in the form of RS and its later amendments. As a corollary, RS could end up becoming a necessary tool in the field of forensics.

It's indeed crucial to realize that perhaps the potential use of VS, chemometrics and scientific examination is currently actively explored and enhanced. Novel VS techniques will be created as the requirement for additional details from the proof increases. Such techniques have demonstrated their value in forensics so far though and will keep doing so for many decades to come.

References

1. Muro, C.K., Doty, K.C., Bueno, J., Halámková, L., and Lednev, I.K. (2015) Vibrational spectroscopy: Recent developments to revolutionize forensic science. *Anal. Chem.*, **87** (1), 306–327.
2. Doty, K.C., Muro, C.K., Bueno, J., Halámková, L., and Lednev, I.K. (2016) What can Raman spectroscopy do for criminalistics? *J. Raman Spectrosc.*, **47** (1), 39–50.
3. Doty, K.C., and Lednev, I.K. (2018) Raman spectroscopy for forensic purposes: Recent applications for serology and gunshot residue analysis. *TrAC - Trends Anal. Chem.*, **103**, 215–222.
4. Silva, C.S., Braz, A., and Pimentel, M.F. (2019) Vibrational spectroscopy and chemometrics in forensic chemistry: Critical review, current trends and challenges. *J. Braz. Chem. Soc.*, **30** (11), 2259–2290.
5. Khandasammy, S.R., Fikiet, M.A., Mistek, E., Ahmed, Y., Halámková, L., Bueno, J., and Lednev, I.K. (2018) Bloodstains, paintings, and drugs: Raman spectroscopy applications in forensic science. *Forensic Chem.*, **8**, 111–133.
6. Colthup, N.B., Daly, L.H., Wiberley, S.E., Colthup, N.B., Daly, L.H., and Wiberley, S.E. (1990) Chapter 7 – Olefin Groups. *Introd. to Infrared Raman Spectrosc.*, **1**, 247–260.
7. Skoog, D.A., West, D.M., Holler, F.J., and Crouch, S.R. (2014) *Fundamentals of analytical chemistry, 6th ed. Saunders College Pub., Fort Worth, 1992. (882 pp.).*, Cengage Learning.
8. Kobilinsky, L. (2012) Frontmatter, in *Forensic Chemistry Handbook*, pp. i–xxii.
9. Stiles, P.L., Dieringer, J.A., Shah, N.C., and Van Duyne, R.P. (2008) Surface-enhanced Raman spectroscopy. *Annu. Rev. Anal. Chem.*, **1** (1), 601–626.
10. Hanlan, J., Skoog, D.A., and West, D.M. (1973) Principles of Instrumental Analysis. *Stud. Conserv.*, **18** (1), 45.
11. George, N., Singh, H., Jotaniya, R., and Pandya, S.R. (2022) Raman spectroscopy for the determination of forensically important bio-fluids. *Forensic Sci. Int.*, **340**.

12. Sikirzhytskaya, A., Sikirzhytski, V., and Lednev, I.K. (2017) Determining Gender by Raman Spectroscopy of a Bloodstain. *Anal. Chem.*, **89** (3), 1486–1492.
13. Ganzoury, M.A., Allam, N.K., Nicolet, T., and All, C. (2015) Introduction to Fourier Transform Infrared Spectrometry. *Renew. Sustain. Energy Rev.*, **50**, 1–8.
14. Naseer, K., Ali, S., and Qazi, J. (2021) ATR-FTIR spectroscopy as the future of diagnostics: a systematic review of the approach using bio-fluids. *Appl. Spectrosc. Rev.*, **56** (2), 85–97.
15. Wartewig, S., and Neubert, R.H.H. (2005) Pharmaceutical applications of Mid-IR and Raman spectroscopy. *Adv. Drug Deliv. Rev.*, **57** (8), 1144–1170.
16. Meurens, M., and Yan, S.H. (2006) Applications of Vibrational Spectroscopy in Brewing, in *Handbook of Vibrational Spectroscopy*.
17. Banas, K., Banas, A., Moser, H.O., Bahou, M., Li, W., Yang, P., Cholewa, M., and Lim, S.K. (2010) Multivariate Analysis Techniques in the Forensics Investigation of the Postblast Residues by Means of Fourier Transform-Infrared Spectroscopy. *Anal. Chem.*, **82** (7), 3038–3044.
18. Kwofie, F. (2019) Vibrational Spectroscopy and Chemometrics Applied to the Forensic Analysis of Automotive Paints and Edible Oils.
19. Slutsky, B. (1998) Handbook of Chemometrics and Qualimetrics: Part A By D. L. Massart, B. G. M. Vandeginste, L. M. C. Buydens, S. De Jong, P. J. Lewi, and J. Smeyers-Verbeke. Data Handling in Science and Technology Volume 20A. Elsevier: Amsterdam. 1997. Xvii + 867 pp. ISBN 0-444-89724-0. $293.25. *J. Chem. Inf. Comput. Sci.*, **38** (6), 1254–1254.
20. Kumar, R., and Sharma, V. (2018) Chemometrics in forensic science. *TrAC Trends Anal. Chem.*, **105**, 191–201.
21. Eugene Y. Lien (2015) FORENSIC BIOLOGY SEROLOGY MANUAL Approving Authority: Eugene Y. Lien, Technical Leader, Serology Operations. 1–28.
22. Garvin, D. (2012) Richland County Sheriff's Department: Evidence and Property Handbook, Eds.2.0, 2ed., pp. 1–56.
23. Rosenblatt, R., Halámková, L., Doty, K.C., de Oliveira, E.A.C., and Lednev, I.K. (2019) Raman spectroscopy for forensic bloodstain identification: Method validation vs. environmental interferences. *Forensic Chem.*, **16**, 100175.
24. Fraser, J., and Williams, R. (2013) *Handbook of Forensic Science*, Willan.
25. D'Elia, V., García, G.M., and Ruiz, C.G. (2015) Spectroscopic Trends for the Determination of Illicit Drugs in Oral Fluid. *Appl. Spectrosc. Rev.*, **50** (9), 775–796.
26. Gooch, J., Morillas, A.V., and Frascione, N. (2019) Bioanalytical advancements in the reliable visualization and discrimination of bodily fluids, in *Advanced Sciences and Technologies for Security Applications*, Springer, pp. 75–102.

27. Harbison, S., and Fleming, R. (2016) Forensic body fluid identification: state of the art. *Res. Reports Forensic Med. Sci.*, 11.
28. McLaughlin, G., Doty, K.C., and Lednev, I.K. (2014) Discrimination of human and animal blood traces via Raman spectroscopy. *Forensic Sci. Int.*, **238**, 91–95.
29. Muro, C.K., Doty, K.C., de Souza Fernandes, L., and Lednev, I.K. (2016) Forensic body fluid identification and differentiation by Raman spectroscopy. *Forensic Chem.*, **1**, 31–38.
30. Sikirzhytskaya, A., Sikirzhytski, V., and Lednev, I.K. (2014) Raman spectroscopy coupled with advanced statistics for differentiating menstrual and peripheral blood. *J. Biophotonics*, **7** (1–2), 59–67.
31. Doty, K.C., and Lednev, I.K. (2018) Differentiating Donor Age Groups Based on Raman Spectroscopy of Bloodstains for Forensic Purposes. *ACS Cent. Sci.*, **4** (7), 862–867.
32. Mistek, E., Halámková, L., Doty, K.C., Muro, C.K., and Lednev, I.K. (2016) Race Differentiation by Raman Spectroscopy of a Bloodstain for Forensic Purposes. *Anal. Chem.*, **88** (15), 7453–7456.
33. Fikiet, M.A., and Lednev, I.K. (2019) Raman spectroscopic method for semen identification: Azoospermia. *Talanta*, **194**, 385–389.
34. Al-Hetlani, E., Halámková, L., Amin, M.O., and Lednev, I.K. (2020) Differentiating smokers and nonsmokers based on Raman spectroscopy of oral fluid and advanced statistics for forensic applications. *J. Biophotonics*, **13** (3).
35. Newton, M. (2015) Sexual Offenses, Adult: Sexual Assault - Persistence of Biological Samples. *Encycl. Forensic Leg. Med. Second Ed.*, 328–333.
36. Pizzorno, J.E., Murray, M.T., and Joiner-Bey, H. (2016) Vaginitis. *Clin. Handb. Nat. Med.*, 945–959.
37. Sikirzhytski, V., Sikirzhytskaya, A., and Lednev, I.K. (2011) Multidimensional Raman spectroscopic signatures as a tool for forensic identification of body fluid traces: A review. *Appl. Spectrosc.*, **65** (11), 1223–1232.
38. Ferkin, M.H., delBarco-Trillo, J., and Petrulis, A. (2017) Communication by Chemical Signals: Physiological Mechanisms, Ontogeny and Learning, Function, Evolution, and Cognition. *Horm. Brain Behav. Third Ed.*, **1**, 285–327.
39. Zegarelli, K.A. (2016) Surface-enhanced Raman spectroscopy for the forensic analysis of vaginal fluid.
40. Shrivastava, P., Jain, V.K., and Nagpal, S. (2021) Gunshot residue detection technologies—a review. *Egypt. J. Forensic Sci.*, 2021 11, **11** (1), 1–21.
41. Bueno, J., Sikirzhytski, V., and Lednev, I.K. (2012) Raman spectroscopic analysis of gunshot residue offering great potential for caliber differentiation. *Anal. Chem.*, **84** (10), 4334–4339.
42. Jain, B., and Yadav, P. (2021) Vibrational spectroscopy and chemometrics in GSR: review and current trend. *Egypt. J. Forensic Sci.*, **11** (1), 1–7.

43. Bueno, J., and Lednev, I.K. (2014) Raman microspectroscopic chemical mapping and chemometric classification for the identification of gunshot residue on adhesive tape. *Anal. Bioanal. Chem.*, **406** (19), 4595–4599.
44. Goudsmits, E., Sharples, G.P., and Birkett, J.W. (2015) Recent trends in organic gunshot residue analysis. *TrAC - Trends Anal. Chem.*, **74**, 46–57.
45. Moore, D.S., and Scharff, R.J. (2009) Portable Raman explosives detection. *Anal. Bioanal. Chem.*, **393** (6–7), 1571–1578.
46. Ramasamy, S., Houspian, A., and Knott, F. (2011) Recovery of DNA and fingermarks following deployment of render-safe tools for vehicle-borne improvised explosive devices (VBIED). *Forensic Sci. Int.*, **210** (1–3), 182–187.
47. Kaplan-Sandquist, K., LeBeau, M.A., and Miller, M.L. (2014) Chemical analysis of pharmaceuticals and explosives in fingermarks using matrix-assisted laser desorption ionization/time-of-flight mass spectrometry. *Forensic Sci. Int.*, **235**, 68–77.
48. Skvortsov, L.A. (2012) Laser methods for detecting explosive residues on surfaces of distant objects. *Quantum Electron.*, **42** (1), 1–11.
49. Mou, Y., and Rabalais, J.W. (2009) Detection and identification of explosive particles in fingerprints using attenuated total reflection-Fourier transform infrared spectromicroscopy. *J. Forensic Sci.*, **54** (4), 846–850.
50. Grant, A., Wilkinson, T.J., Holman, D.R., and Martin, M.C. (2005) Identification of recently handled materials by analysis of latent human fingerprints using infrared spectromicroscopy. *Appl. Spectrosc.*, **59** (9), 1182–1187.
51. King, S., Benson, S., Kelly, T., and Lennard, C. (2013) Determining the effects of routine fingermark detection techniques on the subsequent recovery and analysis of explosive residues on various substrates. *Forensic Sci. Int.*, **233** (1–3), 257–264.
52. Kuula, J., Rinta, H.J., Pölönen, I., Puupponen, H.-H., Haukkamäki, M., and Teräväinen, T. (2014) Detecting explosive substances by the IR spectrography. *Chem. Biol. Radiol. Nucl. Explos. Sens. XV*, **9073**, 90730Q.
53. Pacheco-Londoño, L.C., Castro-Suarez, J.R., and Hernández-Rivera, S.P. (2013) Detection of nitroaromatic and peroxide explosives in air using infrared spectroscopy: QCL and FTIR. *Adv. Opt. Technol.*
54. Theses, M., and Singh, A. (2010) Scholars' Mine Scholars' Mine Standoff Raman spectroscopy detection of trace explosives Standoff Raman spectroscopy detection of trace explosives.
55. Bhartia, R., Hug, W.F., Reid, R.D., and Beegle, L.W. (2015) Explosives detection and analysis by fusing deep ultraviolet native fluorescence and resonance raman spectroscopy. *Laser-Based Opt. Detect. Explos.*, 67–97.
56. Wackerbarth, H., Salb, C., Gundrum, L., Niederkrüger, M., Christou, K., Beushausen, V., and Viöl, W. (2010) Detection of explosives based on surface-enhanced Raman spectroscopy. *Appl. Opt.*, **49** (23), 4362–4366.
57. Goudsmits, E., Sharples, G.P., and Birkett, J.W. (2015) Recent trends in organic gunshot residue analysis. *TrAC - Trends Anal. Chem.*, **74**, 46–57.

58. Braz, A., López-López, M., and García-Ruiz, C. (2013) Raman spectroscopy for forensic analysis of inks in questioned documents. *Forensic Sci. Int.*, **232** (1–3), 206–212.
59. Raza, A., and Saha, B. (2013) Application of Raman spectroscopy in forensic investigation of questioned documents involving stamp inks. *Sci. Justice*, **53** (3), 332–338.
60. Sharif, M., Batool, M., Chand, S., Farooqi, Z.H., Tirmazi, S.A.A.S., and Athar, M. (2019) Forensic Discrimination Potential of Blue, Black, Green, and Red Colored Fountain Pen Inks Commercially Used in Pakistan, by UV/Visible Spectroscopy, Thin Layer Chromatography, and Fourier Transform Infrared Spectroscopy. *Int. J. Anal. Chem.*, **2019**.
61. Khofar, P.N.A., Karim, U.K.A., Elias, E., Safian, M.F., and Halim, M.I.A. (2022) Trends of Forensic Analysis of Pen Ink Using Attenuated Total Reflectance Fourier Transform Infrared (ATR-FTIR) Spectroscopy. *Indones. J. Chem.*, **22** (4), 1144–1154.
62. Edwards, H.G.M. (2018) CHAPTER 1 Analytical Raman Spectroscopy of Inks. 1–15.
63. Zięba-Palus, J., and Kunicki, M. (2006) Application of the micro-FTIR spectroscopy, Raman spectroscopy and XRF method examination of inks. *Forensic Sci. Int.*, **158** (2–3), 164–172.
64. Božičević, M.S., Gajović, A., and Zjakić, I. (2012) Identifying a common origin of toner printed counterfeit banknotes by micro-Raman spectroscopy. *Forensic Sci. Int.*, **223** (1–3), 314–320.
65. Di Foggia, M., Boga, C., Micheletti, G., Nocentini, B., and Taddei, P. (2021) Vibrational Raman and IR data on brown hair subjected to bleaching. *Data Br.*, **38**, 107439.
66. Boll, M.S. (2017) Differentiation of Hair Using ATR FT-IR Spectroscopy: A Statistical Differentiation of Hair Using ATR FT-IR Spectroscopy: A Statistical Classification of Dyed and Non-dyed Hairs Classification of Dyed and Non-dyed Hairs.
67. Panayiotou, H. (2014) Vibrational spectroscopy of keratin fibres : A forensic approach SCHOOL OF PHYSICAL AND CHEMICAL SCIENCES. (January 2004).
68. Manheim, J., Doty, K.C., McLaughlin, G., and Lednev, I.K. (2016) Forensic Hair Differentiation Using Attenuated Total Reflection Fourier Transform Infrared (ATR FT-IR) Spectroscopy. *http://dx.doi.org/10.1177/0003702816652321*, **70** (7), 1109–1117.
69. Zapata, F., Ortega-Ojeda, F.E., and García-Ruiz, C. (2022) Forensic examination of textile fibres using Raman imaging and multivariate analysis. *Spectrochim. Acta - Part A Mol. Biomol. Spectrosc.*, **268**.
70. Aljannahi, A., Alblooshi, R.A., Alremeithi, R.H., Karamitsos, I., Ahli, N.A., Askar, A.M., Albastaki, I.M., Ahli, M.M., and Modak, S. (2022) Forensic

Analysis of Textile Synthetic Fibers Using a FT-IR Spectroscopy Approach. *Molecules*, **27** (13), 1–11.
71. Bianchi, F., Riboni, N., Trolla, V., Furlan, G., Avantaggiato, G., Iacobellis, G., and Careri, M. (2016) Differentiation of aged fibers by Raman spectroscopy and multivariate data analysis. *Talanta*, **154**, 467–473.
72. Peets, P., Kaupmees, K., Vahur, S., and Leito, I. (2019) Reflectance FT-IR spectroscopy as a viable option for textile fiber identification. *Herit. Sci.*, **7** (1).
73. Muehlethaler, C., Massonnet, G., and Esseiva, P. (2011) The application of chemometrics on Infrared and Raman spectra as a tool for the forensic analysis of paints. *Forensic Sci. Int.*, **209** (1–3), 173–182.
74. SWGMAT (1999) FBI — Forensic Paint Analysis and Comparison Guidelines by SWGMAT Paint Subgroup, Part 1 (FSC, July 1999). *FBI Fed. Bur. Investig.*, Volume 1 Number 2.
75. Zieba-Palus, J., and Trzcińska, B.M. (2013) Application of infrared and raman spectroscopy in paint trace examination. *J. Forensic Sci.*, **58** (5), 1359–1363.
76. Buzzini, P., and Suzuki, E. (2016) Forensic applications of Raman spectroscopy for the *in situ* analyses of pigments and dyes in ink and paint evidence. *J. Raman Spectrosc.*, **47** (1), 16–27.
77. De Gelder, J., Vandenabeele, P., Govaert, F., and Moens, L. (2005) Forensic analysis of automotive paints by Raman spectroscopy. *J. Raman Spectrosc.*, **36** (11), 1059–1067.
78. Silva, C., Braz, A., and Pimentel, M.F. (2019) Vibrational Spectroscopy and Chemometrics in Forensic Chemistry: Critical Review, Current Trends and Challenges. *J. Braz. Chem. Soc.*, **30**, 2259–2290.
79. Houck, M.M., and Siegel, J.A. (2010) *Fundamentals of forensic science: Second edition*, Academic Press.
80. Harper, L., Powell, J., and Pijl, E.M. (2017) An overview of forensic drug testing methods and their suitability for harm reduction point-of-care services. *Harm Reduct. J.*, **14** (1), 1–13.
81. Muhamadali, H., Watt, A., Xu, Y., Chisanga, M., Subaihi, A., Jones, C., Ellis, D.I., Sutcliffe, O.B., and Goodacre, R. (2019) Rapid detection and quantification of novel psychoactive substances (NPS) using Raman spectroscopy and surface-enhanced Raman scattering. *Front. Chem.*, 7 (JUN), 412.
82. Dong, R., Weng, S., Yang, L., and Liu, J. (2015) Detection and direct readout of drugs in human urine using dynamic surface-enhanced Raman spectroscopy and support vector machines. *Anal. Chem.*, **87** (5), 2937–2944.
83. Han, Z., Liu, H., Meng, J., Yang, L., Liu, J., and Liu, J. (2015) Portable Kit for Identification and Detection of Drugs in Human Urine Using Surface-Enhanced Raman Spectroscopy. *Anal. Chem.*, **87** (18), 9500–9506.
84. Alder, R., Xiao, L., and Fu, S. (2021) Comparison of commercial surface-enhanced Raman spectroscopy substrates for the analysis of cocaine. *Drug Test. Anal.*, **13** (5), 944–952.

85. De Oliveira Penido, C.A.F., Pacheco, M.T.T., Lednev, I.K., and Silveira, L. (2016) Raman spectroscopy in forensic analysis: Identification of cocaine and other illegal drugs of abuse. *J. Raman Spectrosc.*, **47** (1), 28–38.
86. Kranenburg, R.F., Verduin, J., de Ridder, R., Weesepoel, Y., Alewijn, M., Heerschop, M., Keizers, P.H.J., van Esch, A., and van Asten, A.C. (2021) Performance evaluation of handheld Raman spectroscopy for cocaine detection in forensic case samples. *Drug Test. Anal.*, **13** (5), 1054–1067.
87. West, M.J., and Went, M.J. (2011) Detection of drugs of abuse by Raman spectroscopy. *Drug Test. Anal.*, **3** (9), 532–538.
88. Risoluti, R., Materazzi, S., Gregori, A., and Ripani, L. (2016) Early detection of emerging street drugs by near infrared spectroscopy and chemometrics. *Talanta*, **153**, 407–413.
89. Schulz, H., Baranska, M., Quilitzsch, R., and Schütze, W. (2004) Determination of alkaloids in capsules, milk and ethanolic extracts of poppy (Papaver somniferum L.) by ATR-FT-IR and FT-Raman spectroscopy. *Analyst*, **129** (10), 917–920.

4

UV-Vis Spectroscopy in Forensic Sample Investigation

Ashita Anand[1], Palash Kumar Manna[1*] and Shruti Shukla[2†]

[1]*TERI Deakin Nanobiotechnology Centre, TERI Gram, Gwal Pahari, Gurugram, India*
[2]*Department of Nanotechnology, North-Eastern Hill University (NEHU), East Khasi Hills, Shillong, Meghalaya, India*

Abstract
Crimes nowadays are expanding at an exponential rate which is an area of concern. Criminals repeatedly use futuristic mediums to commit crimes, therefore legal laws are persistently being updated and modified to limit the crime rate. The existing law-making sector are promoting the scope of applying forensic science in order to ameliorate the process of the investigation and help to assist court proceedings crucially. Thus forensic science is an important sector for the legislative agencies for criminal investigations for establishing a connection among crimes and the criminals. In criminal investigations, to solve crimes and prosecute the criminal for justice, the forensic investigators employ various scientific practices from the biological, chemical, and physical sectors. They accumulate and analyze concrete evidences including DNA, fingerprints, fibers and hairs. This chapter represents a comprehensive discussion on the use of UV-Vis spectroscopy methods for the determination of forensic exhibits. In the past decade, analytical techniques such as spectrophotometry have been applied for the identification and discrimination of forensic samples which provides informative inspection of the samples. A number of research articles involving to the use of spectroscopic techniques in forensic science discipline have been published. This chapter specifically displays the application of UV-Vis spectroscopy in various disciplines of forensic science. It is suggested here that this method can be efficiently utilized in forensic science investigation to generate statistically confident results.

**Corresponding author*: palash.manna@teri.res.in
†*Corresponding author*: shruti.shukla@teri.res.in

Priyanka Chhabra, Divya Bajpai Tripathy, Anjali Gupta, Rajeev Kumar, Kajol Bhati and Shruti Shukla (eds.) Advances in Analytical Techniques for Forensic Investigation, (93–112) © 2024 Scrivener Publishing LLC

***Keywords*:** UV-Vis spectroscopy, analytical techniques, forensic evidence, DNA, fingerprints, fibers, hairs

4.1 Introduction

Forensic science is an authority where the investigation of complex evidence is carried out using most interpretative applications. For an unbiased verdict in a criminal case, it is very crucial to precisely inspect the samples and categorize them based on their class characteristics to formulate an accurate identification and classification of every forensic evidences [1]. In this regard, the researchers today have expanded their curiosity in the analytical techniques such as spectrophotometric techniques for examining complex mixtures of drugs, inks, paints, glass and other significant evidences [2]. Advanced spectroscopic methods have emerged to analyze the large and complex datasets. Moreover, the spectroscopic techniques display scientifically accurate and significant results in a quick time frame. There are various spectroscopic methods available and each method is used in accordance with the type of study: characterization, model development and discrimination [3].

4.2 Forensic Science

Forensic science plays an important role in criminal investigations. Forensic science is a science that connects criminal activities to people, things and places, where scientific practices aid to investigate and resolve criminal cases [4]. The process of forensic investigation involves a scientific evaluation of the crime scene for concrete and solid clues. It is helpful in determining the time of crime, the means by which the crime was committed and also identifying the criminal. It is a study that employs scientific techniques to identify, individualize and recognize physical evidence in legal matters [5]. Forensic science is said to be a crucial element in criminal justice. It includes collecting logical and physical traces from the crime scene and inspecting them systematically thus helping to point out the prime suspect and time as well as mode of the crime. Forensic science also helps in determining various aspects of the committed crime and provides clues about the culprit, victim, and criminal activity [6]. The process of physical forensic investigation is illustrated in Figure 4.1. In criminal investigation, the evidence of a crime is extracted, the major components of the crime are identified, the suspect is recognized, the testimony of the criminal is

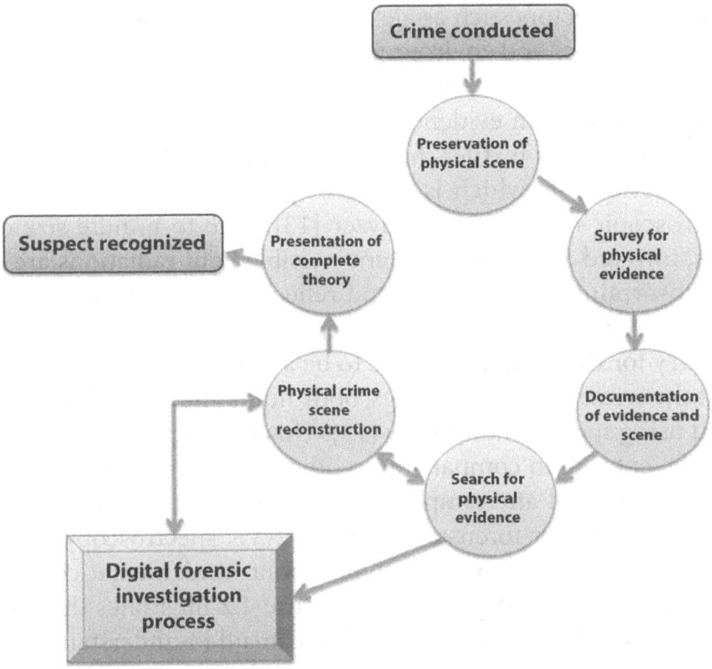

Figure 4.1 The process of crime scene investigation.

confirmed and the innocent is liberated [7]. It includes accelerating criminal investigations by developing forensic databases [8]. Forensic science is incorporated in the Indian Evidence Act, 1872, and contemplated as crucial evidence [9]. The key purpose of forensic science is to prove whether the suspect is guilty or innocent and convert doubt in the case into truth [10].

4.3 UV-Vis Spectroscopy

UV-Vis spectroscopy is an optimum analytical technique that measures a sample by quantifying discrete wavelengths of ultra violet or visible light range that are transmitted across or absorbed by the sample and compared to a blank or reference sample. The composition of sample majorly influences this property and potentially determines the components and concentration of each component in the sample [11]. In this technique, the wavelength that is selected corresponds to the maximum absorbance of the target sample. This way the highest response is collected for a specific analyte concentration thus establishing maximum sensitivity [12].

A number of sectors such as agriculture, food, medicine, pharmaceuticals, forensic science and environmental science thoroughly utilize UV-Vis spectrophotometry. In forensic science, a spectrophotometer is generally used to track down evidence. Particles that is too tiny to be analyzed by naked eye such as textiles, hairs and paints can be investigated using UV-Vis spectroscopy which is a micro-spectrophotometry that consists of a microscopic light source analyzer [13]. Due to minute size of these particles, infrared and more frequently visible light radiations are used to analyze absorption, transmission and reflection properties of these small particles. A well intricate and precise report is generated through spectrophotometry for the samples that are to be analyzed. An array of evidences found at the crime site such as drugs, body fluids and trace materials can be analyzed using spectrophotometry [12]. This technique is contemplated as a time-efficient tool in comparison to other analytical techniques as there is no requirement of any sample preparation. Any criminal investigation is incomplete without forensic science. UV-Vis spectroscopy is a crucial scientific tool that can provide insights about fundamental compositions of materials under investigation [14]. Figure 4.2 illustrates the process of UV-Vis analysis of forensic samples. This can aid in understanding crimes in a comprehensive manner including a number of aspects and thus provides a true and on point judgement of the crime. Micro-spectroscopy is employed in forensic science, where the minute samples as evidence are collected from the crime site and are then analyzed in the microscope [15]. For the analysis the samples are exposed to light radiations in the infrared and visible region. This method collects and determines the transmittance; absorption and reflectance of light characteristics for a specific sample.

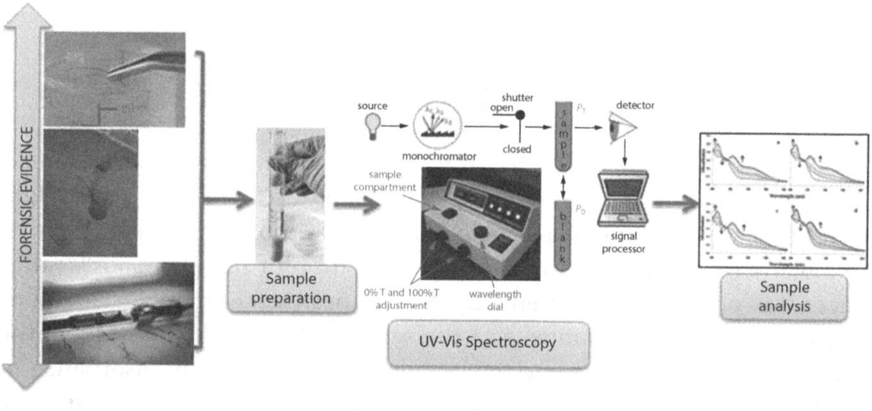

Figure 4.2 UV-Vis spectroscopy for analysis of forensic samples.

This data is considered as fingerprints for that particular material which is documented to be used in future observations [16].

4.4 Applications of UV/Visible Spectroscopy in Forensic Science

4.4.1 Analysis of Narcotics and Drug Testing

Analysis of narcotics and related drugs plays immense importance in forensic science. UV-Vis spectroscopy is regularly used in forensics for drug testing and analysis of narcotics. In this technique the presence of a particular drug is tested by analyzing its λmax (absorption maxima) or by a comparative analysis of the UV-Vis spectra of a drug against the spectra of the reference drug sample. Table 4.1 indicates the values of λmax for some abusive drugs [17].

Forensic drug analysis is an authority that is involved in identification and quantification of illegal drugs. There are generally two key steps in forensic drug testing: screening and confirmation. In this regard, UV-Vis

Table 4.1 Absorption Maxima of some abusive drugs.

S. no.	Drug	Solvent	Absorption maxima (nm)
1.	Cocaine	0.2 N H_2SO_4	233
2.	Codeine	Water	284
3.	Nicotine	0.2 N H_2SO_4	260
4.	Morphine	Acidic solution	285
5.	Methamphetamine	Methanol	259
6.	Caffeine	0.2 N H_2SO_4	271
7.	Phencyclidine	0.1 M HCl	262
8.	Tetra-hydrocannabinol	Methanol	276
9.	MDMA	Ethanol	286
10.	Amphetamine	Methanol	258

spectroscopy plays a significant role as it can help in analyzing drugs quantitatively as well as qualitatively.

A novel quick and selective spectrophotometric technique for the quantification of 4 analgesic drugs: naltrexone (NALT), morphine (MORF), nalbuphine (NALB) and tramadol (TRAM) in pharmaceutical composition has been developed. In this technique a measured amount of N bromosuccinimide (NBS) is added in the acidic solution of the drug to be determined after which the concentration of reacted NBS is measured. NBS reacts with a fixed amount of methyl orange and the absorbance is measured at 508 nm corresponding to the amount of reacted NBS. In a similar method, NBS is allowed to react with orange G and absorbance of the reacted NBS is measured at 478 nm. In both the methods, the amount of reacted NBS corresponds to the amount of drugs present [18].

4.4.2 Determination of Alcohol in Blood

Alcohol or ethanol is a hallucinogenic substance that frequently comes across in forensic toxicology samples owing to the fact that excessive drinking is closely linked to various criminal offences [19] such as drunken driving, domestic violence, sexual assaults, child abuse, homicide and aggravated assaults [20]. There is a quantitative relationship between a person's BAC (blood/alcohol concentration) and the risk of involvement in a road accident or any other criminal offence. A BAC level exceeding 80 mg/dL is considered as an illegal limit to drive a vehicle [21]. There is a well-established significant relation of alcohol consumption with impaired body functions; however it is easier and more relevant to determine the BAC level as compared to measuring diminished performance of an offender. Therefore, in forensics and legal cases where alcohol-related crimes such as drunken driving are investigated, a person's BAC is considered as an important and legal evidence because BAC limits in countries such as England are enforced [22]. For most of the legal purposes, ethanol is majorly determined in the exhaled breath of a person which is a non-invasive and quick method of alcohol sampling as compared to obtaining blood from a vein for analysis [23]. Numerous variety of breath based alcohol analyzers can be found in the market which includes handheld analyzers to determine a driver's sobriety at roadside as well as advanced evidential devices which can be used as a solid evidence for the prosecution of traffic offenders [24].

In this regard, UV-Vis spectroscopy can aid as a quantitative estimation of alcohol in blood utilizing the breath-analyzer test. In developed countries like the US, Australia and Canada, the breath-analyzers were the first instruments to be legally used for law enforcement purposes on an international basis [25]. In this process the person to be tested is asked to forcefully exhale through a mouthpiece tube. The breath then enters a heated cylinder and a specific volume of the exhaled breath is recorded. The breath sample of the offender passes through a glass ampoule which is filled with an acidic solution of potassium dichromate having an orange color. Potassium dichromate in an acidic solution acts as an oxidizing agent which oxidizes the ethanol in breath to acetic acid and the dichromate ions (orange in color) gets reduced to chromate ions (green in color). Thus the concentration of ethanol in the sample is quantified by measuring the decrease in absorbance at 440 nm. This value is then used for Beer's-Lambert law to determine the concentration of alcohol in the exhaled breath [26].

Back in 1920s when the earliest drink and driving legal laws were enforced, the breath and blood alcohol estimation techniques were one of the most classic forensic tests that served as evidence in legal medicine and forensic science disciplines [23]. Alcohol determination in blood is a time consuming and invasive process as it requires blood to be drawn from a vein however, sampling and analysis of breath saves time and is much less time invasive. Furthermore, breath analyzers provide on-the-spot results of alcohol consumption and therefore allows the legal authorities to make decisions on legal actions to be taken [27].

4.4.3 Ink Analysis

A document is made up of a lot of materials out of which the primary materials are usually paper, polymer or cardboard, and the text is deposits of ink, photocopier toner, carbon copy, or pencil (lead). Secondary materials that a document can consist of are erasure residues, correcting materials, stains and fingerprints. A scientific characterization of these materials can be critically significant in a criminal investigation. Ink contains frequently analyzed materials undoubtedly [28].

In forensic science, ink analysis is an area where ink collected from a writing device used to write on a questioned document is compared, identified, characterized and discriminated. Ink analysis can help in discovering the specific pen that was used to prepare a questionable document and therefore reveal critical information about falsification of that particular questioned document [29].

The determination of whether two sections of a written text were derived from the same pen or not is one of the key objectives of most ink analysis [30]. There are various writing devices on a document out of which ballpoint pen is the most commonly used device. Inks in ballpoint pens consist of combinations of coloring agents such as dyes as well as non-coloring agents like additives and solvents [31]. The coloring agents in pen inks can be determined using UV-Vis spectroscopy. The UV–Visible spectroscopy provides crucial information where the spectrum from 200 to 700 nm is reliable and quantifies the mixture of dyes in a sample specifically for ballpoint pen. This approach furnishes rapid and reproducible results in a straightforward manner and is fairly easy to implement [32]. Ink can serve as important evidence in criminal investigations when it is used to write on a suspect that can be linked to criminal offences including insurance frauds, threatening letters and will frauds. Different inks can be straightforwardly examined and classified with UV-Vis spectra of pen inks. This technique isway simpler and time efficient to perform in comparison to other techniques of ink analysis like chromatography [33].

4.4.4 Analysis of Carbon Monoxide Poisoning in Forensic Blood Samples

Carbon monoxide (CO) is a gas that does not have a taste, color and odor, and is non-irritating due to which its intake and exposure in human cells is not feasible to detect [34]. CO is a highly toxic gas and is immediately absorbed by the bloodstream from the lungs and binds to hemo-globin reversibly with an affinity of more than 300 times that of oxygen. Therefore, human exposure to an atmosphere with only 0.1% CO gas can convert more than 50% Hb to COHb [35]. CO causes anemic hypoxia in victims where the appearance of symptoms is highly affected by factors such as exposure time, concentration, and a person's level of exertion. Recently mortalities due to CO poisoning have increased which is a pressing concern. In the U.S, CO poisoning was one of the major causes of deaths over a period of 9 years from 1979 to 1988 [36]. In England and Wales, CO poisoning was the paramount cause of death in children due to poisoning and till now yearly around 1000 people die due to CO poisoning [37]. Traditionally COHb have been measured using spectrophotometric methods employing absorbance at two wavelengths [34, 38–40].

Carbon monoxide (CO) poisoning is difficult to detect and therefore causes a challenge for postmortem toxicology laboratories. A standard UV-Vis spectroscopy is a simple and quick analysis technique offering sufficiently precise and accurate data for the quantification of percentage carboxyhemoglobin in blood samples during postmortem [41].

There are usually 4 stages of human blood hemoglobin (Hb) which is to be considered while determining carboxyhemoglobin in blood samples

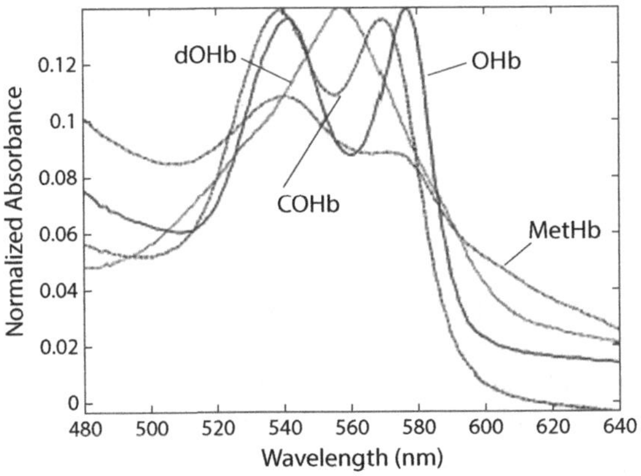

Figure 4.3 Normalized absorbance spectra of different types of hemoglobin: Ohb = oxyhemoglobin, COHb = carboxyhemoglobin, dOHb = deoxyhemoglobin, and MetHb = methemoglobin. Spectra were normalized to unit length [42, 43].

which are: oxyhemoglobin, deoxyhemoglobin, carboxyhemoglobin, and methemoglobin. Figure 4.3 illustrates the UV-Vis spectra of the four hemoglobin stages [42, 43]. For this carbon monoxide can be made to bind with hemechromophore which affect its absorption in ultraviolet-visible region. Therefore, the COHb concentrations of can be estimated using UV-Vis spectra of the blood sample collected from a victim suspected to have died due to CO poisoning [43].

4.4.5 Forensic Determination of Metals by UV/Visible Spectroscopy

Objects of daily use are mostly fabricated using three key metals including aluminium, iron, and copper [44]. Almost every tool, weapon and metal shards found at a crime site are made of these metals thus metal pieces collected from a crime site play a crucial piece of evidence in criminal investigations [44]. The forensic investigation of these metals is thus an important area of evaluation. Various weapons are frequently used by criminals suspected in robberies and in murders. Previously, the forensic investigation of crime spots has often encountered the presence of these metal ions mostly on clothing of the suspect [45]. Sometimes other metal ions like arsenic and lead are often found at industrial workplaces and many times also used as poisons [46]. In houses, salt of arsenic metal ions is usually used as insecticides [47]. Additionally these metal ions are also found in dyes, paints, and explosives like gunpowder [48]. UV-Vis spectroscopy can

Table 4.2 UV-Vis spectroscopy of some important metals.

Metal	Method	λ in nm	Reference
Aluminium	Aluminium ions react with eriochrome cyanine R dye at a pH of 6 to form a red colored complex.	535	[49]
Arsenic	Arsenic (III) reacts with potassium iodate in acid medium to liberate iodine which bleaches the blue color of toluidine blue. The decrease in absorbance is directly proportional to arsenic concentration.	628	[50]
Cadmium	The reagent 2-hydroxy-4-n-butoxy-5bromopropiophenone thiosemicarbazone (HBBrPT) reacts with Cd(II) to give an intense yellow color in the basic medium.	440	[51]
Chromium	Cr (VI) reacts with diphenylcarbazide reagent to give a red-violet colored complex.	540	[52]
Lead	On reaction with chloroform solution of dithizone in presence of NH_3 ions gives a cherry red complex.	510	[53]
Mercury	Mercuric ions react with chloroform solution of dithizone under acidic conditions and gives a orange colored complex.	492	[54]
Copper	Copper(II) react with neocuproine in neutral to slightly acid solution and extract into CHC_{13}/CH_3OH and forms a yellow complex.	457	[55]

be easily used to determine the concentration and presence of these metal ions employing various procedures as outlined in Table 4.2.

4.4.6 Examination of Blood Stains by UV/Visible Spectroscopy

Blood stains are one of the most significant and easily noticeable evidence for crime scene investigators especially in case of murders. Presently discrete and specific genetic information about a person can be obtained from blood stains collected at a crime scene by using straightforward forensic biochemistry analytical techniques [56]. A suspect's identity can be verified along with pattern analysis to reconstruct a crime can be efficiently executed by DNA-profiling of the blood sample obtained from a crime scene [57, 58]. There is a limitation in establishing a timeline of events occurred in criminal cases as it only relies on eyewitness or victim accounts. In case of murders it is occasionally possible to determine the time of death by analyzing certain pathological clues collected from the corpse [59]. However, in most of the criminal cases there is a deficit of eyewitnesses and/or bodies to determine the time of deaths therefore forensic evidence collected from a crime site plays a significant role as they are mostly found in the form of tissues and dried biological stains [60]. A few authentic and accurate techniques are available to determine an approximate time of accumulation of these dried biological stains or tissues [61–64]. Blood stains can be studied using UV-visible spectroscopy technique to detect the presence or absence of certain specific enzymatic activities in the collected stain samples [60].

In this three enzymes plays a major role including glutamic oxaloacetic transaminase (GOT), lactate dehydrogenase (LDH), and glutamic pyruvic transaminase (GPT) as these enzymes have a higher activity in blood stains as compared to serum along with a similar activity in fully hemolyzed blood [65]. This approach forms the basis for employing the UV-Vis spectroscopy technique to analyze blood stains from crime sites [66]. Previously an age estimation of up to 3 months after deposition of blood stain has been confirmed and documented by using combined ratios of LDH/GOT and GOT/GPT. This method involves the collection of blood stain which is followed by using saline solution to extract the blood. Afterwards the enzymes are labelled from the collected blood sample and are detected using UV-Vis spectrophotometer at a wavelength of 340nm. The crucial observation to note here is that the GOT:GPT ratio remains stable over the first month, whereas the LDH:GOT ratio is high (>10) at first, and then reduces to a ratio of 5 after 2 months [67].

4.4.7 Forensic Discrimination of Dyed Fiber Collected from the Incident Site

Fibers generally come across as trace evidence in criminal offences involving personal contact like assault, homicide and sexual offences also including hit-and-run road accidents and other crimes [68–70]. Fibers can also be collected from objects indirectly associated with crimes including weapons and cars or vehicles used in armed robberies [69].

In order to understand the justification of fiber analysis and relevance of fiber-dye combinations in forensic science, a precise knowledge on the biochemistry of fibers and fiber dyes is crucial [71–74]. The integrity of the original samples collected can be efficiently maintained by using non-destructive spectroscopic techniques along with prevention of sample contamination, minimal sample handling, and reduction in overall time of analysis. Dyes fibers can be characterized directly in a relatively inexpensive and informative manner using the UV-Vis spectroscopy [70, 75–80]. Suzuki *et al.* [77] conducted a study to analyze single cotton fibers dyed with vat dyes like indigo and indigo derivatives by using UV-Vis micro-spectroscopy. Reference spectrum of known dyes and fibers can be

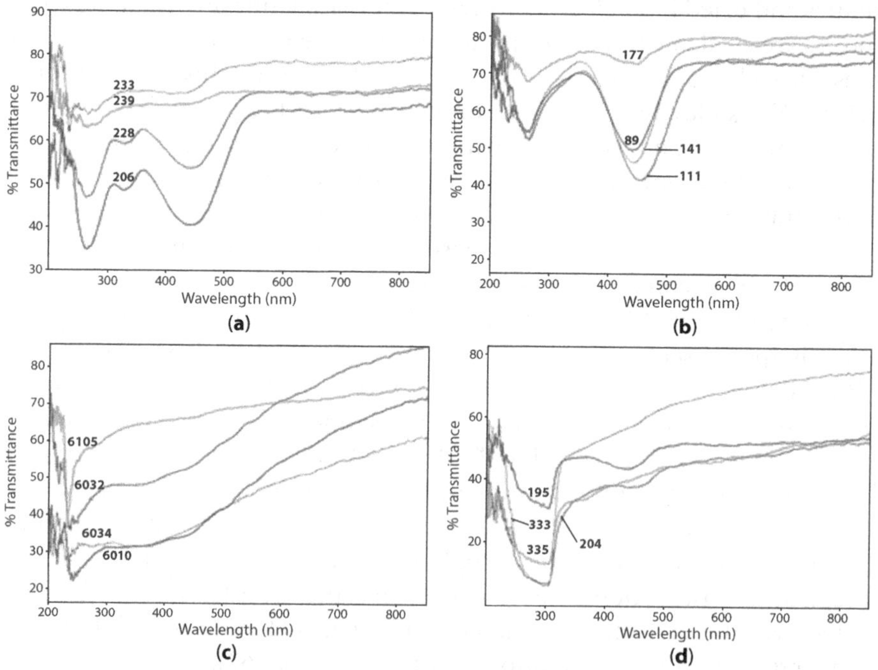

Figure 4.4 UV-VIS spectrum of yellow fibers mounted in glycerin using quartz slides and cover slips: (a) cotton; (b) acrylic, (c) nylon; (d) polyester [81].

easily used to compare and match with the UV-Vis spectra of fibers as trace evidence collected from a crime spot. For instance Figure 4.4 illustrates the UV-Vis spectra of various dyed fibers [81].

4.5 Future Perspective

The Federal Bureau of Investigation (FBI) and the American Hazardous Material Response Unit efficiently use spectrophotometry which has become a gold standard in forensic investigations [82]. For distinguishing between two samples that are essentially indistinguishable, spectrophotometric analysis is required. The majority of forensic examinations analyze inks and fibers using UV-Vis spectroscopy, and then use thin-layer chromatography as a supportive technique. Numerous other analytical methods can be used in addition to spectroscopy to detect forensic materials. Portable HSI, FTIR, and Raman [83] devices are available for the standard detection of forensic evidence at crime scenes [84]. Due to the large number of chemicals that are currently available in libraries, portable and miniature equipment can be employed to identify explosives and narcotics [85–87]. In order to accurately identify a substance based on the automatic matching of the measured spectrum to the spectra in the library; these portable instruments essentially require a library of standard spectra. But spectral data of some forensic materials such as body fluids is not currently available in the libraries [85]. Because they don't emerge as distinct particles like narcotics and explosives do, body fluids present a challenge for forensic investigators because they leave behind stains on various surfaces or even penetrate into fabrics, which also affect the vibrational spectra. Additionally, compared to laboratory instruments, these portable instruments typically offer fewer benefits, services, and performance. Thus, it is necessary to conclude the study on these procedures in the lab first, followed by the research on their miniaturization and use at the crime scene.

4.6 Conclusion

Hairs, fibers, and glass are examples of trace evidence that can be quickly and accurately analyzed using spectroscopy. To ascertain the chemical make-up and whether they are natural or synthetic, even samples as small as a single 10–30 mm fiber can be studied. Spectroscopic analysis is the ideal choice for forensic ink tests. Inks found at the scene can be identified by their distinctive colors using a wavelength analysis, which can also determine whether they resemble particular store-bought pen brands. Spectrophotometry is a non-invasive and less hazardous substitute to chromatography for identifying forensic samples.

In the field of forensics, spectroscopic methods have been investigated for the recognition and distinguishing of human body fluids and other crucial evidence for comprehending a crime scene and attempting to pin the perpetrators down.

Despite their use in forensic laboratories all over the world to locate forensic samples, UV-Vis light sources have some limitations when it comes to sample identification because not all evidence will glow differently under UV light. As a result, this method is only employed as a preliminary assay. Through the larger and broader spectral spectrum of NIR, NIR-HSI partially overcomes the restrictions of selectivity from UV-Vis spectroscopy. Additionally, HSI integrates the geographical data from the captured specimen with the spectral data.

Raman spectroscopy and FTIR appear to be two other viable methods because they have more selectivity than UV-Vis and NIR-HSI and are hence more effective at identifying bodily fluids. These approaches really provide a distinct characterization of evidence due to their clear IR and Raman spectra, which are connected to the unique chemical makeup of each forensic evidence. Additionally, the analysis performed using these procedures is quick, solvent-free, affordable, and non-invasive, all of which are essential for achieving a successful DNA analysis in the forensic investigation of a piece of evidence. However, to be employed in actual forensic investigations, further thorough studies and research geared toward optimization and validation of these techniques for the detection of forensic samples are required. In this regard, it is important to thoroughly research the best instruments for each function, such as preliminary identification at the crime scene or supportive identification in the lab [87]. Additionally, it is important to research the impact of a wide range of variables associated to bodily fluid stains, including the kind of substrate or fabric and the combination of different body fluids.

Consent for Publication

Consent of all authors

Conflict of Interest

No conflicts

Acknowledgement

All the authors have contributed to the chapter with interest.

References

1. Siegel, J.A. and K. Mirakovits, *Forensic science: the basics*. 2015: CRC Press.
2. Kumar, R. and V. Sharma, Chemometrics in forensic science. *TrAC, Trends Anal. Chem.*, 2018. **105**: p. 191-201.
3. Feldman, R., *The role of science in law*. 2009: Oxford University Press.
4. De Forest, P.R. and P. DeForest, *Forensic science: an introduction to criminalistics*. 1983: McGraw-Hill Humanities/Social Sciences/Languages New York.
5. Adhikary, J., DNA technology in administration of justice. 2007: LexisNexis Butterworths.
6. Carrier, B. and E.H. Spafford, Getting physical with the digital investigation process. *International Journal of digital evidence*, 2003. **2**(2): p. 1-20.
7. McEwen, T., The role and impact of forensic evidence in the criminal justice system. National Institute of Justice, 2010.
8. Ghosh, P., Evidentiary Value of Expert Evidence under Indian Evidence Act, 1872.
9. Patel, N., V.K. Gautaman, and S. Jangir, The role of DNA in criminal investigation–Admissibility in Indian legal system and future perspectives. *Int. J. Humanit. Soc. Sci. Invent.*, 2013. **2**(7): p. 15-21.
10. Harris, D.C., *Quantitative chemical analysis*. 2010: Macmillan.
11. Ghasemi, H.I., *et al.*, Interstrand crosslinking of homologous repair template DNA enhances gene editing in human cells. *Nat. Biotechnol.*, 2023: p. 1-7.
12. Weckhuysen, B., Ultraviolet-Visible Spectroscopy. 2004.
13. Weckhuysen, B.M., P. Voort, and G. Catana, *Spectroscopy of transition metal ions on surfaces*. 2000: Leuven University Press.
14. Groothaert, M.H., *et al.*, An operando optical fiber UV–vis spectroscopic study of the catalytic decomposition of NO and N2O over Cu-ZSM-5. *J. Catal.*, 2003. **220**(2): p. 500-512.
15. Weckhuysen, B.M., *et al.*, In situ UV–Vis diffuse reflectance spectroscopy—on line activity measurements of supported chromium oxide catalysts: relating isobutane dehydrogenation activity with Cr-speciation via experimental design. *J. Mol. Catal. A: Chem.*, 2000. **151**(1-2): p. 115-131.
16. Federici, J.F., *et al.*, THz imaging and sensing for security applications—explosives, weapons and drugs. *Semicond. Sci. Technol.*, 2005. **20**(7): p. S266.
17. El-Didamony, A.M., M.Z. Saad, and N.O. Saleem, Spectrophotometric determination of some analgesic drugs in pharmaceutical formulations using

N-bromosuccinimide as an oxidant. *J. Assoc. Arab Univ. Basic Appl. Sci.*, 2015. **17**: p. 43-50.
18. Felson, R.B. and J. Staff, The effects of alcohol intoxication on violent versus other offending. *Crim. Justice Behav.*, 2010. **37**(12): p. 1343-1360.
19. Holmgren, A. and A.W. Jones, Demographics of suicide victims in Sweden in relation to their blood–alcohol concentration and the circumstances and manner of death. *Forensic Sci. Int.*, 2010. **198**(1-3): p. 17-22.
20. Blomberg, R.D., *et al.*, The long beach/fort lauderdale relative risk study. *J. Saf. Res.*, 2009. **40**(4): p. 285-292.
21. Jones, A.W., Enforcement of drink-driving laws by use of "per se" legal alcohol limits: Blood and/or breath concentration as evidence of impairment. Alcohol, Drugs & Driving, 1988.
22. Wigmore, J. and R. Langille, Six generations of breath alcohol testing instruments: Changes in the detection of breath alcohol since 1930. An historical overview. *J. Can. Soc. Forensic Sci.*, 2009. **42**(4): p. 276-283.
23. Jones, A., Alcohol, its analysis in blood and breath for forensic purposes, impairment effects, and acute toxicity. *Wiley Interdiscip. Rev.: Forensic Sci.*, 2019. **1**.
24. Jones, A., Measuring alcohol in blood and breath for forensic purposes-a historical review. *Forensic Sci. Rev.*, 1996. **8**: p. 13-44.
25. Borkenstein, R.F. and H. Smith, The breathalyzer and its applications. *Med. Sci. Law*, 1961. **2**(1): p. 13-22.
26. Jones, A.W., Medicolegal alcohol determination-blood-or breath-alcohol concentration? *Forensic Sci. Rev.*, 2000. **12**(1-2): p. 23-47.
27. Roux, C., *et al.*, A study to investigate the evidential value of blue and black ballpoint pen inks in Australia. *Forensic Sci. Int.*, 1999. **101**(3): p. 167-176.
28. Kher, A., *et al.*, Forensic classification of ballpoint pen inks using high performance liquid chromatography and infrared spectroscopy with principal components analysis and linear discriminant analysis. *Vibrational spectroscopy*, 2006. **40**(2): p. 270-277.
29. Weyermann, C., *et al.*, Statistical discrimination of black gel pen inks analysed by laser desorption/ionization mass spectrometry. *Forensic Sci. Int.*, 2012. **217**(1-3): p. 127-133.
30. Hofer, R., Dating of Ballpoint Pen Ink. *J. Forensic Sci.*, 2004. **49**: p. 1353-7.
31. Senior, S., *et al.*, Characterization and dating of blue ballpoint pen inks using principal component analysis of UV–Vis absorption spectra, IR spectroscopy, and HPTLC. *J. Forensic Sci.*, 2012. **57**(4): p. 1087-1093.
32. Sharma, V. and R. Kumar, Dating of ballpoint pen writing inks via spectroscopic and multiple linear regression analysis: A novel approach. *Microchem. J.*, 2017. **134**: p. 104-113.
33. Lee, L.C., *et al.*, Forensic analysis of blue ballpoint pen inks using ultraviolet-visible spectrometer and ultra-performance liquid chromatograph. *Malaysian J. Anal. Sci.*, 2015. **19**(2): p. 397-401.

34. Hirschler, M., Carbon monoxide and human lethality: fire and non-fire studies. 1993: CRC Press.
35. Cobb, N. and R.A. Etzel, Unintentional carbon monoxide—Related deaths in the United States, 1979 through 1988. *JAMA*, 1991. **266**(5): p. 659-663.
36. Meredith, T. and A. Vale, Carbon monoxide poisoning. *British Medical Journal (Clinical research Ed.)*, 1988. **296**(6615): p. 77.
37. Klendshoj, N.C., M. Feldstein, and A.L. Sprague, The spectrophotometric determination of carbon monoxide. *J. Biol. Chem.*, 1950. **183**(1): p. 297-303.
38. Egan, W.J., W.E. Brewer, and S.L. Morgan, Measurement of carboxyhemoglobin in forensic blood samples using UV-visible spectrometry and improved principal component regression. *Appl. Spectrosc.*, 1999. **53**(2): p. 218-225.
39. Rodkey, F., *et al.*, Spectrophotometric measurement of carboxyhemoglobin and methemoglobin in blood. *Clin. Chem.*, 1979. **25**(8): p. 1388-1393.
40. Katsumata, Y., *et al.*, A simple spectrophotometry for determination of carboxyhemoglobin in blood. *J. Forensic Sci.*, 1982. **27**(4): p. 928-934.
41. Lichtman, M.A., *et al.*, Editors, in Williams Manual of Hematology, *8e*. 2011, McGraw-Hill Education: New York, NY.
42. Klaassen, C. and D. Eaton, Casarett and Doulls Toxicology (Edited by MO Amdur, J. Doull and CD Klaassen). 1991, Pergamon Press, New York.
43. Beutler, S. and K. Blume, Williams Hematology, Edited by Ernest Beutler, Mar-shall A. Lichtman, Barry S. Coller, and Thomas J. Kipps. *Am. J. Hum. Genet.*, 1995. **57**(514).
44. Pirk, G.W., Metallurgical examinations in criminal cases. *Police J.*, 1941. **14**(1): p. 84-102.
45. Hamann, C.R. and D. Hamann, Metals in Everyday Life. *Metal Allergy: From Dermatitis to Implant and Device Failure*, 2018: p. 137-162.
46. Bencko, V., Yan Li Foong F 2017. The history of arsenical pesticides and health risks related to the use of Agent Blue. *Ann Agric Environ Med.* **24**(2): p. 312-316.
47. Siriangkhawut, W., S. Tontrong, and P. Chantiratikul, Quantitation of aluminium content in waters and soft drinks by spectrophotometry using eriochrome cyanine R. *Res. J. Pharm. Biol. Chem. Sci.*, 2013. **4**(3): p. 1154-1161.
48. Narayana, B., *et al.*, Spectrophotometric determination of arsenic in environmental and biological samples. 2006.
49. Parikh, K., R. Patel, and K. Patel, New spectrophotometric method for determination of cadmium. *E- J. Chem.*, 2009. **6**(S1): p. S496-S500.
50. Wiryawan, A., *et al.*, Method of analysis for determination of the chromium (Cr) species in water samples by spectrophotometry with diphenylcarbazide. *J. Environ. Eng. Sustain. Technol.*, 2018. **5**(1): p. 37-46.
51. Nagaraj, P., *et al.*, Spectrophotometric method for the determination of chromium (VI) in water samples. *Environ. Monit. Assess.*, 2009. **157**(1-4): p. 575-82.

52. Murcia, N.S., *et al.*, Quincy meets Perry Mason: An experience in chemistry and law: A simple spectrophotometric method for the determination of traces of mercury (II) and lead (II). *J. Chem. Educ.*, 1990. **67**(7): p. 608.
53. Sari, I., *et al.*, The Differences of the Result of Copper Test Using UV-Vis Spectrophotometry with Neocuproine Complexing Agent and AAS. 2018.
54. Butler, J.M., Genetics and genomics of core short tandem repeat loci used in human identity testing. *J. Forensic Sci.*, 2006. **51**(2): p. 253-265.
55. Anderson, S., *et al.*, A method for determining the age of a bloodstain. *Forensic Sci. Int.*, 2005. **148**(1): p. 37-45.
56. Andrasko, J., The estimation of age of bloodstains by HPLC analysis. *J. Forensic Sci.*, 1997. **42**(4): p. 601-607.
57. Inoue, H., *et al.*, A new marker for estimation of bloodstain age by high performance liquid chromatography. *Forensic Sci. Int.*, 1992. **57**(1): p. 17-27.
58. Inoue, H., *et al.*, Identification of fetal hemoglobin and simultaneous estimation of bloodstain age by high-performance liquid chromatography. *Int. J. Leg. Med.*, 1991. **104**: p. 127-131.
59. Funao, T. and I. Maeda, Studies on the determination of the age of bloodstains. *Jpn. J. Leg. Med.*, 1959. **13**: p. 735-740.
60. Kind, S., D. Patterson, and G. Owen, Estimation of the age of dried blood stains by a spectrophotometric method. *Forensic Sci.*, 1972. **1**(1): p. 27-54.
61. Kumagai, R., Analysis of hemoglobin in bloodstains using high-performance liquid chromatography. Nihon hoigaku zasshi= *Jpn. J. Leg. Med.*, 1993. **47**(3): p. 213-219.
62. Matsuoka, T., T. Taguchi, and J. Okuda, Estimation of bloodstain age by rapid determinations of oxyhemoglobin by use of oxygen electrode and total hemoglobin. *Biol. Pharm. Bull.*, 1995. **18**(8): p. 1031-1035.
63. Rajamannar, K., Determination of the age of bloodstains using immunoelectrophoresis. *J. Forensic Sci.*, 1977. **22**(1): p. 159-164.
64. Bauer, M., S. Polzin, and D. Patzelt, Quantification of RNA degradation by semi-quantitative duplex and competitive RT-PCR: a possible indicator of the age of bloodstains? *Forensic Sci. Int.*, 2003. **138**(1-3): p. 94-103.
65. Schaffert, R.R., G.R. Kingsley, and G. Getchell, Automated determination of serum glutamic oxalacetic and glutamic pyruvic transaminase. *Clin. Chem.*, 1964. **10**(6): p. 519-532.
66. Kind, S. and M. Watson, The estimation of blood stain age from the spectrophotometric properties of ammoniacal blood stain extracts. *Forensic Sci.*, 1973. **2**: p. 325-332.
67. Magrot, T., Activity Of Serum Sorbit Dehydrogenase, Glutamic-Oxalacetic And Glutamic Pyruvic Traminase After Partial Hepatectomy. *Ceskoslovenska Gastroenterologie a Vyziva*, 1963. **17**: p. 343-346.

68. Gaudette, B.D., The forensic aspects of textile fiber examination. *Forensic science handbook,* 1988. **2**: p. 209-272.
69. David, S.K. and M.T. Pailthorpe, Classification of textile fibres: production, structure, and properties. Forensic examination of fibres, 1999. **2**.
70. Adanur, S., Wellington Sears Handbook Of Indsutrial Textiles, *Technomic Pub., Basel.* 1995, ISBN 1-56676-340-1.
71. White, P.C. and I. Tebbett, Chromatographic Analysis for Fiber Dyes. 1992: Ellis Horwood, New York, NY.
72. Vigo, T.L., Textile processing and properties: Preparation, dyeing, finishing and performance. 2013: Elsevier.
73. Frank, R.S. and S.P. Sobol, Fibres and their examination in forensic science. *Forensic science progress*, 1990: p. 41-125.
74. Adolf, F.-P. and J. Dunlop, Microspectrophotometry/colour measurement. Forensic examination of fibres, 1999. **2**.
75. Suzuki, S., *et al.*, Microspectrophotometric discrimination of single fibres dyed by indigo and its derivatives using ultraviolet-visible transmittance spectra. *Sci. Justice*, 2001. **41**(2): p. 107-111.
76. Macrae, R., R. Dudley, and K. Smalldon, The characterization of dyestuffs on wool fibers with special reference to microspectrophotometry. *J. Forensic Sci.*, 1979. **24**(1): p. 117-129.
77. Carroll, G.R., Forensic fibre microscopy. 1992: Ellis Horwood: New York, NY.
78. Cantrell, S., *et al.*, A textile fibre survey as an aid to the interpretation of fibre evidence in the Sydney region. *Forensic Sci. Int.*, 2001. **123**(1): p. 48-53.
79. Sharma, V., R. Kumar, and P. Kaur, Forensic examination of textile fibers using UV-Vis spectroscopy combined with multivariate analysis. *J. Appl. Spectrosc.*, 2019. **86**: p. 96-100.
80. Morgan, S.L., *et al.*, Forensic discrimination of dyed textile fibers using UV-VIS and fluorescence microspectrophotometry. *Proceedings of the European Fibres Group*, 2004: p. 1-11.
81. Rendle, D. and K. Wiggins, Forensic analysis of textile fibre dyes. *Rev. Prog. Color. Relat. Top.*, 1995. **25**(1): p. 29-34.
82. Narejo, N. and M.A. Avais, Examining the Role of Forensic Science for the Investigative-Solution of Crimes. *Sindh Univ. Res. Jour.(Sci. Ser.)* Vol, 2012. **44**(2): p. 251-254.
83. Mojica, E.-R. and Z. Dai, New Raman spectroscopic methods' application in forensic science. *Talanta Open*, 2022. **6**: p. 100124.
84. Lin, A.C.Y., *et al.*, Forensic applications of infrared imaging for the detection and recording of latent evidence. *J. Forensic Sci.*, 2007. **52**(5): p. 1148-1150.
85. Sorak, D., *et al.*, New developments and applications of handheld Raman, mid-infrared, and near-infrared spectrometers. *Appl. Spectrosc. Rev.*, 2012. **47**(2): p. 83-115.

86. Chalmers, J.M., H.G. Edwards, and M.D. Hargreaves, Infrared and Raman Spectroscopy in Forensic Science. 2012.
87. Izake, E.L., Forensic and homeland security applications of modern portable Raman spectroscopy. *Forensic Sci. Int.*, 2010. **202**(1-3): p. 1-8.

5

Nuclear Magnetic Resonance Spectroscopy: A Versatile Tool for Forensic Sample Analysis

Devi Deepti Attinti[1], Kwasi Kantanka Safo[1], M. Balakrishna[1], Noble George[1,2] and Shivani Pandya[1,2*]

[1]*Dept. of Forensic Science, PIAS, Parul University, Vadodara (Gujarat), India*
[2]*Centre of Research for Development, Parul University, Vadodara (Gujarat), India*

Abstract
Nuclear Magnetic Resonance (NMR) spectroscopy has become a foremost analytical tool in forensic science due to its ability to come up with molecular level information on a wide range of chemicals. In this book chapter, we present a complete introduction of the applications of NMR spectroscopy in forensic sample analysis. We begin with an overview of the fundamental principles of NMR spectroscopy, followed by a discussion of the gear and sample preparation techniques required for successful analysis. We next go over the various NMR spectroscopy techniques, such as one- and two-dimensional NMR, solid-state NMR, and dynamic nuclear polarization (DNP)-enhanced NMR. Following that, we address the forensic uses of NMR spectroscopy in drug analysis, forensic toxicology, fire debris analysis, paint and polymer analysis, and fiber analysis, as well as offer case studies proving the utility of NMR spectroscopy in forensic investigations. We also cover the data processing and interpretation techniques required for successful NMR analysis, such as spectral processing, interpretation, and chemometrics. Finally, we cover accomplishments and future objectives in the field of NMR spectroscopy for forensic analysis, including high-field NMR spectroscopy, innovations in hardware and software, integration with other analytical techniques, and novel forensic applications.

***Keywords*:** Nuclear magnetic resonance, forensic sample analysis, spectroscopy, drug analysis, body fluid identification, fiber analysis

**Corresponding author*: shivpan02@gmail.com

Priyanka Chhabra, Divya Bajpai Tripathy, Anjali Gupta, Rajeev Kumar, Kajol Bhati and Shruti Shukla (eds.) Advances in Analytical Techniques for Forensic Investigation, (113–148) © 2024 Scrivener Publishing LLC

5.1 Introduction to NMR in Forensic Science

5.1.1 Overview of NMR Spectroscopy

NMR spectroscopy is widely utilized analytical tool for revealing the molecular structure of both micro and macro molecules [1]. NMR spectroscopy focuses on specific atomic nuclei and how they behave when exposed to a magnetic field [2, 3]. Because all nuclei are electrically charged and have some degree of spin, when subjected to a magnetic field, energy may be transferred from a low energy state to a high energy one. When it returns to its low energy state, it emits energy at the same frequency as same as when energy is transferred at a wavelength corresponding to radio frequency. These signals that correspond to this transfer is detected in various ways and analyzed in the form of NMR spectrum [4, 5]. NMR can be entirely ascertaining the structure of compound. The most used isotopes in NMR are "^{1}H, ^{13}C, ^{19}F, ^{15}N, ^{31}P" and so on. It is an effective instrument that allows for both quantitative and qualitative analysis [6]. Consequently, it has been utilized in a numerous disciplines of science including chemical, biological, medicine, biochemistry, geology, and material sciences. Recently NMR is gaining its attention in the field of forensics due to its specific characteristics like non-invasiveness, least sample requirement and reveals both structural and dynamic data with accurate results [7–9]. The rising popularity of the NMR application is a result of several advancements in its technology and methodology that have made it possible to analyze complicated mixtures while significantly reducing the sample volume required. Progress made in the last few decades may be seen in the development of pulse patterns, accessibility of high-power solenoids and the development of cryogenic probes with high sensitivity. With the emergence of computerized equipment's, NMR has evolved into a fascinating quantitative instrument with capabilities equivalent to frequently used chromatographic approaches. NMR has also demonstrated to be an intriguing method for obtaining fingerprints from various matrices, resulting in excellent sample differentiation [3, 10]. Ultimately, the combination of chemometrics with NMR spectroscopy enabled the discovery of concealed correlations in complicated data (for example food analysis). For instance, supervised multivariate data analysis has been developed via calibration, classification and prediction [11]. Despite of its advantages, NMR has even drawbacks includes high cost, low sensitivity, less resolution and overlapping signals. However, regardless of its disadvantages, NMR is still an effective method for analyzing substances without causing any damage to the samples [3, 6].

5.1.2 Importance of NMR in Forensic Analysis

Forensic science is a multidisciplinary field, mainly based on analysis of evidences obtained from scene of crime. Structural, composition and analysis of the evidences with the help of sophisticated instruments plays a mighty role in the investigations [6, 12]. NMR is one among those instruments that gives structural determination of compound without pre-treatment of sample. NMR has acquired prominence primarily in the field of forensic chemistry (Figure 5.1) [13], which enables to examine the illicit drugs [14], petroleum products, psychoactive substances [15], chemicals and analysis of illicit capsules [5, 16]. Even it has been used to identify body fluids [17], post mortem interval (through NMR metabolomics) [18], poisoning cases (by analysis of its metabolites and xenobiotics) [5, 19], pharmaceuticals [20], explosives, toxins, examination of electrical tapes [10] and examination of condoms [21]. NMR has a vital significance in the investigation of arson cases by analyzing the fire debris [22]. NMR is widely used in

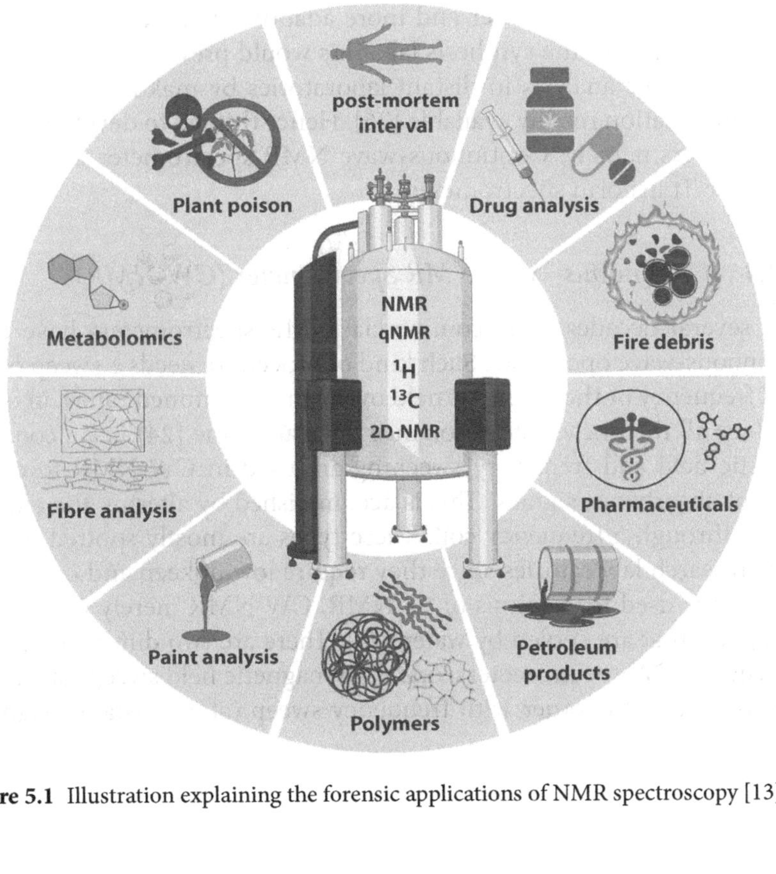

Figure 5.1 Illustration explaining the forensic applications of NMR spectroscopy [13].

forensics due to its high reproducibility, non-destructible nature, simple sample preparation and ease of use [13]. Hence NMR is said to be scientific tool for extensive information which can provide chemical structure and composition of forensic evidences that can be used to identify chemicals and establish the time of death [23].

5.2 NMR Instrumentation and Sample Preparation

5.2.1 Types of NMR Spectrometers

In 1951, onset of NMR chemical shift brought about the idea that NMR spectroscopy might be helpful for chemical characterization, and even this resulted in the initial run of spectrometers [24]. There are different types of magnets in order to characterize the spectrometers includes permanent, resistive and super conducting magnets. Magnets with a superconducting high field are used in NMR spectrometers [25]. When elucidation of structures is needed during and after chemical transformations, the utilization of NMR might become easier and more adaptive if an NMR spectrometer was accessible in the synthesis lab. This would prevent prolonged wait times for sample analysis in distant laboratories by making the spectroscopic information readily available [26]. Hence this led to development of spectrometers namely, Continuous-wave NMR spectrometer and pulsed or Fourier-Transform spectrometer.

5.2.1.1 Continuous-Wave NMR Spectrometer (CW-NMR)

From several decades most commercial NMR spectrometers have used "continuous-wave operation". Such kind of procedure needs a sweep of the NMR frequency or the magnetic field over a predetermined range, in order to induce all the nuclei into resonance once at a time [24] i.e., a constant magnetic field and frequency sweeping are used in CW-NMR to create resonant absorbance signals. This is accomplished by altering the current flowing through a frequency coil. These types are mostly spotted in academic research laboratories since they require low upkeep and operation. Usually, it is used for analysis of ^1H NMR. CW-NMR merely needs electromagnets that are cooled by water [27]. There are two different types of constructive CW spectrometers: one with magnetic field sweep (at a given frequency), and the other with frequency sweep (at a constant magnetic field) [28]. CW-NMR typically consists of sample holder, permanent magnet, magnetic coils, sweep generator, Radio frequency generator and receiver and a spectrum signal [5]. CW-NMR is more effective method in which a analyte is stimulated by a strong, brief RF pulse [29, 30]. But the major drawback is lack of sensitivity, which is caused by relatively low magnetogyric ratio. Significant progress has already been made in improving the signal-to-noise ratio attainable from NMR spectrometers by using signal-averaging methods and by utilizing proton noise-decoupling techniques [31, 32]. Since to increase sensitivity and accurate data based on mathematical calculation led to the rise of pulsed or Fourier transform spectrometer.

5.2.1.2 Fourier-Transform NMR Spectrometer (FT-NMR)

FT-NMR is also known as pulsed spectrometer. Fourier Transform (FT) is a standard type of spectrometer which is based on mathematical calculation of data [28]. The magnet is one of the core components whereas the field strength of a magnet is an essential component of FT-NMR. The fact that the magnets don't require the magnetic field to fluctuate through time makes FT-NMR techniques superior to CW-NMR spectrometers. This enables the use of superconductive coils, which can generate extraordinarily powerful static magnetic fields [33, 34]. It is based on radiofrequency (RF) radiation that is applied in the form of a short and effective pulse for nucleus excitation, which is accompanied by the measurement of the induced magnetism in the detector coil when all stimulated nucleus is able to get back to their original states. Free induction decay (FID) is used to describe the relaxation. FID a time-dependent signal that is decaying, is then transformed using FT-function from time domain to the typical frequency domain spectrum [24, 27]. The main advantages of FT-NMR spectrometer are, compared to using the traditional spectral sweep technique, it is possible to collect spectra in a less time, sensitivity is higher and the technique enables the study of internal Overhauser effects and it is simple to calculate the integration and high moments of the spectrum impulse responses and gives accurate frequency [29]. The FT-NMR is frequently used spectrometer due to its major benefit that the free induction decay signal may be quickly generated, allowing for the application of the pulse repeatedly and the coherent addition of the FID signals in a computer program within a specified amount of time [31]. Hence it is widely used spectrometer for NMR spectra.

5.2.2 Sample Preparation Techniques

Sample preparation is an important stage in NMR spectroscopy and it can affect the nature of the spectra and structure elucidation. So, proper sample preparation technique should be employed to yield reproducible spectra with minimal variation in chemical shift between samples, have a high signal-to-noise ratio and enable the identification of the most metabolites possible. The technique to be ideally quick, reliable, non-selective and compatible with large output analyses [35]. The basic sample preparation techniques of NMR include solvent selection (it should be easily detachable, having a low ionic strength, being effective at neutralizing and removing macromolecules, and being non-reactive), metabolite quenching (if samples are not instantly quenched, metabolite might swiftly change at the time of sampling so it should be stored in dry ice or liquid N_2), concentration, volume of sample and selective detection (via chemical derivatization) [36]. The important thing to consider while sample preparation is in order to prevent metabolite degradation, samples should be stored at the lowest temperature as soon as is feasible after collection. Freeze-thaw cycles should also be avoided. The sample preparation is influenced by the pH (especially body fluids) has a substantial impact on the chemical shifts in the NMR spectrum. The pH must be adjusted, which is commonly accomplished by adding a phosphate buffer at pH 7.4. Each sample may also be individually brought to a certain PH by adding NaOH and HCl [37]. Solvent selection which plays a crucial rôle in sample preparation depends on factors like thermal behavior, solubility, reactivity and frequency of signal [33]. Hence proper sample preparation technique is obtained depending upon the type of analyte and to its subsequent NMR.

5.2.3 Quantitative NMR (qNMR) Spectroscopy

NMR is well known potent structural technique for determining the identity of chemical species, but with organized research, it may also be utilized for precise quantitative measurement, known as quantitative NMR spectroscopy (qNMR) [38]. qNMR is the discipline of NMR spectroscopy, focuses on quantifying compounds employing the strength of signal and its link to analyte concentration [39]. It has proven to be a useful method for assay determination, or precise purity evaluations of pharmacological reference standards. Using information from an NMR spectrum, specifically the area or integral of an NMR peak, qNMR measures the concentration of a chemical in a solution. Under specific experimental circumstances, the integral is proportional to amount of substrate and the quantity of nuclei from the equivalent signal. Although proton NMR studies are quite popular, qNMR can also use other nuclei like ^{31}P, ^{19}F and ^{13}C. The molecule must require an NMR-active nucleotide that is unique to the target analyte. Utilizing either an internal or an external calibration standard can be utilized for quantification [38]. qNMR has been used extensively in different contexts including medicines, organic products, metabolomics, nutritional science, isotopomics and forensic science as a result of several methodological advancements [40]. The toxicity of drugs, disease diagnostics, tumor, pathophysiology of disease, anxiety, controlled substances, botanical and microbial reactions have all advantages from the widespread use of qNMR spectroscopy [1, 41]. One major application of qNMR in pharmaceutical studies includes pathways for degradation, residual solvents, to identify isomeric composition and molar ratios of analytes [1, 42, 43]. Although it has low sensitivity but employing qNMR can increase efficiency by speeding up the preparation and analysis processes. As it uses less solvents and produces less waste, qNMR is also environmentally beneficial. Hence applications of qNMR are growing rapidly in pharmaceutical and associated industries [38].

5.3 NMR Spectroscopy Techniques

5.3.1 One Dimensional NMR Spectroscopy

One dimensional NMR spectroscopy (1D NMR) is a technique which is more utilized to increase signal-to-noise ratio and determining a FID signal by a factor with the same decay time constant [44]. The chemical surroundings of nuclei in compounds are investigated using the 1D NMR, which records data on the chemical shift of the molecules, these chemical changes of the nucleus reveal the structural data of a compound [45]. 1D NMR can provide information by line shape variations that can be examined by just noticing variations in the physical attributes of the NMR spectra as a result of time [46–49] and gives a spectra after 1D Fourier transformation (FT) [50]. 1D NMR has broad range of applications, especially in the areas of chemistry and biochemistry, includes reaction kinetics, structural inter-conversion and protein folding and in-vivo process due to advancements in sensitivity that made it possible to quickly acquire pulsed NMR spectrum and its potency for real-time quantitative examinations of slow dynamic phenomena. Recently, in accordance with the standard 1D pulse sequences, ^{1}H NMR has been utilized in metabolomics. Nevertheless, due to its ultimately low spectral resolution 1D NMR provides extremely poor atomic resolution when employed on macromolecules [40, 48, 51–53] and difficult to detect molecular structure as it overlaps signals. In order to tackle this problem, it led to the development of 2D NMR spectroscopy.

5.3.2 Two-Dimensional NMR Spectroscopy (2D NMR)

The discoveries with the idea of multidimensional NMR of Jeener in 1971, led to the development of 2-dimensional NMR spectroscopy (2D NMR). 2D NMR is considerably more effective technique of distinguishing resonances at significantly greater fields than 1D traces and creates opportunity far more extensive array of methods for obtaining structural and dynamic data, of a sort that is unattainable for conventional spectroscopic approaches based on 1D scans [54, 55]. Formally, 2D NMR appears to be a logical progression from one-dimensional time-domain spectroscopy which composes the signal with respect to two-time variables [50]. 2D NMR has a pivotal part in the majority of chemical and biological fields incorporating the utilization of NMR [56–58]. They are typically employed to correlate the chemical changes of two equivalent or two distinct nuclei. Thus, there are homo- and heteronuclear 2D correlation experiments which includes nuclear Over Hauser effect spectroscopy [55, 59] and correlation spectroscopy (COSY) [54, 55], heteronuclear single-quantum correlation (HSQC) [55, 60], heteronuclear multiple-quantum correlation (HMQC) [55, 61], and heteronuclear multiple-bond correlation (HMBC) [55, 62]. The potential of 2-D NMR resides in its capability to deal with overlapping signals, boost sensitivity and reveal data that are not accessible by 1-D approaches. In accordance to that, 2D NMR has proven it feasible to quantify internuclear distances and scalar coupling [63]. Even 2D NMR approaches show significant potential for precisely identifying and quantifying metabolites in complicated biological samples, which is a prerequisite for attaining the full potential of metabolomics [64]. Although it has potential uses, but its long acquisition time and signal issue limits their application. Hence to overcome these issues, diffusion-ordered NMR and ultrafast 2D NMR are developed, which are extremely resistant to hardware instabilities because the entire 2-D NMR database is captured in a single scan and a repeatability of very little has been reported [40, 65]. Additionally, 2-D NMR can be used to analyze ^{13}C and ^{15}N by increasing the sensitivity of detection by up to two orders of magnitude while also offering relevant connective data [63]. Hence it is also useful for the continuous tracking of chemical and biological reactions, from advancements in hyphenated technologies and in quantitative fields [55].

5.3.3 Solid State NMR Spectroscopy

Solid state NMR (SSNMR) spectroscopy is an essential analytical technique and an atomic-level tool for identifying the composition, chemical structure, 3D structures and dynamic characteristics of semi-solids and solids. SSNMR is used to examine a variety of material systems, such as polymers, organic and inorganic crystals, biomolecules, glasses and other amorphous solids. It is based on the principle of Zeeman interactions (specific to nuclear isotope) between the magnetic field and nuclear spin. However, due to orientation dependent of nuclear spin interactions in solid NMR, most of the high-resolution SSNMR spectra are acquired using magic-angle spinning (MAS), which has a solid impact on the specific kind of RF pulse pattern necessary for obtaining structural and dynamical data [66, 67]. SSNMR have potential uses in the domain of forensics, includes examination of pharmaceutical solids [68], illicit drugs like MDMA, cocaine, cannabinoids [69] and other substances, polymers [70] and determination of composition of glass. ^{13}C solid state NMR is helpful even in photographic development [71]. SSNMR is gaining its attention in forensic science due to its non- invasive, quantitation of solids, crystallinity and to identify the level of API in drug products which is important to characterize the structure of drug [72]. The major advantage of SSNMR in pharmaceuticals is that, it can be used to measure the proportion of crystalline material to amorphous substance in a specific analyte which helps in determining the type and dynamics of compound [72–75] and can even distinguish between different compounds and detect molecular miscibility and interactions. There are different types of SSNMR based on isotopes like ^{13}C SSNMR, ^{19}F and ^{1}H SSNMR for quantification of solid samples [68]. Despite its benefits, it also has certain disadvantages, such as high cost and lack of accessibility [72]. To address these fundamental challenges in the assessment of solid materials, novel procedures were implemented [76, 77] which includes Magic angle spinning (MAS) and cross polymerization, both techniques help to minimize the line broadening seen in SSNMR. This enables the high-resolution processing of NMR spectra from solid state materials, which makes it possible to view the NMR spectrum of an API in the amount form itself, in its natural state. Polymorphic forms can be distinguished and identified on the basis of chemical shift of the individual resonances [76]. Hence it is an effective and adaptable spectroscopic method for analyzing pharmaceutical compounds.

5.3.4 Dynamic Nuclear Polarization (DNP)-Enhanced NMR Spectroscopy

DNP enhanced NMR spectroscopy is a technique which substantially enhances the NMR signals of solids and liquids and serves as a potential method for structural and dynamic studies of even biological components and complexes [78]. It is based on using a paramagnet-doped diamagnetic sample and transfer of strong polarization of electrons to adjacent nucleus through microwave irradiation of electron-nuclear transitions [78–80]. Subsequently, it is acknowledged that microwave-driven DNP analyses are effective tools for boosting signals in imaging and solid-state and solution NMR. DNP increases the sensitivity of NMR spectra by an exponent of 100, thereby minimizes the time in multivariate NMR studies by about 10^4 [81, 82]. The majority of modern DNP investigations on insulating substances are based on mechanisms such as thermal mixing, solid effect, Over Hauser effect and cross effect [78, 80]. DNP have a numerous use in the field of chemistry, physics and biological contexts [83, 84]. Even it has been utilized in the field of investigation for purpose of analysis of pharmaceuticals [85, 86] and controlled substances and polymers [87]. Although it has major advantage in the field of pharmacy, its low sensitivity limits its application. Hence in order to overcome those problems, DNP enhanced solid state NMR (SSNMR) and dissolution DNP (D-DNP) techniques have been developed. DNP-enhanced SSNMR is being used more frequently for analyzing API (active pharmaceutical ingredient) polymorphism and structure and even it improves the structure identification of polymers by providing the NMR signals of comparatively high molecular weight polymers, because of the optimized signal-to-noise ratio of the NMR spectrum offered by DNP [87, 88]. Hence DNP's significant increases in sensitivity make solid-state NMR investigations conceivable that were previously extremely difficult or unattainable [86]. The major application of D-DNP is using highly polarized imaging tracers for analysis of *in vivo* metabolic MRI [83, 89, 90]. Although, relatively few uses for mixtures has been established, despite the fact that D-DNP would offer a wide range of potential ways to measure low-concentrated analytes in intricate biological samples like extracts or biofluids [40, 91]. Hence, relying on current assessment, potential future equipment and technique advancements will be produced with the goal of enhancing D-DNP in order to make it more efficient, universal, or transferable [83].

5.4 Forensic Applications of NMR Spectroscopy

5.4.1 Drug Analysis

Due to the rampant use of controlled substances, scientists are required to provide efficient and rapid methods for detecting and analyzing abused drugs. Though there are conventional drug detection and analysis methods in the laboratory which includes Gas chromatography (GC), High performance liquid chromatography (HPLC), Gas chromatography-Mass spectrometry (GC-MS), Liquid chromatography-Mass spectrometry, Immunoassay, etc., NMR is an important investigative tool used in drug analysis to determine and characterize drugs and illicit drug molecules, evaluate their purity and study their interactions, and it is even confirmed that NMR can be used to qualitatively analyze new drugs at very low concentrations, thus, can be used for the identification of unknown drug or substances during investigations [92] (Figure 5.2). The purity of the drug sample can also be identified using NMR. Deviations from the projected spectral pattern disclose the purity of drugs as well as any possible hazards and also indicate about the presence of adulterants or other chemicals, thereby identifying its source of origin [93]. Determination of the potency of new APIs which initially was a cumbersome process which was made efficient using quantitative NMR (q-NMR) because it's rapidness, selectivity [94]. NMR, due to its high discriminating power is capable of differentiating different classes of drugs [95].

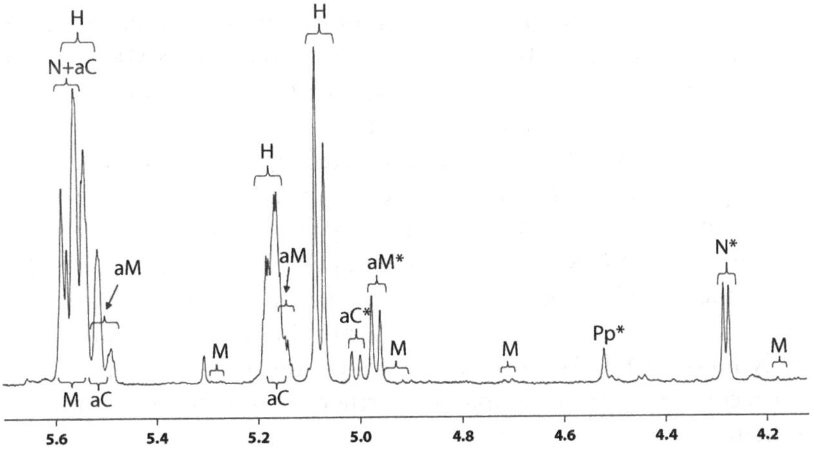

Figure 5.2 Illustrates the NMR spectrum for identifying different type of drugs [92].

5.4.2 Forensic Toxicology

There are many uses for NMR spectroscopy in forensic toxicology. The detection and assessment of substances and their metabolites in biological samples including blood, urine and hair is one such application [97]. It is possible to identify certain substances and gauge their amounts using NMR spectroscopy, which can be used in court proceedings to prove drug use or intoxication. In forensic investigations, NMR have utilized even to identify the toxins like organophosphorus insecticides. In metabolomic research, NMR can also be utilized to find metabolic pathways and biomarkers linked to drug use or other hazardous exposures in which it has better reproducibility [23]. NMR spectroscopy is capable of analyzing biological samples in minute quantities without complex extraction processes [98]. Salicylate, valproic acid, paraquat and tetrahydrofuran are some examples of xenobiotics that can possibly poison people. NMR can be used to detect and measure their levels in the body. As research done by Wahl *et al.* [99], said that methanol and ethylene glycol intoxication can be diagnosed and measured using ^{1}H NMR. The NMR approach not only allowed for speedy diagnosis with a small sample size and no need for extraction, but it can be used for qualitative examination and precise quantification [98, 100–102].

5.4.3 Body Fluid Analysis

In forensic science, determining body fluid traces plays a crucial role at a crime scene. The key phases in the identification of a trace are examination of the type of body fluid, determination of the species (human or animal) and the identification of the individual [18]. Recently NMR has gained more attention towards the investigative analysis, especially body fluids (Figure 5.3). ^{1}H NMR has a potential use in analysis of body fluids and binary mixtures. Therefore, ^{1}H NMR spectroscopy offers the benefit of not depending on just one chemical character but rather on a variety of single features that are unique to a particular body fluid, producing a "metabolite fingerprint" [17]. NMR has proved in analysis of binary mixtures of fluids like blood-saliva, blood-urine, saliva-semen, urine-semen with proper and accurate results and even it helps in identifying the metabolites present in body fluids [103]. Additionally, NMR is non-destructive, it is accessible to recover the entire sample for further analysis following the NMR examination.

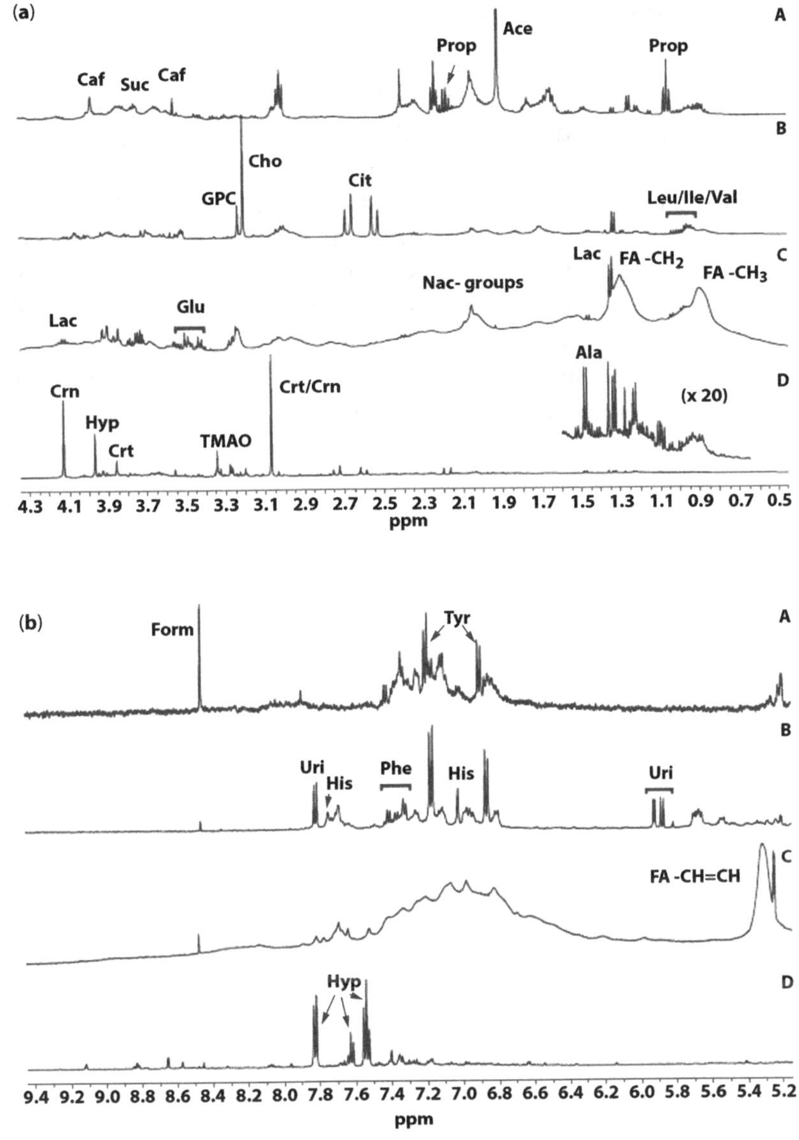

Figure 5.3 Illustration explaining about ^{1}H NMR of (A) saliva (B) seminal fluid (C) serum and (D) urine samples for analysis of different types of compounds and Amino acids. (a) 0.5 to 4.3 ppm and (b) 5.2 to 9.4 ppm [17].

5.4.4 Fire Debris Analysis

Despite not being utilized frequently as a principal technique in the examination of fire debris, NMR can sometimes yield useful data on the origin of fire and source by identifying and quantifying organic components in samples of fire debris [104]. Accelerants used in arson instances can be identified and characterized with the aid of NMR. Using the NMR spectra of fire debris samples, forensic investigators can pinpoint specific chemical substances connected to accelerants, such as petroleum-based chemicals, solvents, or volatile organic compounds. The distinctive NMR signals of the chemicals can reveal the presence or absence of accelerants. The chemical make-up of each accelerant varies and NMR can reveal details about the spectrum patterns and distinctive chemical shifts of these substances

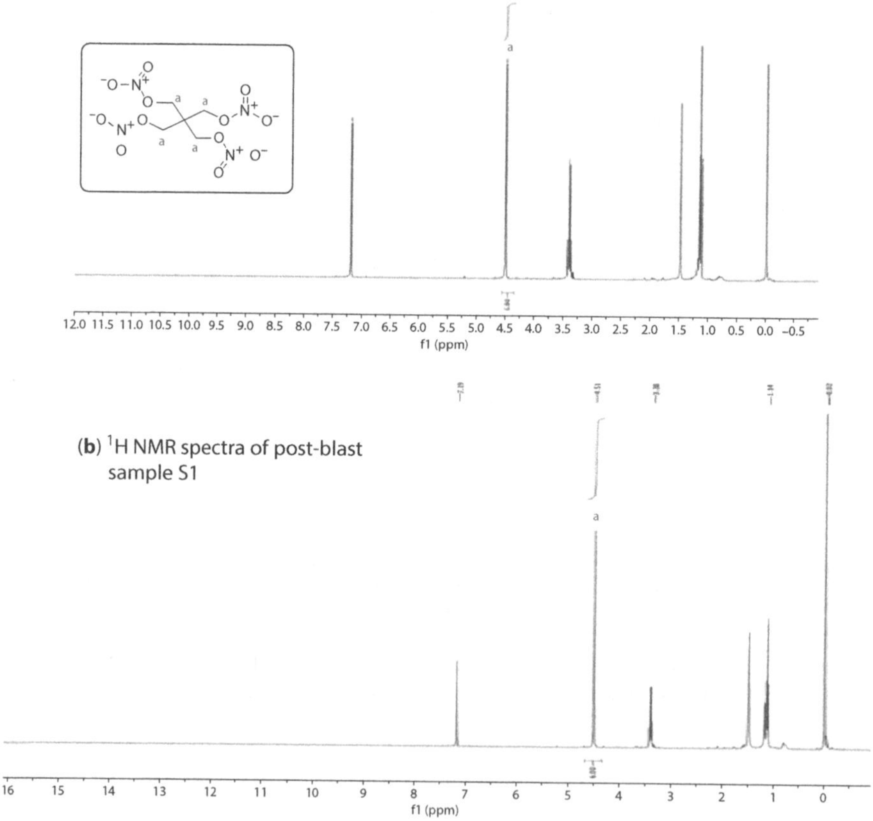

Figure 5.4 Showing ^{1}H NMR of PETN explosive (a) standard sample of PETN (b) sample from post-blast residue [110].

[105–108]. Even NMR helps to identify the presence of compounds and explosives from the post blast residues (Figure 5.4). The kind of accelerant used can be identified by relating the NMR spectra of the fire debris samples to reference spectra of well-known accelerants [109].

5.4.5 Polymer and Paint Analysis

NMR is one of the most advanced method for polymer identification that can be applied for the instant identification of cyanoacrylate monomers [111]. Molecular weight of polymers, characterization of polymers (Figure 5.5) [10], quantification of monomer content, distinguishing bonds holding polymers together and composition analysis of copolymers can be performed by NMR spectroscopy [112–116]. The particular chemical structures of the existing binders or resins, chemical structure of the pigments and components, as well as, distinguishing between different paint samples, assessing aging effects on paints, detecting and identifying additives and contaminants can be ascertained by examining the NMR spectra of paint samples. Considering that these details make it easy to compare known and unknown paint samples, connect disparate data sets, and discover common origins. It's worthy to note that combining NMR along with further analytical tools such as FTIR and MS provide in-depth examination and verification of findings.

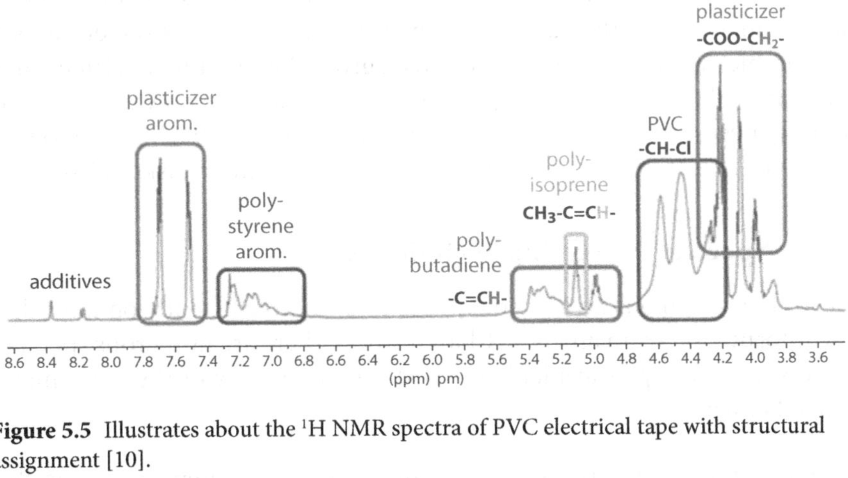

Figure 5.5 Illustrates about the ^{1}H NMR spectra of PVC electrical tape with structural assignment [10].

5.4.6 Fiber Analysis

It is possible to utilize NMR spectroscopy to determine the molecular make-up and measure contaminants in fibers. A study conducted on poly ethylene terephthalate (PET) fiber by Farah *et al.* (2014) [117] using ^{1}H NMR spectroscopy revealed differences in spectra analysis; among the changes were peak shifts, distinct peak splitting and the emergence of new peaks. The causes of degradation in polypropylene fiber were determined by evaluating the thermal, chemical and mechanical properties using ^{13}C solid-state NMR [118]. Natural fibers like cotton, wool and silk can be distinguished from synthetic fibers like polyester, nylon and acrylic by their distinctive NMR spectra. Also, forensic experts can identify any extra or alien components in the fiber by comparing the NMR spectra of a known pure fiber to an unidentified sample [117, 118].

5.5 Data Processing and Interpretation

NMR interpretation and analysis is based on collection of data handling after experiments, including NMR spectrum analysis, processing, data prior processing and evaluation of data, is essential to acquire excellent outcome. To aid this process several software applications have developed includes "AMIX (Bruker Biospin, Germany), Chenomx NMR Suite (Chenomx, Canada) and a popular classical NMR data processing tool is NMR Pipe". These techniques offer numerous features involving spectrum processing, via identification, quantification and features for fundamental data analysis. Further data assessment methods, such as screening out undesirable variations, are required (background noise, uncorrelated variation) in a dataset, developing and employing statistical evaluation, are typically necessary because of the complexity of NMR data. This led to rise of chemometrics and statistical methods to achieve these tasks [119–121].

5.5.1 Spectral Processing Techniques

Spectral processing is an essential phase in order to efficiently obtain valuable information from any NMR-based study. There are numerous spectral processing techniques available for NMR analysis. Few of them are mentioned below:

i. ***Fourier transform***: The frequency domain signal, often known as the spectrum, is produced by the Fourier transformation of a signal. These

NMR signals are transformed from time domain to frequency domain [120]. Similar to the time domain signal, frequency domain has a real and an imaginary component i.e. absorption mode line (absorption mode Lorentzian) is visible in the actual part of the spectra and the dispersion mode Lorentzian line shape is produced by the imaginary portion of the spectrum. Furthermore, "FT works with a certain line broadening factor and removal of a potential digital filter imposed on FID" (for example Bruker Advance spectrometer) [122].

ii. ***Zero filling***: The FID needs to be transformed into a digital format before processing so that it may be saved to computer memory. Once the FID is Fourier converted, the spectrum is characterized by a number of values(data). To these data points, equal set of zeros are added which is known as 'zero filling', so that the corresponding spectrum carried double the number of points. Obviously, this does not increase resolution because the measured signal remains the same, but the spectral lines will be more clearly delineated [122].

iii. ***Phase correction***: Phasing is a method of NMR spectral correction that aims to maximize the linearity and absorptive quality of all NMR peaks over the whole NMR spectrum. Especially phasing errors can have an impact on observed peak regions, spectral binning and spectral alignment. Although most modern NMR spectrometers have automatic phasing capabilities, manual phasing is frequently necessary in metabolomics because many automatic phasing techniques deform low-intensity peaks and is crucial for managing the residual water signal. Despite these limitations, it continues to make extensive use of auto-phasing, because it is quick and operator-bias-free [123, 124].

iv. ***Baseline correction***: It is an essential method for reducing spectral aberrations resulted from electrical errors, insufficient digitized sorting and sampling. But when it done effectively, it produces a spectrum with a better appearance and signal-free portions that are entirely flat, horizontal lines with zero intensity [123]. However, present version of Atomics offers two techniques for baseline correction: non-parametric recognition (based on Sergey algorithm which includes recognition of base through data points and smooth construction of baseline using those data points) and linear fitting (it uses pre-set points of the spectra to calculate parameters of a linear function and then baseline is generated [120, 125]. However, for appropriate peak integration and spectrum alignment, accurate baselines are essential and even small inaccuracies in the baseline structure can quickly cause errors in the assessment of low-abundance (by orders of magnitude) [123].

v. ***Spectral and peak alignment***: it is a process that continuously shifts positions of the peak in different spectra so that peaks pertaining to similar components can be directly aligned. Spectral alignment is required to enable the comparison and quantification of the same peaks across many NMR spectra from the same molecules. Although spectrum alignment is frequently employed in NMR spectral evaluation, and it's also vital to know that arrangement might obscure crucial details such as "sample pH, metal ion concentrations, ionic strengths, and temperature" that are recorded in chemical shift data [123]. Peak alignment is another crucial step to eliminate the influence of fluctuations from the spectral datasets. One easy step is that spectral referencing, that lowers the inner reference peak of each spectrum to 0 ppm. Using the same technique, the whole spectrum is shifted by same reference peak. As a result, all of the spectra that have peak imbalances are properly aligned [120, 126].

vi. ***Normalization:*** Once NMR peaks have been arranged, recognized and their corresponding intensity is known, the followed by the adjusting for inherent concentration discrepancies. Hence, the most effective method for accomplishing these concentration and intensity differences is normalization, a prominent processing of information method which seeks to produce the samples equivalent to one another. Hence it is considered as an important step in the processing which can provide reliable data [123].

5.5.2 Spectral Interpretation and Analysis

Interpretation and analysis of data plays a key role in NMR spectroscopy. Interpretation, compound recognition and statistical evaluation may start once the entire NMR data have been adequately analyzed via careful execution of phase and baseline correction, zero filling, normalization, and scaling. Spectral interpretation and analysis in NMR help to clarify the molecule setup, composition and dynamics of a compound. It can be interpreted using chemical shifts, coupling constants, spin multiplicity and integration [123].

a) ***Chemical shift***: Chemical shifts reveal important details on the chemical environment and molecular connectivity of a molecule's nucleus. Chemical shifts could be employed to characterize the structure and dynamics of a wide number of compounds, particularly functional groups can be inferred using ^{1}H chemical shifts, ^{13}C (organic compounds containing carbon) and ^{15}N(nitrogen based compounds) chemical shifts [127]. Even it can provide information regarding secondary structure sidechain conformations, dynamics, solvation, and hydrogen bonding [128–132]. These chemical shifts depend on the shielding and de-shielding of protons. Usually 3, (trimethylsilyl)-2,2′,3,3′-tetradeuteropropionic acid (TSP) and 4,4-dimethyl-4-silapentane-1-sulfonic acid (DSS) are frequently utilized as chemical shift reference standards in the metabolomics [123, 133] but it is pH sensitive [134]. Therefore, standard Deuterated DSS, is employed for quantification, particularly if the quantity of the reference chemical is specifically known [123, 135], even Sodium formate and acetate is used as an alternate way for referencing chemical shift. Although, chemical shifts signal position depends on a number of sample characteristics, such as temperature, pH, exchangeable moieties, salts, and effects of the demagnetization field [136, 137]. Yet it is well defined and essential technique used to elucidate the molecular structure of compounds.

b) ***Coupling constants and spin multiplicities***: when the spins of two nuclei that are coupled by interaction of few chemical bonds, a process known as scalar coupling (splitting of signals) is occurred. Usually, this connection is apparent only when there are no more than four chemical bonds between the two nuclei. These splitting signals follow a pattern that is influenced by the number of connected nuclei as well as a coupling constant (J) [kind of nuclei and the distance (measured in chemical bonds) between them [138–143]. The distinct form of a split signal is referred to be multiplicity, which reveals more information regarding the molecule. There are different forms of multiplicities, includes HH multiplets (gives data for spatial proximity of protons that are involved) and CH (multiplets of ^{13}C signals occur due to $^{1}J_{CH}$ bonding which provides data bout the bonding of C atoms). Interpretation of coupling constants like HH [through germinal ($^{2}J_{HH}$) and vicinal coupling ($^{3}J_{HH}$] and CH ($^{1}J_{CH}$) provides data about the interaction of magnetic moment of nuclei and bonding electrons. The N+1 rule can be used to estimate this multiplicity [127]. Hence multiplicities are essential to provide a skeletal structure of compound.

c) ***Integration***: Peak integration is one of essential method to determine quantitative accuracy, which is significantly impacted by the integral zone spectrum, the magnitude of the slope, and the bias (zero and first order coefficients of a linear line provides the baseline in the integral zone). Hence error can be easily identified in integration particularly when determining the slope and bias. The integrals are more vulnerable to baseline defect. For proper quantitation, manual corrections of slope and bias are needed. To minimize errors, it is preferable to execute integration more than five times and take the mean of all the data points [1, 144].

d) ***2-D NMR methods***: Because macromolecules like proteins possess a lot of NMR-active nuclei, whose NMR spectra are complicated and include a lot of overlapping peaks. Large molecules also exhibit a quicker rate of relaxation, which results in widening of peak and a reduction in resolution. In order to overcome these drawbacks, 2D NMR operations produce spectra with signals that correlate combinations of various nuclei that are characterized by two chemical shift axes (rather than one, as in 1D spectra). It includes correlation spectroscopy (COSY- display peaks with correlation of coupled protons), Nuclear Overhauser effect spectroscopy (NOESY- essential for structure elucidation of macromolecules that give data about spatial organization) and Total correlated spectroscopy (TOCSY- spectrum display correlation signals between nuclear couples that are a part of the same spin system. Therefore, these methods are very efficient in interpreting the spectra of NMR in complex molecules [139–143].

e) ***Software analysis***: Recently, software tools have gained popularity in analysis and interpretation of NMR data even in the field of metabolomics. These tools are extensively utilized, well-assessed, and freely accessible. These include MVAPACK for multivariate analysis [123, 145], MetaboAnalyst [123, 146–148] for both analysis and metabolite annotation, and biological interpretation and many more. Additionally, there are a variety of paid resources including the NMR Suite from Chenomx, the AMIX software from Bruker etc. [123].

5.5.3 Chemometrics and Statistical Analysis

Johnels *et al.* presented the initial study on the use of chemometrics to NMR in 1983 [149, 150]. Chemometrics is a discipline of multivariate data analysis that employs statistics to develop equations for obtaining chemical information from huge 2D multivariate collection of data [151]. The fundamental principles of most chemometric approaches are based on hidden factors or principal components, which are displayed in the same space as the initial data [152]. For the development of chemometric data, minimal number of parameters are necessary, and also allows for the visualization of correlations through simple graphs using graphic computer interface [151]. Chemometrics have numerous uses in the area of chemical and biological sciences, especially in pharmaceutical area which has already provided solutions to many analytical issues including those relating to the reliability of herbal remedies, the examination of the chiral centers of medications, the detection of counterfeit medicines, and many more [153–157]. The application of chemometrics for frequency domain data has successfully developed, owing to metabolomics techniques that aim to analyze metabolic processes through NMR of biofluids [149, 158]. The examination of complicated 1-D and 2-D NMR structures of complex biological and medicinal composites served as a catalyst for new discoveries in incorporating chemometric data evaluation to high-resolution NMR signals [149, 159, 160]. This comprises effective and dependable techniques for solving and analyzing intricate chemical and biological information that result in understandable and valid models equipped to handle illegible, noisy, and collinear data structures [161]. Pattern recognition methods like principal component analysis and discriminant analysis [156, 162–164], multivariate calibration techniques include principal component regression, orthogonal partial least square discriminant analysis (OPLS-DA) and partial least squares (PLS) [156, 165, 166] and deconvolution methods like multivariate curve resolution- alternating least squares (MCR-ALS) [156, 165] and neural networks. It's also critical to emphasize that statistical experimental design (SED), a tool used in chemometrics, offers a way to gather pertinent data [161, 167, 168]. The approaches for chemometric identification presented here contribute significantly to the method validation necessary for the growing popularity of low field NMR I n forensics.

5.6 Conclusion

5.6.1 Challenges and Opportunities

The significance of nuclear magnetic resonance (NMR) spectroscopy in forensic investigation has tremendous prospects for offering indispensable data for legal decisions and criminal investigation. NMR spectroscopy is a potent technique for identifying chemical structure and composition of compound, recognizing the source of a sample, and giving precise time-of-death analyses, enabling scientists to recognize and perhaps quantify unidentified molecules. Although they are numerous techniques, it provides accurate information regarding the molecular and dynamics of compound. One major challenge of NMR spectroscopy in the field of forensics is time-consuming, sensitive sample preparation and high cost. Additionally, small or complicated sample matrices, low concentrate analytes like those seen in forensic evidence, might make it difficult to obtain high-quality spectra. Hence to overcome those challenges numerous methods of NMR like solid state NMR, one dimensional and 2-dimensional NMR, chemometrics and DNP enhanced NMR creates more opportunities for the analysts to use NMR in the forensic setting which provides accurate and sensitive information., which make it more versatile tool in investigative field.

5.6.2 Future Outlook and Potential Advancements

Recently, the advancement in NMR spectroscopy for metabolomic studies in the field of forensics, has received more attention- which examine a variety of metabolites in a sample to find diagnostic biomarkers and these metabolites can be detected using it. NMR would prove to predict the enormous impact of the technology if its sensitivity could be increased by several orders of magnitude, which seems feasible given the most recent developments in the hyperpolarization sector. As NMR technology develops, it might become more easy and rapid to produce high-quality spectra from more complex sample matrices especially combination of drugs. Additionally, novel approaches to forensic material analysis, like solid-state NMR, quantitative and diffusion-ordered NMR spectroscopy, may open up new possibilities for forensic analysis.

References

1. S. K. Bharti and R. Roy, "Quantitative 1H NMR spectroscopy," *TrAC - Trends Anal. Chem.*, vol. 35. pp. 5–26, May 2012. doi: 10.1016/j.trac.2012.02.007.
2. J. Keeler, *Understanding NMR spectroscopy*. 2010. doi: 10.5860/choice.43-5896.
3. A. D. C. Santos, L. M. Dutra, L. R. A. Menezes, M. F. C. Santos, and A. Barison, "Forensic NMR spectroscopy: Just a beginning of a promising partnership," *TrAC - Trends Anal. Chem.*, vol. 107. Elsevier B.V., pp. 31–42, Oct. 01, 2018. doi: 10.1016/j.trac.2018.07.015.
4. B. M. Ham, "Analytical Chemistry in the Life Sciences and Medicine," *Kirk-Othmer Encycl. Chem. Technol.*, pp. 1–29, Sep. 2016, doi: 10.1002/0471238961.2018051413151420.A01.PUB2.
5. J. Sanz and D. Massiot, "Nuclear Magnetic Resonance Spectroscopy," in *Developments in Clay Science*, 2013, pp. 233–274. doi: 10.1016/B978-0-08-098259-5.00010-X.

6. C. Hussain, D. Rawtani, G. Pandey, and M. Tharmavaram, *Handbook of Analytical Techniques for Forensic Samples: Current and Emerging Developments*. 2020. Accessed: May 13, 2023. [Online]. Available: https://books.google.com/books?hl=en&lr=&id=MMULEAAAQBAJ&oi=fnd&pg=PP1&dq=handbook+of+analytical+techniques+for+forensic+samples&ots=CKl4FANQK7&sig=KsBHticB7Il6XuYy8mMpv7kNIqQ
7. T. D. Claridge, E. Amsterdam, N. York, P. San Diego, and S. Francisco, *High-resolution NMR techniques in organic chemistry*. 2016. Accessed: May 13, 2023. [Online]. Available: https://books.google.com/books?hl=en&lr=&id=uPUeBgAAQBAJ&oi=fnd&pg=PP1&dq=High-Resolution+NMR+Techniques+in+Organic+Chemistry%3B+Elsevier&ots=feqEo0edQn&sig=Q6DdRXtY7PLrfIAerO0jSsUU5Iw
8. H. Gunther and H. Gunther, *NMR spectroscopy: basic principles, concepts, and applications in chemistry*. 1994. Accessed: May 13, 2023. [Online]. Available: https://analyticalscience.wiley.com/do/10.1002/sepspec.9783527330003/full/
9. H. Y. Yu, S. Myoung, and S. Ahn, "Recent applications of benchtop nuclear magnetic resonance spectroscopy," *Magnetochemistry*, vol. 7, no. 9. MDPI, 2021. doi: 10.3390/magnetochemistry7090121.
10. T. Schoenberger, U. Simmross, and C. Poppe, "Forensic examination of electrical tapes using high resolution magic angle spinning 1H NMR spectroscopy," *Anal. Bioanal. Chem.*, vol. 408, no. 1, pp. 123–129, Jan. 2016, doi: 10.1007/S00216-015-9126-Z.
11. P. Dais and A. Spyros, "Nuclear Magnetic Resonance," in *Chemical Analysis of Food: Techniques and Applications*, Elsevier, 2012, pp. 91–115. doi: 10.1016/B978-0-12-384862-8.00004-2.
12. G. Pandey, M. Tharmavaram, D. Rawtani, S. Kumar, and Y. Agrawal, "Multifarious applications of atomic force microscopy in forensic science investigations," *Forensic Sci. Int.*, vol. 273. Elsevier, pp. 53–63, Apr. 01, 2017. doi: 10.1016/j.forsciint.2017.01.030.
13. S. L. Draper and E. R. McCarney, "Benchtop nuclear magnetic resonance spectroscopy in forensic chemistry," *Magn. Reson. Chem.*, vol. 61, no. 2. John Wiley and Sons Ltd, pp. 106–129, Feb. 01, 2023. doi: 10.1002/mrc.5197.
14. U. Holzgrabe, R. Deubner, C. Schollmayer, and B. Waibel, "Quantitative NMR spectroscopy - Applications in drug analysis," *J. Pharm. Biomed. Anal.*, vol. 38, no. 5 SPEC. ISS. Elsevier, pp. 806–812, May 2005. doi: 10.1016/j.jpba.2005.01.050.
15. J. N. P. Serrano, L. E. C. Benedito, M. P. de Souza, A. O. Maldaner, and A. L. de Oliveira, "Quantitative NMR as a tool for analysis of new psychoactive substances," *Forensic Chem.*, vol. 21, Dec. 2020, doi: 10.1016/j.forc.2020.100282.

16. G. S. H. Lee *et al.*, "Analysis of 3,4-Methylenedioxy- N -Methylamphetamine (MDMA) in 'Ecstasy' Tablets by 13 C Solid State Nuclear Magnetic Resonance (NMR) Spectroscopy," *J. Forensic Sci.*, vol. 44, no. 4, p. 14550J, Jul. 1999, doi: 10.1520/jfs14550j.
17. P. Scano *et al.*, "1H NMR metabolite fingerprinting as a new tool for body fluid identification in forensic science," *Magn. Reson. Chem.*, vol. 51, no. 8, pp. 454–462, Aug. 2013, doi: 10.1002/mrc.3966.
18. E. Locci *et al.*, "Forensic NMR metabolomics: one more arrow in the quiver," *Metabolomics*, vol. 16, no. 11. Springer, Nov. 01, 2020. doi: 10.1007/s11306-020-01743-6.
19. M. Imbenotte, N. Azaroual, B. Cartigny, G. Vermeersch, and M. Lhermitte, "Identification and quantitation of xenobiotics by 1H NMR spectroscopy in poisoning cases," *Forensic Sci. Int.*, vol. 133, no. 1–2, pp. 132–135, Apr. 2003, doi: 10.1016/S0379-0738(03)00059-8.
20. U. Holzgrabe, "Quantitative NMR spectroscopy in pharmaceutical applications," *Prog. Nucl. Magn. Reson. Spectrosc.*, vol. 57, no. 2. pp. 229–240, 2010. doi: 10.1016/j.pnmrs.2010.05.001.
21. G. S. H. Lee, K. M. Brinch, K. Kannangara, M. Dawson, and M. A. Wilson, "A Methodology Based on NMR Spectroscopy for the Forensic Analysis of Condoms," *J. Forensic Sci.*, vol. 46, no. 4, p. 15052J, Jul. 2001, doi: 10.1520/jfs15052j.
22. K. Bryce, I. Stone, and K. Daugherty, *Analysis of fire debris by nuclear magnetic resonance spectroscopy*. 1981. Accessed: May 13, 2023. [Online]. Available: https://www.ojp.gov/ncjrs/virtual-library/abstracts/analysis-fire-debris-nuclear-magnetic-resonance-spectroscopy
23. M. Szeremeta, K. Pietrowska, A. Niemcunowicz-Janica, A. Kretowski, and M. Ciborowski, "Applications of metabolomics in forensic toxicology and forensic medicine," *Int. J. Mol. Sci.*, vol. 22, no. 6. MDPI AG, pp. 1–16, Mar. 02, 2021. doi: 10.3390/ijms22063010.
24. J. C. Lindon, "NMR spectrometers," in *Encyclopedia of Spectroscopy and Spectrometry*, 2016, pp. 224–231. doi: 10.1016/B978-0-12-803224-4.00079-0.
25. C. Deleanu and J. R. Jocelyn Paré, "Chapter 6 Nuclear magnetic resonance spectroscopy (NMR): Principles and applications," *Tech. Instrum. Anal. Chem.*, vol. 18, no. C, pp. 179–237, 1997, doi: 10.1016/S0167-9244(97)80015-7.
26. K. Singh and B. Blümich, "NMR spectroscopy with compact instruments," *TrAC Trends Anal. Chem.*, vol. 83, pp. 12–26, May 2016, doi: 10.1016/J.TRAC.2016.02.014.
27. Deepak, "Advantages of FT – NMR over Continuous Wave NMR," *lab-training.com*, 2015. https://lab-training.com/advantages-of-ft-nmr-over-continuous-wave-nmr/ (accessed May 25, 2023).
28. C. Deleanu and J. R. Jocelyn Paré, "Chapter 6 Nuclear magnetic resonance spectroscopy (NMR): Principles and applications," *Tech. Instrum. Anal. Chem.*, vol. 18, no. C, pp. 179–237, 1997, doi: 10.1016/S0167-9244(97)80015-7.

29. R. R. Ernst and W. A. Anderson, "Application of fourier transform spectroscopy to magnetic resonance," *Rev. Sci. Instrum.*, vol. 37, no. 1, pp. 93–102, 1966, doi: 10.1063/1.1719961.
30. J. C. Korte, K. J. Layton, B. Tahayori, P. M. Farrell, S. M. Moore, and L. A. Johnston, "NMR spectroscopy using Rabi modulated continuous wave excitation," *Biomed. Signal Process. Control*, vol. 33, pp. 422–428, May 2017, doi: 10.1016/J.BSPC.2016.10.006.
31. T. C. Farrar, "Pulsed and Fourier Transform NMR Spectroscopy," *Anal. Chem.*, vol. 42, no. 2, Feb. 1970, doi: 10.1021/ac60286a805.
32. H. J. Reich, M. Jautelat, M. T. Messe, F. J. Weigert, and J. D. Roberts, "Nuclear Magnetic Resonance Spectroscopy. Carbon-13 Spectra of Steroids," *J. Am. Chem. Soc.*, vol. 91, no. 26, pp. 7445–7454, 1969, doi: 10.1021/ja01054a037.
33. A. Tampieri, M. Szabó, F. Medina, and H. Gulyás, "A brief introduction to the basics of NMR spectroscopy and selected examples of its applications to materials characterization," *Phys. Sci. Rev.*, vol. 6, no. 1, Jan. 2021, doi: 10.1515/psr-2019-0086.
34. R. S. Macomber and G. S. Harbison, "A Complete Introduction to Modern NMR Spectroscopy," *Phys. Today*, vol. 52, no. 1, pp. 68–68, 1999, doi: 10.1063/1.882558.
35. B. En Edict Yanibada *et al.*, "Evaluation of sample preparation methods for NMR-based metabolomics of cow milk," *Heliyon*, vol. 4, p. 856, 2018, doi: 10.1016/j.heliyon.2018.
36. T. W. M. Fan and A. N. Lane, "Applications of NMR spectroscopy to systems biochemistry," *Prog. Nucl. Magn. Reson. Spectrosc.*, vol. 92–93. Elsevier B.V., pp. 18–53, Feb. 01, 2016. doi: 10.1016/j.pnmrs.2016.01.005.
37. A. Zhang, H. Sun, P. Wang, Y. Han, and X. Wang, "Recent and potential developments of biofluid analyses in metabolomics," *J. Proteomics*, vol. 75, no. 4, pp. 1079–1088, May 2012, doi: 10.1016/J.JPROT.2011.10.027.
38. John Tobin, "Quantitative NMR Spectroscopy - Acanthus Research," *acanthus research*, Jun. 24, 2022. https://acanthusresearch.com/generalblog/quantitative-nmr-spectroscopy/ (accessed May 19, 2023).
39. A. A. Crook and R. Powers, "Quantitative NMR-Based Biomedical Metabolomics: Current Status and Applications," *Molecules*, vol. 25, no. 21, Nov. 2020, doi: 10.3390/MOLECULES25215128.
40. P. Giraudeau, "Challenges and perspectives in quantitative NMR," *Magn. Reson. Chem.*, vol. 55, no. 1, pp. 61–69, Jan. 2017, doi: 10.1002/mrc.4475.
41. F. Malz, H. J.-J. of pharmaceutical and biomedical analysis, and undefined 2005, "Validation of quantitative NMR," *Elsevier*, vol. 38, pp. 813–823, 2005, doi: 10.1016/j.jpba.2005.01.043.
42. U. Holzgrabe, "Quantitative NMR spectroscopy in pharmaceutical applications," *Prog. Nucl. Magn. Reson. Spectrosc.*, vol. 57, no. 2. pp. 229–240, Aug. 2010. doi: 10.1016/j.pnmrs.2010.05.001.

43. S. Mahajan and I. P. Singh, "Determining and reporting purity of organic molecules: why qNMR," *Magn. Reson. Chem.*, vol. 51, no. 2, pp. 76–81, May 2013, doi: 10.1002/MRC.3906.
44. R. G. Spencer, "Equivalence of the time-domain matched filter and the spectral-domain matched filter in one-dimensional NMR spectroscopy," *Concepts Magn. Reson. Part A Bridg. Educ. Res.*, vol. 36 A, no. 5, pp. 255–265, Sep. 2010, doi: 10.1002/cmr.a.20162.
45. L. Yan, Y. Hu, X. Zhang, and B. Yue, "Applications of NMR Techniques in the Development and Operation of Proton Exchange Membrane Fuel Cells," in *Annual Reports on NMR Spectroscopy*, Academic Press Inc., 2016, pp. 149–213. doi: 10.1016/bs.arnmr.2015.11.003.
46. M. Gal, M. Mishkovsky, and L. Frydman, "Real-time monitoring of chemical transformations by ultrafast 2D NMR spectroscopy," *J. Am. Chem. Soc.*, vol. 128, no. 3, pp. 951–956, Jan. 2006, doi: 10.1021/ja0564158.
47. M. Mizuguchi, G. J. Kroon, P. E. Wright, and H. J. Dyson, "Folding of a β-sheet protein monitored by real-time NMR spectroscopy," *J. Mol. Biol.*, vol. 328, no. 5, pp. 1161–1171, 2003, doi: 10.1016/S0022-2836(03)00349-8.
48. N. A. J. Van Nuland, V. Forge, J. Balbach, and C. M. Dobson, "Real-Time NMR Studies of Protein Folding," *Acc. Chem. Res.*, vol. 31, no. 11, pp. 773–780, 1998, doi: 10.1021/AR970079L.
49. M. Zeeb and J. Balbach, "Kinetic Protein Folding Studies using NMR Spectroscopy," in *Protein Folding Handbook*, 2008, pp. 536–572. doi: 10.1002/9783527619498.ch16.
50. L. Frydman, A. Lupulescu, and T. Scherf, "Principles and features of single-scan two-dimensional NMR spectroscopy," *J. Am. Chem. Soc.*, vol. 125, no. 30, pp. 9204–9217, Jul. 2003, doi: 10.1021/ja030055b.
51. J. Balbach, V. Forge, W. Lau, N. van Nuland, K. B.- Science, and undefined 1996, "Protein folding monitored at individual residues during a two-dimensional NMR experiment," *science.org*, vol. 274, no. 5290, pp. 1161–1163, Nov. 1996, doi: 10.1126/science.274.5290.1161.
52. J. Sanders and B. Hunter, "Modern NMR spectroscopy: a guide for chemists," 1988, Accessed: May 15, 2023. [Online]. Available: https://www.osti.gov/biblio/5277235
53. P. Schanda and B. Brutscher, "Very fast two-dimensional NMR spectroscopy for real-time investigation of dynamic events in proteins on the time scale of seconds," *J. Am. Chem. Soc.*, vol. 127, no. 22, pp. 8014–8015, Jun. 2005, doi: 10.1021/ja051306e.
54. W. P. Aue, E. Bartholdi, and R. R. Ernst, "Two-dimensional spectroscopy. Application to nuclear magnetic resonance," *J. Chem. Phys.*, vol. 64, no. 5, pp. 2229–2246, May 1976, doi: 10.1063/1.432450.
55. P. Giraudeau and L. Frydman, "Ultrafast 2D NMR: An emerging tool in analytical spectroscopy," *Annu. Rev. Anal. Chem.*, vol. 7. Annual Reviews Inc., pp. 129–161, 2014. doi: 10.1146/annurev-071213-020208.

56. J. Cavanagh, W. J. Fairbrother, A. G. Palmer, M. Rance, and N. J. Skelton, *Protein NMR Spectroscopy: Principles and Practice*. 2006. doi: 10.1524/zpch.1997.202.part_1_2.297.
57. Y. Shrot, B. Shapira, and L. Frydman, "Ultrafast 2D NMR spectroscopy using a continuous spatial encoding of the spin interactions," *J. Magn. Reson.*, vol. 171, no. 1, pp. 163–170, Nov. 2004, doi: 10.1016/j.jmr.2004.08.001.
58. T. M. Barbara, "Principles of Nuclear Magnetic Resonance in One and Two Dimensions. Richard R. Ernst , Geoffrey Bodenhausen , Alexander Wokaun," *Q. Rev. Biol.*, vol. 63, no. 1, pp. 131–132, 1988, doi: 10.1086/415835.
59. J. Jeener, B. H. Meier, P. Bachmann, and R. R. Ernst, "Investigation of exchange processes by two-dimensional NMR spectroscopy," *J. Chem. Phys.*, vol. 71, no. 11, pp. 4546–4553, 1979, doi: 10.1063/1.438208.
60. G. Bodenhausen and D. J. Ruben, "Natural abundance nitrogen-15 NMR by enhanced heteronuclear spectroscopy," *Chem. Phys. Lett.*, vol. 69, no. 1, pp. 185–189, 1980, doi: 10.1016/0009-2614(80)80041-8.
61. A. Bax and B. H.- Griffey, "Correlation of proton and nitrogen-15 chemical shifts by multiple quantum NMR," *J. Magn. Reson.*, 1983, Accessed: May 15, 2023. [Online]. Available: https://www.sciencedirect.com/science/article/pii/002223648390241X
62. A. Bax and M. F. Summers, "1H and 13C Assignments from Sensitivity-Enhanced Detection of Heteronuclear Multiple-Bond Connectivity by 2D Multiple Quantum NMR," *J. Am. Chem. Soc.*, vol. 108, no. 8, pp. 2093–2094, 1986, doi: 10.1021/ja00268a061.
63. A. Bax and L. Lerner, "Two-dimensional nuclear magnetic resonance spectroscopy," *Science (80-.).*, vol. 232, no. 4753, pp. 960–967, 1986, doi: 10.1126/SCIENCE.3518060.
64. C. Ludwig and M. R. Viant, "Two-dimensional J-resolved NMR spectroscopy: Review of a key methodology in the metabolomics toolbox," *Phytochem. Anal.*, vol. 21, no. 1. pp. 22–32, 2010. doi: 10.1002/pca.1186.
65. A. Le Guennec *et al.*, "Fast determination of absolute metabolite concentrations by spatially encoded 2D NMR: Application to breast cancer cell extracts," *Anal. Chem.*, vol. 84, no. 24, pp. 10831–10837, Dec. 2012, doi: 10.1021/AC3033504.
66. M. Leskes, "Nuclear magnetic resonance spectroscopy | solid-state," in *Encyclopedia of Analytical Science*, Elsevier, 2019, pp. 403–413. doi: 10.1016/B978-0-12-409547-2.14529-9.
67. B. Reif, S. E. Ashbrook, L. Emsley, and M. Hong, "Solid-state NMR spectroscopy," *Nat. Rev. Methods Primers*, vol. 1, no. 1. Springer Nature, Dec. 01, 2021. doi: 10.1038/s43586-020-00002-1.
68. M. Li, W. Xu, and Y. Su, "Solid-state NMR spectroscopy in pharmaceutical sciences," *TrAC - Trends Anal. Chem.*, vol. 135. Elsevier B.V., Feb. 01, 2021. doi: 10.1016/j.trac.2020.116152.
69. N. K. Burns *et al.*, "The identification of synthetic cannabinoids surface coated on herbal substrates using solid-state nuclear magnetic resonance

spectroscopy," *Anal. Chim. Acta*, vol. 1104, pp. 105–109, Apr. 2020, doi: 10.1016/j.aca.2019.12.051.

70. G. Foran, N. Verdier, D. Lepage, C. Malveau, N. Dupré, and M. Dollé, "Use of solid-state NMR spectroscopy for the characterization of molecular structure and dynamics in solid polymer and hybrid electrolytes," *Polymers*, vol. 13, no. 8. MDPI AG, Apr. 02, 2021. doi: 10.3390/polym13081207.
71. F. Bertocchi, R. Nepravishta, W. Mandaliti, and M. Paci, "A Forensic Application of Solid-State 13C NMR Spectroscopy: the Date of a Photographic Development," *Appl. Magn. Reson.*, vol. 47, no. 9, pp. 1015–1019, Sep. 2016, doi: 10.1007/s00723-016-0807-3.
72. R. T. Berendt, D. M. Sperger, E. J. Munson, and P. K. Isbester, "Solid-state NMR spectroscopy in pharmaceutical research and analysis," *TrAC - Trends Anal. Chem.*, vol. 25, no. 10, pp. 977–984, Nov. 2006, doi: 10.1016/j.trac.2006.07.006.
73. P. Gao, "Determination of the composition of delavirdine mesylate polymorph and pseudopolymorph mixtures using 13C CP/MAS NMR," *Pharm. Res.*, vol. 13, no. 7, pp. 1095–1104, 1996, doi: 10.1023/A:1016027212156.
74. A. R. Sheth, J. W. Lubach, E. J. Munson, F. X. Muller, and D. J. W. Grant, "Mechanochromism of piroxicam accompanied by intermolecular proton transfer probed by spectroscopic methods and solid-phase changes," *J. Am. Chem. Soc.*, vol. 127, no. 18, pp. 6641–6651, May 2005, doi: 10.1021/JA045823T.
75. T. J. Offerdahl *et al.*, "Quantitation of crystalline and amorphous forms of anhydrous neotame using 13C CPMAS NMR spectroscopy," *J. Pharm. Sci.*, vol. 94, no. 12, pp. 2591–2605, Dec. 2005, doi: 10.1002/JPS.20469.
76. K. C. Bynum, *Preformulation and early phase method development*, vol. 10, no. C. 2011. doi: 10.1016/B978-0-12-375680-0.00009-7.
77. T. and M. E. Offerdahl, "Solid-state NMR spectroscopy of pharmaceutical materials," vol. Rev. 7(1), pp. 109–112, 2004.
78. T. Maly *et al.*, "Dynamic nuclear polarization at high magnetic fields," *J. Chem. Phys.*, vol. 128, no. 5, 2008, doi: 10.1063/1.2833582.
79. K. N. Hu, H. H. Yu, T. M. Swager, and R. G. Griffin, "Dynamic nuclear polarization with biradicals," *J. Am. Chem. Soc.*, vol. 126, no. 35, pp. 10844–10845, Sep. 2004, doi: 10.1021/ja039749a.
80. Q. Z. Ni *et al.*, "High frequency dynamic nuclear polarization," *Acc. Chem. Res.*, vol. 46, no. 9, pp. 1933–1941, Sep. 2013, doi: 10.1021/ar300348n.
81. E. A. Nanni, A. B. Barnes, R. G. Griffin, and R. J. Temkin, "THz dynamic nuclear polarization NMR," *IEEE Trans. Terahertz Sci. Technol.*, vol. 1, no. 1, pp. 145–163, Sep. 2011, doi: 10.1109/TTHZ.2011.2159546.
82. A. B. Barnes *et al.*, "High-field dynamic nuclear polarization for solid and solution biological NMR," *Appl. Magn. Reson.*, vol. 34, no. 3–4, pp. 237–263, Aug. 2008, doi: 10.1007/s00723-008-0129-1.
83. S. Jannin, J. N. Dumez, P. Giraudeau, and D. Kurzbach, "Application and methodology of dissolution dynamic nuclear polarization in physical,

chemical and biological contexts," *J. Magn. Reson.*, vol. 305, pp. 41–50, Aug. 2019, doi: 10.1016/j.jmr.2019.06.001.
84. W. C. Liao, B. Ghaffari, C. P. Gordon, J. Xu, and C. Copéret, "Dynamic Nuclear Polarization Surface Enhanced NMR spectroscopy (DNP SENS): Principles, protocols, and practice," *Curr. Opin. Colloid Interface Sci.*, vol. 33. Elsevier Ltd, pp. 63–71, Jan. 01, 2018. doi: 10.1016/j.cocis.2018.02.006.
85. A. J. Rossini *et al.*, "Dynamic nuclear polarization enhanced NMR spectroscopy for pharmaceutical formulations," *J. Am. Chem. Soc.*, vol. 136, no. 6, pp. 2324–2334, Feb. 2014, doi: 10.1021/ja4092038.
86. L. Zhao, A. C. Pinon, L. Emsley, and A. J. Rossini, "DNP-enhanced solid-state NMR spectroscopy of active pharmaceutical ingredients," *Magn. Reson. Chem.*, vol. 56, no. 7. John Wiley and Sons Ltd, pp. 583–609, Jul. 01, 2018. doi: 10.1002/mrc.4688.
87. D. Le *et al.*, "Up to 100% Improvement in Dynamic Nuclear Polarization Solid-State NMR Sensitivity Enhancement of Polymers by Removing Oxygen," *Macromol. Rapid Commun.*, vol. 36, no. 15, pp. 1416–1421, Aug. 2015, doi: 10.1002/marc.201500133.
88. O. Ouari *et al.*, "Improved structural elucidation of synthetic polymers by dynamic nuclear polarization solid-state NMR spectroscopy," *ACS Macro Lett.*, vol. 2, no. 8, pp. 715–719, Aug. 2013, doi: 10.1021/MZ4003003.
89. S. J. Nelson *et al.*, "Metabolic imaging of patients with prostate cancer using hyperpolarized [1-13C]pyruvate," *Sci. Transl. Med.*, vol. 5, no. 198, Aug. 2013, doi: 10.1126/SCITRANSLMED.3006070.
90. D. Wilson, J. K.-J. of N. Medicine, and undefined 2014, "Hyperpolarized 13C MR for molecular imaging of prostate cancer," *Soc. Nucl. Med.*, vol. 55, no. 10, pp. 1567–1572, Oct. 2014, doi: 10.2967/jnumed.114.141705.
91. J. N. Dumez *et al.*, "Hyperpolarized NMR of plant and cancer cell extracts at natural abundance," *Analyst*, vol. 140, no. 17, pp. 5860–5863, Aug. 2015, doi: 10.1039/C5AN01203A.
92. Y. Zhong *et al.*, "The application of a desktop NMR spectrometer in drug analysis," *Int. J. Anal. Chem.*, vol. 2018, 2018, doi: 10.1155/2018/3104569.
93. U. Holzgrabe, R. Deubner, C. Schollmayer, and B. Waibel, "Quantitative NMR spectroscopy - Applications in drug analysis," *J. Pharm. Biomed. Anal.*, vol. 38, no. 5 SPEC. ISS. Elsevier, pp. 806–812, Aug. 10, 2005. doi: 10.1016/j.jpba.2005.01.050.
94. G. K. Webster and S. Kumar, "Expanding the analytical toolbox: Pharmaceutical application of quantitative NMR," *Anal. Chem.*, vol. 86, no. 23, pp. 11474–11480, May 2014, doi: 10.1021/ac502871w.
95. D. Antic, "Illicit Drug Analysis Using Benchtop NMR: Amphetamines," 2014. [Online]. Available: www.thermoscientific.com
96. S. Balayssac *et al.*, "Characterization of heroin samples by 1H NMR and 2D DOSY 1H NMR," *Forensic Sci. Int.*, vol. 234, no. 1, pp. 29–38, 2014, doi: 10.1016/j.forsciint.2013.10.025.

97. G. A. (Graham A. Webb, Ed., *Annual reports on NMR spectroscopy. Volume 56*, 1st ed. Elsevier Academic Press, 2005. [Online]. Available: https://shop.elsevier.com/books/annual-reports-on-nmr-spectroscopy/webb/978-0-12-505456-0#full-description
98. J. Liu, J. Decatur, G. Proni, and E. Champeil, "Identification and quantitation of 3,4-methylenedioxy-N-methylamphetamine (MDMA, ecstasy) in human urine by 1H NMR spectroscopy. Application to five cases of intoxication," *Forensic Sci. Int.*, vol. 194, no. 1–3, pp. 103–107, May 2010, doi: 10.1016/j.forsciint.2009.10.022.
99. A. Wahl *et al.*, "Poisoning with methanol and ethylene glycol: 1 H NMR spectroscopy as an effective clinical tool for diagnosis and quantification," *Toxicology*, vol. 128. pp. 73–81, 1998.
100. B. Cartigny *et al.*, "Determination of glyphosate in biological fluids by 1H and 31P NMR spectroscopy," in *Forensic Science International* , May 2004, pp. 141–145. doi: 10.1016/j.forsciint.2004.03.025.
101. M. Imbenotte, N. Azaroual, B. Cartigny, G. Vermeersch, and M. Lhermitte, "Identification and quantitation of xenobiotics by 1H NMR spectroscopy in poisoning cases," in *Forensic Science International*, Elsevier Ireland Ltd, May 2003, pp. 132–135. doi: 10.1016/S0379-0738(03)00059-8.
102. A. J. Simpson and S. A. Brown, "Purge NMR: Effective and easy solvent suppression," *J. Magn. Reson.*, vol. 175, no. 2, pp. 340–346, May 2005, doi: 10.1016/j.jmr.2005.05.008.
103. F. Zapata, M. Á. Fernández de la Ossa, and C. García-Ruiz, "Emerging spectrometric techniques for the forensic analysis of body fluids," *TrAC - Trends Anal. Chem.*, vol. 64. Elsevier B.V., pp. 53–63, Jan. 01, 2015. doi: 10.1016/j.trac.2014.08.011.
104. C. Martín-Alberca, F. E. Ortega-Ojeda, and C. García-Ruiz, "Analytical tools for the analysis of fire debris. A review: 2008-2015," *Anal. Chim. Acta*, vol. 928. Elsevier B.V., pp. 1–19, May 2016. doi: 10.1016/j.aca.2016.04.056.
105. D. L. Flumignan, N. Boralle, and J. E. De Oliveira, "Screening Brazilian commercial gasoline quality by hydrogen nuclear magnetic resonance spectroscopic fingerprintings and pattern-recognition multivariate chemometric analysis," *Talanta*, vol. 82, no. 1, pp. 99–105, May 2010, doi: 10.1016/J.TALANTA.2010.04.002.
106. C. R. Kaiser, J. L. Borges, A. R. dos Santos, D. A. Azevedo, and L. A. DAvila, "Quality control of gasoline by 1H NMR: Aromatics, olefinics, paraffinics, and oxygenated and benzene contents," *Fuel*, vol. 89, no. 1, pp. 99–104, May 2010, doi: 10.1016/j.fuel.2009.06.023.
107. V. S. Pinto, "Use of 1H nuclear magnetic resonance and chemometrics to detect the percentage of ethanol anhydrous in Brazilian type C premium gasoline," *Fuel*, vol. 276, May 2020, doi: 10.1016/j.fuel.2020.118015.
108. R. M. R. Tainara, L. F. Danilo, B. Nivaldo, and E. D. O. José, "1H NMR fingerprinting of brazilian commercial gasoline: Pattern-recognition analyses for

origin authentication purposes," *Energy and Fuels*, vol. 23, no. 8, pp. 3954–3959, May 2009, doi: 10.1021/EF8010977.
109. R. Meusinger, "Qualitative and quantitative determination of oxygenates in gasolines using 1H nuclear magnetic resonance spectroscopy," *Anal. Chim. Acta*, vol. 391, no. 3, pp. 277–288, May 1999, doi: 10.1016/S0003-2670(99)00250-0.
110. P. Munjal, B. Sharma, J. R. Sethi, A. Dalal, and S. L. Gholap, "Identification and analysis of organic explosives from post-blast debris by nuclear magnetic resonance," *J. Hazard. Mater.*, vol. 403, no. August 2020, p. 124003, 2021, doi: 10.1016/j.jhazmat.2020.124003.
111. F. B. I. Quantico, Va.)Laboratory., *Proceedings of the International Symposium on the Analysis and Identification of Polymers*. U.S. Dept. of Justice, Federal Bureau of Investigation, 1984.
112. D. Kaczmarek *et al.*, "Response of block copolyelectrolyte complexes to addition of ionic surfactants," *Colloids Surfaces A Physicochem. Eng. Asp.*, vol. 532, pp. 290–296, May 2017, doi: 10.1016/J.COLSURFA.2017.04.078.
113. S. T. Knox, S. Parkinson, R. Stone, and N. J. Warren, "Benchtop flow-NMR for rapid online monitoring of RAFT and free radical polymerisation in batch and continuous reactors," *Polym. Chem.*, vol. 10, no. 35, pp. 4774–4778, May 2019, doi: 10.1039/C9PY00982E.
114. J. Rönnols, E. Danieli, H. Freichels, and F. Aldaeus, "Lignin analysis with benchtop NMR spectroscopy," *Holzforschung*, vol. 74, no. 2, pp. 226–231, May 2020, doi: 10.1515/HF-2018-0282.
115. M. Rubens, J. Van Herck, and T. Junkers, "Automated Polymer Synthesis Platform for Integrated Conversion Targeting Based on Inline Benchtop NMR," *ACS Macro Lett.*, vol. 8, no. 11, pp. 1437–1441, May 2019, doi: 10.1021/ACSMACROLETT.9B00767.
116. Mauricio, "Spinsolve Benchtop NMR for Polymer Characterization," *Magritek*, 2021. https://magritek.com/2021/10/08/quantitative-microplastic-analysis-with-spinsolve-benchtop-nmr/#:~:text=It describes how benchtop NMR can be used,used demonstrating its outstanding sensitivity and solvent suppression.
117. S. Farah, T. Tsach, A. Bentolila, and A. J. Domb, "Morphological, spectral and chromatography analysis and forensic comparison of PET fibers," *Talanta*, vol. 123, pp. 54–62, 2014, doi: 10.1016/j.talanta.2014.01.041.
118. I. C. Escobar and B. Van Der Bruggen, "Microfiltration and ultrafiltration membrane science and technology," *J. Appl. Polym. Sci.*, vol. 132, no. 21. John Wiley and Sons Inc, May 2015. doi: 10.1002/app.42002.
119. F. Delaglio, S. Grzesiek, G. W. Vuister, G. Zhu, J. Pfeifer, and A. Bax, "NMRPipe: A multidimensional spectral processing system based on UNIX pipes," *J. Biomol. NMR*, vol. 6, no. 3, pp. 277–293, Nov. 1995, doi: 10.1007/BF00197809.

120. T. Wang *et al.*, "Automics: An integrated platform for NMR-based metabonomics spectral processing and data analysis," *BMC Bioinf.*, vol. 10, Mar. 2009, doi: 10.1186/1471-2105-10-83.
121. Q. Zhao, R. Stoyanova, S. Du, P. Sajda, T. B.- Bioinformatics, and Undefined, "HiRes—a tool for comprehensive assessment and interpretation of metabolomic data," *academic.oup.com*, 2006, Accessed: May 16, 2023. [Online]. Available: https://academic.oup.com/bioinformatics/article-abstract/22/20/2562/218603
122. J. Keeler, "Understanding NMR Spectroscopy," 2002.
123. A. H. Emwas *et al.*, "Recommended strategies for spectral processing and post-processing of 1D 1 H-NMR data of biofluids with a particular focus on urine," *Metabolomics*, vol. 14, no. 3. Springer New York LLC, Mar. 01, 2018. doi: 10.1007/s11306-018-1321-4.
124. D. S. Wishart, "Quantitative metabolomics using NMR," *TrAC - Trends Anal. Chem.*, vol. 27, no. 3, pp. 228–237, Mar. 2008, doi: 10.1016/J.TRAC.2007.12.001.
125. S. Golotvin and A. Williams, "Improved Baseline Recognition and Modeling of FT NMR Spectra," *J. Magn. Reson.*, vol. 146, no. 1, pp. 122–125, 2000, doi: 10.1006/jmre.2000.2121.
126. J. Forshed, I. Schuppe-Koistinen, and S. P. Jacobsson, "Peak alignment of NMR signals by means of a genetic algorithm," *Anal. Chim. Acta*, vol. 487, no. 2, pp. 189–199, Jul. 2003, doi: 10.1016/S0003-2670(03)00570-1.
127. E. Breitmaier, "Front Matter," in *Structure Elucidation by NMR in Organic Chemistry*, John Wiley & Sons, Ltd, 2003, pp. i–xii. doi: 10.1002/0470853069.fmatter.
128. S. P. Mielke and V. V. Krishnan, "Characterization of protein secondary structure from NMR chemical shifts," *Prog. Nucl. Magn. Reson. Spectrosc.*, vol. 54, no. 3–4, pp. 141–165, Apr. 2009, doi: 10.1016/J.PNMRS.2008.06.002.
129. S. Nerli, A. C. McShan, and N. G. Sgourakis, "Chemical shift-based methods in NMR structuredetermination," *Prog. Nucl. Magn. Reson. Spectrosc.*, vol. 106–107, p. 1, Jun. 2018, doi: 10.1016/J.PNMRS.2018.03.002.
130. H. Saitô, I. Ando, and A. Ramamoorthy, "Chemical shift tensor - The heart of NMR: Insights into biological aspects of proteins," *Prog. Nucl. Magn. Reson. Spectrosc.*, vol. 57, no. 2, pp. 181–228, Aug. 2010, doi: 10.1016/J.PNMRS.2010.04.005.
131. G. Wagner, A. Pardi, and K. Wüthrich, "Hydrogen Bond Length and 1H NMR Chemical Shifts in Proteins," *J. Am. Chem. Soc.*, vol. 105, no. 18, pp. 5948–5949, 1983, doi: 10.1021/JA00356A056.
132. D. S. Wishart, "Interpreting protein chemical shift data," *Prog. Nucl. Magn. Reson. Spectrosc.*, vol. 58, no. 1–2, pp. 62–87, 2011, doi: 10.1016/J.PNMRS.2010.07.004.
133. A. C. Dona *et al.*, "A guide to the identification of metabolites in NMR-based metabonomics/metabolomics experiments," *Comput. Struct. Biotechnol. J.*, vol. 14, pp. 135–153, 2016, doi: 10.1016/j.csbj.2016.02.005.

134. D. S. Wishart *et al.*, "1H, 13C and 15N chemical shift referencing in biomolecular NMR," *J. Biomol. NMR*, vol. 6, no. 2, pp. 135–140, Sep. 1995, doi: 10.1007/BF00211777.
135. P. Mercier, M. J. Lewis, D. Chang, D. Baker, and D. S. Wishart, "Towards automatic metabolomic profiling of high-resolution one-dimensional proton NMR spectra," *J. Biomol. NMR*, vol. 49, no. 3–4, pp. 307–323, Apr. 2011, doi: 10.1007/s10858-011-9480-x.
136. HT Edzes, "The nuclear magnetization as the origin of transient changes in the magnetic field in pulsed NMR experiments," *Elsevier Journal Magn. Reson. 1990,* 1969, doi: https://doi.org/10.1016/0022-2364(90)90261-7.
137. M. H. Levitt, "Demagnetization field effects in two-dimensional solution NMR," *Concepts Magn. Reson.*, vol. 8, no. 2, pp. 77–103, 1996, doi: 10.1002/(SICI)1099-0534(1996)8:2<77::AID-CMR1>3.0.CO;2-L.
138. R. Bible, *Interpretation of NMR spectra: An empirical approach.* 2013. Accessed: May 17, 2023. [Online]. Available: https://books.google.com/books?hl=en&lr=&id=8EnUBwAAQBAJ&oi=fnd&pg=PA1&dq=+++10.+++++Bible+RH.+Interpretation+of+NMR+spectra:+an+empirical+approach.+Springer+Science+%26+Business+Media.+2013.&ots=t07xc2dorh&sig=rjPAeib3uNyoDDMBofWzD86fCAo
139. A. Derome, *Modern NMR techniques for chemistry research.* 2013. Accessed: May 17, 2023. [Online]. Available: https://books.google.com/books?hl=en&lr=&id=sEYXBQAAQBAJ&oi=fnd&pg=PP1&dq=+Derome+AE.+Modern+NMR+techniques+for+chemistry+research.+Elsevier.+2013.&ots=i-jRHjpnxCE&sig=fFc1_HLe6-3umBRah4oGgKV5MJs
140. H. Friebolin and J. Becconsall, *Basic one-and two-dimensional NMR spectroscopy.* 2005. Accessed: May 17, 2023. [Online]. Available: https://analyticalscience.wiley.com/do/10.1002/sepspec.9783527327829/
141. P. Héctor Zamora Carreras, "NMR Spectroscopy Principles, Interpreting an NMR Spectrum and Common Problems," *Anal. Sep.*, Oct. 2021.
142. Hore PJ. : ., "Nuclear magnetic resonance. ," *Oxford Univ. Press USA*, 2015.
143. N. Jacobsen, *NMR data interpretation explained: understanding 1D and 2D NMR spectra of organic compounds and natural products.* 2016. Accessed: May 17, 2023. [Online]. Available: https://books.google.com/books?hl=en&lr=&id=OxQWCgAAQBAJ&oi=fnd&pg=PR13&dq=++Jacobsen+NE.+NMR+data+interpretation+explained:+understanding+1D+and+2D+NMR+spectra+of+organic+compounds+and+natural+products.+John+Wiley+%26+Sons.+2016.&ots=3iCVTVGBXs&sig=g2MmX
144. N. K. Srivastava, S. Pradhan, B. Mittal, R. Kumar, C. M. Pandey, and G. A. Nagana Gowda, "Novel corrective equations for complete estimation of human tissue lipids after their partial destruction by perchloric acid pre-treatment: High-resolution 1H-NMR-based study," *NMR Biomed.*, vol. 21, no. 2, pp. 89–100, Feb. 2008, doi: 10.1002/NBM.1159.

145. B. Worley and R. Powers, "MVAPACK: A complete data handling package for NMR metabolomics," *ACS Chem. Biol.*, vol. 9, no. 5, pp. 1138–1144, May 2014, doi: 10.1021/CB4008937.
146. J. Xia, N. Psychogios, ... N. Y.-N. acids, and undefined 2009, "MetaboAnalyst: a web server for metabolomic data analysis and interpretation," *academic.oup.com*, vol. 37, 2009, doi: 10.1093/nar/gkp356.
147. J. Xia and D. S. Wishart, "MSEA: A web-based tool to identify biologically meaningful patterns in quantitative metabolomic data," *Nucleic Acids Res.*, vol. 38, no. SUPPL. 2, 2010, doi: 10.1093/nar/gkq329.
148. J. Xia, I. V. Sinelnikov, B. Han, and D. S. Wishart, "MetaboAnalyst 3.0-making metabolomics more meaningful," *Nucleic Acids Res.*, vol. 43, no. W1, pp. W251–W257, 2015, doi: 10.1093/nar/gkv380.
149. P. Ebrahimi, N. Viereck, R. Bro, and S. B. Engelsen, "Chemometric Analysis of NMR Spectra," in *Modern Magnetic Resonance*, Springer International Publishing, 2017, pp. 1–20. doi: 10.1007/978-3-319-28275-6_20-1.
150. D. Johnels *et al.*, "Clustering of aryl carbon-13 nuclear magnetic resonance substituent chemical shifts. A multivariate data analysis using principal components," *J. Chem. Soc. Perkin Trans. 2*, no. 6, pp. 863–871, 1983, doi: 10.1039/P29830000863.
151. H. Winning, F. H. Larsen, R. Bro, and S. B. Engelsen, "Quantitative analysis of NMR spectra with chemometrics," *J. Magn. Reson.*, vol. 190, no. 1, pp. 26–32, Jan. 2008, doi: 10.1016/j.jmr.2007.10.005.
152. Y. B. Monakhova, T. Kuballa, and D. W. Lachenmeier, "Chemometric methods in NMR spectroscopic analysis of food products," *J. Anal. Chem.*, vol. 68, no. 9. pp. 755–766, Sep. 2013. doi: 10.1134/S1061934813090098.
153. Chmielewska ABaczek T, "Comparative analysis of chiral drugs in view of chemometrics," *J. AOAC Int.*, 2012, doi: 10.5740/jaoacint.SGE_Chmielewsk.
154. H. A. Gad, S. H. El-Ahmady, M. I. Abou-Shoer, and M. M. Al-Azizi, "Application of chemometrics in authentication of herbal medicines: A review," *Phytochem. Anal.*, vol. 24, no. 1, pp. 1–24, Jan. 2013, doi: 10.1002/PCA.2378.
155. B. Krakowska, D. Custers, E. Deconinck, and M. Daszykowski, "Chemometrics and the identification of counterfeit medicines—A review," *J. Pharm. Biomed. Anal.*, vol. 127, pp. 112–122, Aug. 2016, doi: 10.1016/J.JPBA.2016.04.016.
156. Y. B. Monakhova, U. Holzgrabe, and B. W. K. Diehl, "Current role and future perspectives of multivariate (chemometric) methods in NMR spectroscopic analysis of pharmaceutical products," *J. Pharm. Biomed. Anal.*, vol. 147. Elsevier B.V., pp. 580–589, Jan. 05, 2018. doi: 10.1016/j.jpba.2017.05.034.
157. A. Rahman, "APPLICATION OF FOURIER TRANSFORM INFRARED SPECTROSCOPY FOR QUALITY CONTROL OF PHARMACEUTICAL PRODUCTS: A REVIEW," *Indones. J. Pharm.*, vol. 23, no. 1, pp. 1–8, Jan. 2012, doi: 10.14499/INDONESIANJPHARM23ISS1PP1-8.
158. Lindon JNicholson JHolmes E *et al.*, "Metabonomics: metabolic processes studied by NMR spectroscopy of biofluids," *Concepts Magn.*

Reson. Part A Bridg. Educ. Res., vol. 12(5), pp. 289–320, 2000, Accessed: May 16, 2023. [Online]. Available: https://onlinelibrary.wiley.com/doi/abs/10.1002/1099-0534(2000)12:5%3C289::AID-CMR3%3E3.0.CO;2-W

159. H. Grahn, F. Delaglio, M. Delsuc, and G. L.- J, "Multivariate data analysis for pattern recognition in two-dimensional NMR," *J. Magn. Reson.*, vol. 77(2), pp. 294–307, 1988, Accessed: May 16, 2023. [Online]. Available: https://www.sciencedirect.com/science/article/pii/0022236488901795
160. R. E. Hoffman and G. C. Levy, "Modern methods of N M R data processing and data evaluation," *Prog. Nucl. Magn. Reson. Spectrosc.*, vol. 23, no. 3, pp. 211–258, 1991, doi: 10.1016/0079-6565(91)80005-M.
161. J. Trygg, E. Holmes, and T. Lundstedt, "Chemometrics in metabonomics," *J. Proteome Res.*, vol. 6, no. 2. pp. 469–479, Feb. 2007. doi: 10.1021/pr060594q.
162. Kumar NBansal ASarma, "Chemometrics tools used in analytical chemistry: An overview," *Talanta*, 2014, doi: DOI: 10.1016/j.talanta.2014.02.003.
163. M. Jd. Jw. J. Et, "Analysis of complex mixtures using high-resolution nuclear magnetic resonance spectroscopy and chemometrics," *Prog. Nucl. Magn. Reson. Spectrosc.*, 2011, Accessed: May 16, 2023. [Online]. Available: https://eprints.ncl.ac.uk/258035
164. P. G. Svante Wold *, Kim Esbensen, "Principal component analysis," *Chemom. Intell. Lab. Syst.*, vol. 2, no. 1–3, pp. 37–52, 1987, doi: https://doi.org/10.1016/0169-7439(87)80084-9.
165. A. de Juan and R. Tauler, "Multivariate Curve Resolution (MCR) from 2000: Progress in concepts and applications," *Crit. Rev. Anal. Chem.*, vol. 36, no. 3–4, pp. 163–176, Jul. 2006, doi: 10.1080/10408340600970005.
166. P. Geladi and B. K.- Acta, "Partial least-squares regression: a tutorial," *Anal. Chim. Acta*, 1986, Accessed: May 16, 2023. [Online]. Available: https://www.sciencedirect.com/science/article/pii/0003267086800289
167. G. Box, W. Hunter, and S. Hunter, *Statistics for experimenters*. 1978. Accessed: May 16, 2023. [Online]. Available: https://hwbdocuments.env.nm.gov/Los Alamos National Labs/TA 54/11528.pdf
168. T. Lundstedt, E. Seifert, L. Abramo, and … B. T.-… and, "Experimental design and optimization," *Intell. Lab.*, 1998, Accessed: May 16, 2023. [Online]. Available: https://www.sciencedirect.com/science/article/pii/S0169743998000653

6

Forensic Aspects of Mass Spectroscopy and Isotope Ratio Mass Spectroscopy

Elipe Arjun[1], Priyanka Chhabra[2] and Priyanka Singh[1]*

[1]Amity Institute of Forensic Sciences, Amity University, Noida, Uttar Pradesh, India
[2]Center for Medical Biotechnology, Amity Institute of Biotechnology, Amity University, Noida, Uttar Pradesh, India

Abstract
The forensic uses of Mass Spectrometry (MS) and Isotope Ratio Mass Spectrometry (IRMS) are discussed in this chapter. By detecting and measuring chemical constituents in challenging materials, MS revolutionized forensic analysis, whereas IRMS improves precision in calculating isotopic compositions. It is described the ideas, instruments, and benefits of integrating MS with IRMS. Real-world examples show how important they are in drug analysis, toxicology, arson investigations, and counterfeit detection. Problems including equipment limits and contamination sources are addressed. The prospects of MS and IRMS in forensic science are discussed, with ongoing advances in resolving complex cases and delivering justice on the horizon.

Keywords: Mass spectrometry (MS), isotope ratio mass spectrometry (IRMS), isotope, forensic

6.1 Introduction

Mass spectrometry is a technique that separates and analyses the components of a sample based on their mass-to-charge ratio. It is often used in forensic investigations to identify the chemical composition of a substance, determine its purity, and compare it to known standards.

**Corresponding author*: prawal50@gmail.com

Priyanka Chhabra, Divya Bajpai Tripathy, Anjali Gupta, Rajeev Kumar, Kajol Bhati and Shruti Shukla (eds.) Advances in Analytical Techniques for Forensic Investigation, (149–188) © 2024 Scrivener Publishing LLC

Mass spectrometry can also be used to identify unknown compounds by comparing their mass spectra with reference to spectra in a database. [1] Isotope mass ratio analysis involves measuring the ratios of isotopes of an element in a sample. This can be useful in forensic investigations because different sources of a substance may have different isotopic ratios. For example, the isotopic ratio of carbon in drugs synthesized from plant sources will differ from that of synthetic drugs. This can be used to help identify the origin of the substance and traces it back to its source [2].

In addition to identifying substances, mass spectrometry, and isotope mass ratio analysis can also be used to establish timelines and identify potential suspects. For example, the analysis of isotopic ratios in hair or nails can provide information about the geographical origin and diet of a person, which may be useful in identifying them or establishing an alibi.

Overall, mass spectrometry and isotope mass ratio analysis are powerful tools in forensic science, providing valuable information to investigators and helping to solve crimes.

The isotopic profile or "signature" of a material refers to the ratios of the stable isotopes of elements, such as 2 H/1 H, 13C/12C, 15N/14N, and 18O/16O. Biological, chemical, and physical processes that cause variations in the ratios of stable isotopes, measuring their relative abundance by IRMS can reveal information about a material's history. Forensic investigators have used IRMS techniques to measure a variety of materials, including illegal drugs, explosives, counterfeit currency, food, beverages, animal tissues ivory, and human remains. For instance, the isotopes in human hair protein can reveal an individual's death date, what she/he ate, and how often and where she/he travelled. This Chapter discusses the applications of the two common instrument configurations that are used for the gas source IRMS dual-inlet IRMS (DI-IRMS) and the continuous flow of IRMS (CF-IRMS) and how they are useful in the field of forensics [3].

6.1.1 Overview of Isotopes and Mass Spectroscopy

Hydrogen, Carbon, Nitrogen, and Oxygen are some of examples of bio-elements found in the materials like illegal substances Human Hair, Drugs, and Water. Many bio-elements exist in multiple forms called isotopes. Element Carbon has six protons in the nucleus, defining its atomic number (6) and placed in the periodic table. Most carbon atoms have six neutrons in the nucleus; the shorthand for this isotope form of carbon is 12C, which is derived from the total number of protons and neutrons. In some rare cases, a carbon atom may contain an additional neutron, giving rise to the 13C isotope, with a different mass: 13C is slightly heavier than 12C because of the additional neutron. The rare 13C form of carbon is a stable isotope that doesn't undergo radioactive decay, which behaves a little differently than 12C in biological, chemical, and physical processes because of the mass difference. (Another form of carbon has two additional neutrons in the nucleus and is called 14C or radiocarbon; this isotope form of carbon is radioactive and is often used in age dating applications.).

As shown in Table 6.1 abundances of stable isotopes of light elements are typically measured with an isotope ratio mass spectrometer. Stable isotopes should not be confused with radioactive isotopes of an element, such as "C (also referred to as radioactive carbon) or 'H (also called tritium). Radioactive isotopes have limited lifetimes and undergo decay to form a different element, although the time required for this decay may vary widely ranging from nanoseconds to many thousands of years. For instance, carbon has five very short-lived radioactive isotopes ('C, "C, "C, "C, and ^{1}C) with lifetimes of seconds to minutes and one longer-lived radioactive isotope ("C) with a half-life of 5710 years. Radioactive "C" is

Table 6.1 Stable isotopes of light elements [1].

Element	Isotope	Abundance (%)
Hydrogen	"H	99.985
	"H	0.015
Carbon	"C	98.89
	"C	1.11
Nitrogen	"N	99.63
	"N	0.37
Oxygen	"O	99.759
	"O	0.037
	"O	0.204
Sulphur	"S	95.00
	"S	0.76
	"S	4.22
	"S	0.014

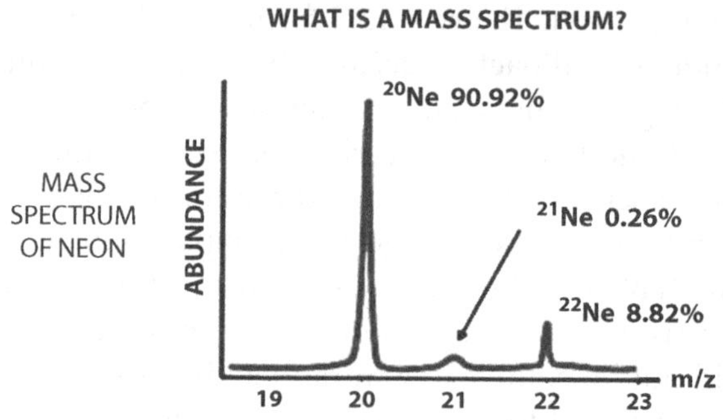

Figure 6.1 Mass spectrometer [2].

perhaps best known because of its utility in dating biological materials that are less than 50,000 years old and as a tracer in metabolic studies.

A mass spectrum is a plot that represents the distribution of ions based on their mass-to-charge ratio (m/z) as shown in Figure 6.1. It provides valuable information about the masses and relative abundances of ions present in a sample. Each peak in the mass spectrum corresponds to an ion with a specific m/z value, and the height of the peak indicates the abundance of that ion in the sample. Mass spectra are crucial in identifying unknown compounds, elucidating molecular structures, and quantifying the composition of mixtures [4].

6.1.2 The Importance of Stable Isotope Analysis Assists Forensic Cases

Stable isotope ratio analyses yield potentially unique information for forensic investigations, complementing other approaches by adding a "stable isotope signature" to compounds or materials that are identified as identical by other methods. Key applications of the stable isotope ratios that include the sample matching, sample processing information, and the source location identification. Several samples of the material of interest (e.g., counterfeit money, Illicit Drugs, and toxins) can be obtained by investigators with the intent of identifying groups that are related or the sources of the material. Biological samples obtained from the same location and time will have experienced the same environmental conditions, they will therefore have similar stable isotope ratios [5]. Chemical processing of the materials can also be result in the distinctive stable isotope ratios and the impurities which are left behind during the production of derived products. Because of this, samples may readily be grouped based on their stable isotope ratio signatures.

In addition to matching samples, forensic scientist can compare individual sample to databases of stable isotope ratio information obtained from authentic samples. In this case, a sample of an unknown origin that could be assigned to a probable source location by comparison with an authentic stable isotope ratio database and or a previously made assignment of origin. It could be corroborated by the database comparison. By using first principle models and by utilizing of the stable isotope fractionation in organisms and the spatial modelling capacity of the Geographic Information Systems, it is possible to create spatial maps of the predicted stable isotope ratios. Comparing a sample stable isotope ratio to the map predictions can help identify potential source locations. These innovative applications of stable isotope ratios in forensic work will continue to evolve in the future as databases and for understanding of stable isotope ratios expand [6].

Three primary classes of information can be provided for seized samples based on stable isotope ratio data Samples can be matched either to other samples seized or to samples previously obtained and recorded in a database as shown in Figure 6.2. If the database is sufficiently extensive or if another modelling has been completed (see text), then two additional classes of questions can be addressed: What are the expected stable isotope ratios of samples from a given location and given a sample stable isotope ratio, from where that sample might have originated.

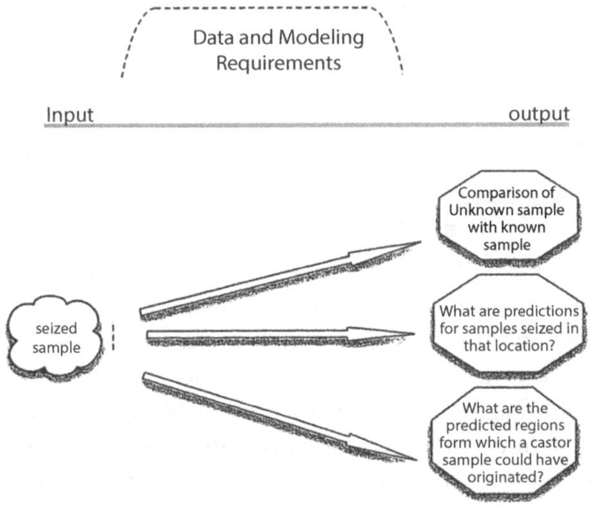

Figure 6.2 Stable isotope ratio analysis of forensic samples [1].

6.1.3 Stable Isotope Abundances in Forensic Evidence

In the process of creating various products, natural isotope fractionation occurs, which leads to a broad range of stable isotope ratio values. In forensic cases, three types of biological samples may be examined: human hair, drugs, and food. These materials often display a wide range of values, providing an opportunity to detect differences in stable isotope ratios between samples. For instance, depending on an individual's diet, carbon isotope ratios in human hair can vary from 10% to 25%. On the other hand, carbon isotopes in food can range from 30% to 10%, depending on the plant's photosynthetic pathway [7]. However, if plants are grown indoors with a carbon dioxide supply (such as indoor-grown tomatoes), the carbon isotope ratios can be as low as 50%. In drugs, biologically derived drugs often have carbon isotope ratio values that overlap with the carbon isotope values of foods, but when synthetic drugs are included, the range of values can be much greater and is dependent on the starting materials that are used for the synthesis. Stable isotope analyses can provide valuable information for identifying forensic, biological, and commercial samples. Variations in stable isotope ratios allow for further characterization of a sample or group of samples. The issue of within-sample heterogeneity is a concern, as it can make it difficult to differentiate between samples with similar ratios. In general, the precision of a single measurement from a mass spectrometer is more reliable than that of the entire sample due to heterogeneity. Biological samples are often more heterogeneous than synthetic samples due to variations in the composition of different tissues. It is important to understand the expected heterogeneity in a set of samples before interpreting any stable isotope ratio data.

6.2 Mass Spectroscopy Principle Instrumentation

6.2.1 Mass Spectrometry

Mass spectrometry (MS) is a highly effective analytical technique used to measure known materials, discover unknown compounds within a sample, and understand the structure and chemical properties of various molecules. The process involves transforming the sample into gaseous ions, with or without fragmentation, which are then analyzed based on their mass-to-charge ratio (m/z) and relative abundances. This technique is dependent on chemical reactions that occur in the Gas Phase.

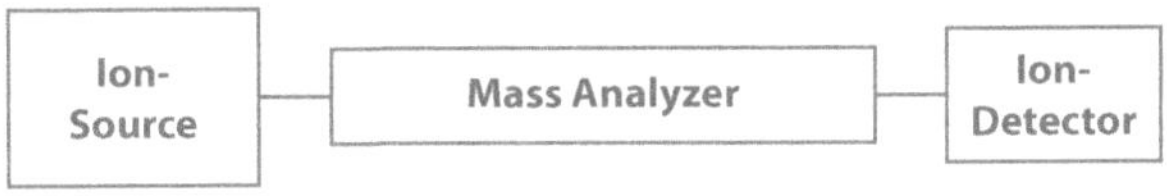

Figure 6.3 Mechanism of working of mass spectroscopy [3].

6.2.2 Principle

A mass spectrometer is a tool that creates various ions from a sample being studied. It then separates them based on their mass-to-charge ratio (m/z) and records the abundance of each ion type. The three main parts of a mass spectrometer are the ion source, which produces gaseous ions from the substance that is being studied; and the mass analyzer, which separates the ions into their individual mass components based upon their m/z i.e. Charge to Mass ratio; and the detector system, which detects the ions and then records the abundance of each resolved ionic species as shown in Figure 6.3. The detector system includes a conversion dynode with a secondary electron multiplier and a multichannel plate.

6.2.3 Instrumentation

An isotope ratio mass spectrometry (IRMS) system includes a sample introduction setup like elemental analyzers (EA-IRMS), gas chromatographs (GC-IRMS), and liquid chromatographs (LC-RMS), along with an electron ionization source, a magnetic sector analyzer, a Faraday-collector detector array, and a computer-controlled data acquisition system, shown in Figure 6.4. These tools need high sensitivity to detect small mass differences and rare isotopes. Typically, they use a single magnet to guide ions toward a set of Faraday collector detectors, which capture the ions and convert their energy into electric current.

6.3 Ion Source

The ion source is a crucial element in mass spectrometry as it initiates the process of ionization. During ionization, the sample is subjected to a high-energy source, which causes the conversion of neutral atoms or molecules into charged ions. This step is essential because it makes the compounds in the sample detectable and measurable by the mass spectrometer (Figure 6.4) [8].

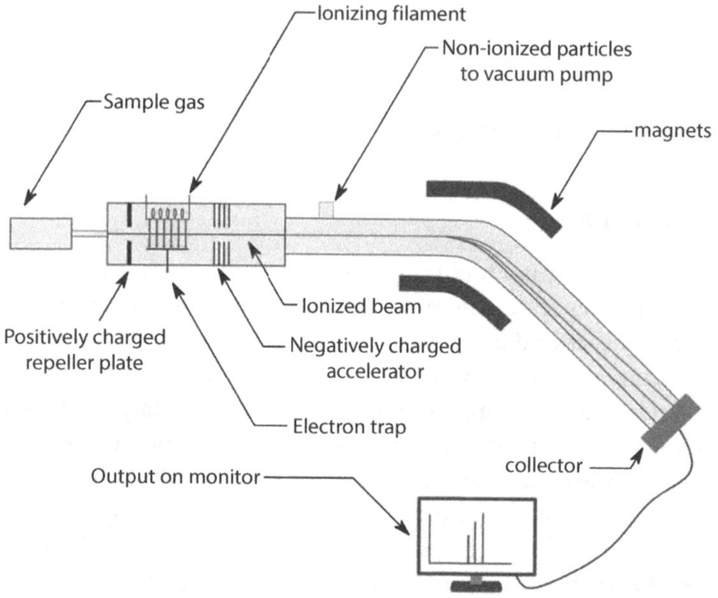

Figure 6.4 Isotope ratio mass spectrometry: Instrumentation. *Credit: Adobe Stock.*

6.3.1 Electron Impact (EI)

In the Electron Impact ionization technique, the sample is bombarded with high-energy electrons, which knock out electrons from the sample's molecules, resulting in the formation of positively charged ions. EI is commonly used for analyzing volatile organic compounds and small molecules. EI is widely used for relatively volatile samples that are insensitive to heat and relatively low molecular weight. Usually, electrons with energies of 70 eV are used. The spectra usually contain many fragmentation peaks and are useful for structural characterization and identification [9].

6.3.2 Electrospray Ionization (ESI)

ESI is commonly used for biomolecules, such as proteins and peptides. In this technique, the sample is dissolved in a liquid and sprayed through a fine needle under high voltage. As the solvent evaporates, the charged droplets convert the molecules into ions, which are then introduced into the mass spectrometer. a solution is nebulized under atmospheric pressure and exposed to a high electrical field (3-5 kV), which creates a charge on the surface of the sample droplets. Droplets that are rapidly become smaller through the solvent vaporization and produce molecular ions. ESI is extremely useful for accurate mass measurement, and by producing multiple charged ions to high molecular mass substances [10].

6.3.3 Matrix-Assisted Laser Desorption/Ionization (MALDI)

MALDI is often used for large biomolecules, such as proteins and nucleic acids. The amount of sample needed is very low (moles or less) MALDI is a great choice when it comes to coupling it with Time-of-flight (TOF) mass analyzers. Lately, MALDI is also coupled to the Orbitrap analyzers with applications (among others) on MS imaging. A very important novel route is seen in the application of MALDI in the analysis of bacteria and microorganisms providing superior performance compared to the conventional methods [11].

6.3.4 Chemical Ionization

CI is applied to similar samples, and analytes and is used to enhance the abundance of the molecular ion that permits calculation of the molecular mass of a compound. The process of ionization starts with the ionization of the reagent gas through electron impact [12]. This reaction then results in the creation of analyte ions through the interaction with the analyte molecules. CI is a lower-energy option compared to EI, which generates simpler mass spectra with less fragmentation. These ionization techniques are widely applied to gas chromatography separation techniques coupled to mass spectrometry (GC–MS) [13].

6.4 Mass Analyzer

The mass analyzer is responsible for separating ions based on their mass-to-charge ratio (m/z). Different types of mass analyzers are employed in mass spectrometers, depending on the specific application and analytical requirements.

6.4.1 Quadrupole Mass Analyzer

The quadrupole mass analyzer utilizes a combination of radiofrequency (RF) and direct current (DC) voltages to filter ions based on their m/z values. By varying these voltages, specific ions can be allowed to pass through the quadrupole mass filter, while others are excluded. This technique is widely used for quantitative analysis and selective ion monitoring [14].

6.4.2 Time-of-Flight (TOF) Mass Analyzer

In the TOF mass analyzer, ions are accelerated through an electric field, and the time taken for ions of different masses to reach the detector is measured. Lighter ions travel faster, while heavier ions take longer, allowing for their separation based on their m/z values. TOF analyzers are known for their high sensitivity and accurate mass determination [15].

6.4.3 Magnetic Sector Mass Analyzer

This type of mass analyzer uses a magnetic field to bend ions based on their m/z values. The degree of deflection depends on the mass and charge of the ions, allowing for their separation and subsequent detection. Magnetic sector analyzers are renowned for their high resolution and precision [16].

6.5 Detector

The detector is a critical component that receives the separated ions from the mass analyzer and converts them into measurable signals. These signals are then processed to construct mass spectra, which represent the abundance of ions at different m/z values.

6.5.1 Electron Multiplier Detector

The electron multiplier is a common type of detector used in mass spectrometry. It works by amplifying the electrical signals generated by the ions, enhancing the sensitivity of the mass spectrometer [17].

6.5.2 Time-to-Digital Converter (TDC) Detector

TDC detectors are often used in time-of-flight mass spectrometers. They measure the time taken by ions to reach the detector, which corresponds to their m/z values. This information is then converted into digital signals for further analysis [18].

6.5.3 Channeltron Detector

Channeltron detectors are known for their high dynamic range and sensitivity. They operate by converting the kinetic energy of ions into electrons, which are then multiplied and detected [17].

6.5.4 High Mass Detection Detectors

There has been a significant increase in interest in the detection of ions that have high mass. The definition of high mass depends on one's perspective that for those engaged in residual gas analysis, a high mass of ion might be anything more than 200Da. While LC/MS and biomedical applications require the detection of ions from tens and even hundreds of thousands of Daltons and GC/MS applications may require the detection of ions from 700-2000 Daltons. The detection efficiency decreases nearly exponentially with increasing mass of ions and becomes negligible to solve this problem several approaches have been developed, including the use of higher impact energies and high energy conversion dynode [19].

6.6 Applications of Mass Spectrometry in Forensics

Mass spectrometry (MS) is a powerful analytical technique widely used in various fields, including forensic science. It helps to identify and quantify molecules based on their mass-to-charge ratio, providing valuable information about the chemical composition of a sample. In the context of forensics, mass spectrometry has several applications, some of which are listed below.

6.6.1 Toxicology

MS plays a crucial role in toxicology testing by identifying and quantifying drugs, poisons, and other toxic compounds in biological samples (blood, urine, hair, etc.). This is particularly important in cases of drug overdose, poisoning, or driving under the influence. Initial drug screening is performed using mass spectrometry in biological samples like urine, blood, or hair, to identify the presence of drugs and their metabolites [20]. It can identify a wide range of drugs, including illicit substances, pharmaceuticals, and new psychoactive substances (NPS). Mass spectrometry is used in forensic autopsy investigations to analyze postmortem samples to determine the cause of death and identify any toxic substances that may have contributed to it. Mass spectrometry enables the precise quantification of toxic substances in biological samples, which is critical in cases of drug overdose, driving under the influence (DUI), or workplace drug testing. Mass spectrometry is essential in identifying and monitoring new designer drugs and NPS [21]. MS can be used to analyze environmental samples such as water, soil, and air, to detect and quantify pollutants, pesticides, and other toxic chemicals, helping to investigate cases of environmental contamination and exposure. Hair analysis using mass spectrometry can provide a historical record of drug use or toxic exposure over an extended period. Mass spectrometry can detect volatile substances like alcohol and volatile organic compounds (VOCs) in breath, blood, or other biological samples, which is important in DUI investigations and exposure to harmful vapors. MS is used to identify and quantify various poisons and toxins, including heavy metals, pesticides, and naturally occurring toxins in food or biological samples. Mass spectrometry is employed in forensic intelligence and profiling to understand drug trends, patterns of drug use, and trafficking routes based on the analysis of seized drug samples. MS can assist in the interpretation of postmortem redistribution, a phenomenon where drug concentrations may change in the body after death, providing insight into the actual drug exposure during an individual's life [22].

6.6.2 Explosives

MS can detect and analyze trace amounts of explosive residues, such as in post-blast investigations. It can also help analyze gunshot residues in forensic ballistics cases. Mass spectrometry (MS) is a crucial analytical technique for the forensic analysis of explosives. It helps identify and characterize explosive materials, residues, and related compounds. Some of the key forensic applications of mass spectrometry for explosives: Mass spectrometry is used to analyze samples collected from crime scenes, post-blast debris, or suspected explosive devices to detect and identify explosive residues. It can identify trace amounts of explosive compounds left behind after detonation, aiding in determining the type of explosive used [23]. MS is employed in the examination of explosive devices to identify their components, including explosive materials, stabilizers, and additives. This information is vital in understanding the device's construction and potential sources of the materials used. Mass spectrometry-based explosive trace detectors are used at security checkpoints, airports, and other critical locations to detect and identify minute amounts of explosives on surfaces, clothing, or belongings. Mass spectrometry can identify and quantify precursor chemicals used in the manufacturing of explosives, helping law enforcement agencies track the supply chain and sources of explosive materials. After an explosion, mass spectrometry can be used to analyze environmental samples, such as soil, air, and water, to identify and quantify explosive residues [24]. This information aids investigators in understanding the extent of the explosion and reconstructing the event. MS helps in characterizing homemade explosives, which are often composed of readily available or improvised materials. The analysis can reveal the specific composition and possible synthesis methods used. Some explosives are formulated with unique chemical markers known as taggants. Mass spectrometry can detect and identify these taggants, assisting in tracing the origin and manufacturer of the explosives. Mass spectrometry is used to prepare training aids for explosive detection canines by analyzing and identifying the odors associated with different explosive materials. In the aftermath of an explosion, mass spectrometry can be employed to analyze biological samples from victims to detect and identify explosive residues that may have been transferred during the blast. Mass spectrometry is also used in forensic intelligence to analyze and compare explosive residues from different crime scenes, helping investigators link multiple incidents to potential suspects or terrorist organizations [25].

6.6.3 Environmental Forensics

Environmental forensics is an exciting field that utilizes scientific techniques and methods to investigate environmental contamination, identify pollution sources, and assess the extent of environmental damage. With the integration of various scientific disciplines and forensic techniques, environmental forensics offers numerous applications and benefits. Some of the key aspects and applications of environmental forensics include contaminant source identification, historical pollution assessment, fingerprinting techniques, contaminant transport, and fate studies, legal and regulatory support, oil spill investigations, air quality and atmospheric contaminants, waste site remediation, wildlife contamination studies, and ecological risk assessment [26]. By utilizing these techniques, experts can trace pollutants back to their origins, evaluate the effectiveness of remediation efforts, assess potential risks to human health and ecosystems, and provide scientific evidence to support environmental lawsuits and remediation efforts [27]. MS can be used to identify pollutants, contaminants, and toxins in environmental samples, helping to trace their sources and assess their impact on ecosystems and human health.

6.6.4 DNA Sequencing and Proteomics

MS is used in conjunction with other techniques for DNA sequencing and proteomics, which can provide important information in criminal investigations and the identification of human remains. DNA sequencing and proteomics, combined with mass spectrometry, have significant forensic applications, providing valuable information for the identification and characterization of biological evidence in criminal investigations. Mass spectrometry is employed in DNA sequencing to detect and analyze short tandem repeat (STR) markers, which are specific regions of the DNA that vary between individuals [28]. This information is used for DNA profiling, commonly known as DNA fingerprinting, to establish the identity of individuals in criminal cases. In cases where human remains are found, mass spectrometry-based DNA sequencing is used for identifying individuals by comparing their DNA with samples from missing persons or relatives. Mass spectrometry is utilized to generate genetic profiles that can be uploaded to public DNA databases to identify potential relatives of unknown suspects, helping to generate leads in cold cases [29]. DNA sequencing in mass spectrometry is applied to identify the origin of body fluids found at crime scenes, such as blood, semen, or saliva, providing critical information about the events that occurred. Mass spectrometry can detect the presence of biological contaminants, such as bacterial or fungal DNA, in forensic samples, ensuring the accuracy and reliability of DNA analysis. Mass spectrometry-based proteomics can identify characteristic proteins found in various body fluids, aiding in the identification of specific fluids at crime scenes. Proteomic analysis using mass spectrometry can identify proteins from traces of biological stains (e.g., bloodstains) to determine their origin and support crime scene reconstruction [29]. Proteomics allows for the profiling of biological evidence collected at crime scenes, helping forensic experts understand the biological composition of the samples. In forensic autopsies, mass spectrometry-based proteomics can be employed to analyze proteins in post-mortem samples, providing insights into the cause of death or the presence of toxins or drugs. Mass spectrometry-based proteomics can be used to estimate the age of individuals based on changes in protein profiles found in various tissues and body fluids. Proteomics can complement DNA profiling in cases where DNA is degraded or not available, providing an additional means of identification. The integration of DNA sequencing and proteomics with mass spectrometry in forensic applications has significantly improved the capabilities of forensic laboratories, providing more comprehensive and accurate analyses of biological evidence [30]. These techniques play a vital role in identifying suspects, establishing victim identities, and contributing to the resolution of criminal cases.

6.6.5 Forensic Geochemistry

MS can be utilized to analyze soil, minerals, and geological samples to link crime scene evidence to specific geographic locations. Forensic geochemistry, combined with mass spectrometry, is a specialized field that applies analytical techniques to investigate geological materials and trace evidence in criminal investigations. Mass spectrometry plays a crucial role in analyzing and identifying elements, isotopes, and compounds in geological samples. Spectrometry is used to analyze trace elements and isotopes in geological samples found at crime scenes, such as soil, minerals, rocks, and trace metals [31]. By comparing these signatures with reference samples from potential sources, forensic experts can determine the geographical origin of the materials and link them to suspects or crime scenes. Mass spectrometry is employed to analyze the chemical composition of minerals and gemstones, aiding in the identification of valuable and rare specimens, and detecting forgeries or fake gemstones. Mass spectrometry is utilized in forensic seismology to analyze seismic signals from explosions or earthquakes, providing information about their sources, such as underground nuclear tests or industrial blasts [31]. cases of natural disasters or geological events, mass spectrometry can be used to analyze samples from the disaster site to understand the geology and assess the impacts. Mass spectrometry-based geochemical profiling can be used to create databases of geological materials from different regions, aiding in crime scene investigations and providing valuable information for criminal intelligence.

6.6.6 Forensic Chemistry

Mass spectrometry can be used to analyze pigments, dyes, and other materials used in art and artifacts to determine authenticity or detect forgeries.

Mass spectrometry can identify the chemical composition of pigments used in paintings, sculptures, and other artworks. This allows experts to match them with known historical pigments or identify modern pigments that may not be consistent with the supposed age of the artwork. For textiles and ancient artifacts, mass spectrometry helps identify dyes and dyeing techniques used in their creation. It can differentiate between natural and synthetic dyes, aiding in the dating and authentication of the artifacts [32]. Mass spectrometry can analyze the binding media used in artworks, such as oils, resins, and glues. This information is critical in understanding the painting's technique and potential restoration efforts. By comparing the elemental and isotopic compositions of the materials with those of known ancient objects, mass spectrometry can analyze the materials used in ancient artifacts to determine their age and authenticity. This information helps experts establish the object's provenance and genuineness [33]. Mass spectrometry can identify modern materials or contaminants present in artworks, which may indicate forgery or restoration attempts. Mass spectrometry can identify the composition of varnishes and coatings applied to artworks. This analysis helps establish the artwork's condition and the possible use of historical or modern varnishes. Mass spectrometry is applied in provenance studies, where the materials used in artworks are compared to known geological or historical sources to trace their origins and cultural context [34]. Mass spectrometry assists in assessing the compatibility of conservation materials with the original components of an artwork, ensuring the preservation of its integrity.

6.7 Isotope Ratio Mass Spectrometry Principle and Instrumentation

6.7.1 Isotope Ratio Mass Spectrometry (IRMS)

IRMS is a technique used to measure the isotopic composition of elements in a sample. Isotopes are the atoms of same element that have different numbers of neutrons in their nucleus [35]. The technique known as isotope ratio mass spectrometry (IRMS) is highly accurate when it comes to measuring small differences in isotope abundances. This includes isotopes such as 2 H/1 H, 13C/12C, 15N/14N, and 18O/16O. Samples are turned into gases like H2, CO2, N2, and CO depending on their chemical composition. This is achieved through interaction with the electron beam in the ion source. The ions are then focused and accelerated with high voltage before passing through a magnetic field [36]. The Faraday cups detect the ions, and multiple collectors are used to measure several ion ratios at once. Each cup is connected to its own amplifier with a different gain, and the signals are recorded by the IRMS data system to produce a chromatogram for ions of a given m/z. Additionally, cups can also be used to determine the isotopic ratios of sulphur and chlorine. IRMS is used to measure the relative abundance of stable isotopes in a material, A measure of isotopic differences, called "delta" (δ) notation, is used to present stable isotope ratios of the materials for example, carbon-12, carbon-13, and carbon-14 are three isotopes of the element carbon. The ratio of the isotopes in a sample can provide information about the origin and history of the sample. It's fascinating to think about how the isotopic profile of materials can provide valuable information about their origin. That's why measuring small differences in isotope abundances using techniques like isotope ratio mass spectrometry (IRMS) is such an important tool [37]. IRMS has a wide range of applications in fields like forensic sciences, food authenticity and traceability, archaeology/geochemistry, and biological sciences. By analyzing the isotopic ratios of different elements, we can learn so much about the world around us [38].

IRMS is used in many different fields, including geology, environmental science, biology, and forensic science, to name a few. It can provide valuable information about the history and origins of a sample, such as its age, location, and the conditions under which it formed.

6.7.2 Principle

The ions pass through a magnetic field prior detected by the Faraday cups. The accelerating voltage and the strength of the magnetic field determine the trajectory of the ions and eventually which ions will finally reach the detector [38]. Multiple collectors are used for the simultaneous measurement of the intensity of several ion ratios. Each cup is connected to its own amplifier with a different gain and the signals are recorded by the IRMS data system to produce a chromatogram for ions of a given m/z. IRMS works by ionizing the sample and separating the isotopes based on their mass-to-charge ratio (m/z) using a mass spectrometer [39]. The separated isotopes are then detected and quantified. The principles behind IRMS are since isotopes of the same element have slightly different masses, which causes them to behave differently in a mass spectrometer. The ratio of the isotopes is determined by comparing the intensities of their mass peaks in the mass spectrum [40].

6.7.3 Instrumentation

The isotopic profile of different materials can offer valuable insights into their origin. One of the most widely used types of IRMS instruments is the Elemental Analyzer IRMS (EA-IRMS), which has a broad range of applications across various fields like forensic sciences, food authenticity and traceability, archaeology/geochemistry, and biological sciences. The EA-IRMS can be used to analyze both solid and liquid samples by introducing them through tin capsules and an auto-sampler, respectively [41]. The analysis process includes combustion or thermal conversion of the sample, the introduction of gases to the ion source of the IRMS, ionization, separation, and final detection. Another precise method of measuring isotope ratios is the dual inlet IRMS, which uses gas samples. The Gas Bench configuration offers a universal online gas preparation and introduction system for IRMS, allowing for the determination of headspace samples, including water equilibration, carbonates, and moreish requires a specialized mass spectrometer that is capable of separating isotopes with very similar masses Figure 6.5 [42]. The sample is typically introduced into the mass spectrometer as a gas but can also be introduced as a solid or liquid using various sample preparation techniques. The accuracy and precision of IRMS measurements are critical and are dependent on factors such as the quality of the sample, the stability of the instrument, and the calibration standards used [20].

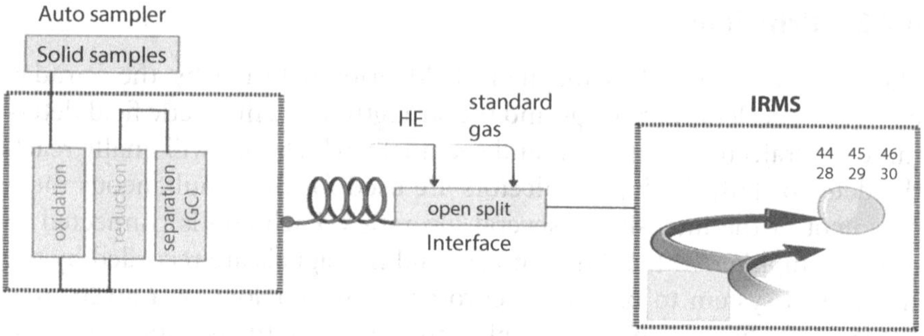

Figure 6.5 Isotope ratio mass spectrometry: Instrumentations [4].

6.7.4 Ion Source

This component ionizes the sample and produces ions for analysis. There are different types of ion sources used in IRMS, such as electron impact ionization (EI), chemical ionization (CI), and field ionization (FI). IRMS, the ion source is selected based on the nature of the sample and the required sensitivity and precision for isotopic analysis [43]. The goal is to ionize the sample efficiently while minimizing fragmentation and isotope fractionation. Isotope fractionation can occur during ionization, leading to isotopic ratios that differ from the original sample's true ratios. For precise and accurate isotopic measurements, modern IRMS instruments commonly use techniques like Continuous Flow Isotope Ratio Mass Spectrometry (CF-IRMS) or Dual Inlet Isotope Ratio Mass Spectrometry (DI-IRMS). CF-IRMS is used for continuous analysis of liquids and gases, while DI-IRMS is used for discrete analysis of solid samples [44]. The selection of the appropriate ion source and isotopic measurement technique is essential in IRMS, as it directly impacts the quality and accuracy of isotopic data obtained from the samples.

6.7.5 Types of Ion Sources in IRMS

6.7.5.1 Electron Impact Ionization (EI)

Electron Impact Ionization (EI) is an ionization method used in mass spectrometry, including traditional mass spectrometers, but it is less commonly used in modern Isotope Ratio Mass Spectrometry (IRMS) instruments. In EI, the sample is bombarded with high-energy electrons, typically generated from a heated filament. These high-energy electrons collide with the sample molecules, causing the ejection of one or more electrons from the molecules, resulting in the formation of positively charged ions (cations) [43]. These ions are then accelerated and focused into the mass analyzer of the mass spectrometer. EI is known for its ability to produce intense ion signals and relatively simple mass spectra. It is particularly useful for the analysis of volatile and thermally stable organic compounds, making it well-suited for various applications in conventional mass spectrometry. However, in the context of Isotope Ratio Mass Spectrometry (IRMS), EI is less favored due to certain limitations. One of the main concerns is that the high-energy electron impact can lead to significant fragmentation of the sample molecules. This fragmentation can cause isotope fractionation, which alters the isotopic ratios of the sample from their true values [45]. In IRMS, accuracy and precision in isotopic measurements are of paramount importance, making it necessary to minimize any sources of fractionation. As a result, modern IRMS instruments typically utilize other ionization techniques, such as Chemical Ionization (CI) or Gas Chromatography-Combustion-Isotope Ratio Mass Spectrometry (GC-C-IRMS), which are better suited for analyzing stable isotopes with minimal fragmentation and isotope fractionation. While EI remains a valuable ionization method in conventional mass spectrometry for various applications, its limited use in modern IRMS instruments is primarily due to the need for precise and accurate isotopic measurements with minimal interference from fragmentation and fractionation effects [46].

6.7.5.2 Chemical Ionization (CI)

Chemical Ionization (CI) is a method used in mass spectrometry, including Isotope Ratio Mass Spectrometry (IRMS). In CI, the sample is ionized through reactions with reagent gas ions, typically generated from a reagent gas such as methane or ammonia. The process of CI involves introducing the sample into the ion source of the mass spectrometer, where it coexists with the reagent gas. The reagent gas is usually ionized by an electron impact, creating reagent gas ions (e.g., methane ions, CH_4^+) [47]. These reagent gas ions then react with the sample molecules, leading to the formation of ions (cations or anions) through a series of chemical reactions. There are several advantages to using Chemical Ionization in Isotope Ratio Mass Spectrometry. Firstly, it leads to less fragmentation of sample molecules compared to Electron Impact Ionization (EI). This is especially beneficial when analyzing stable isotopes in complex samples, as it helps preserve the original molecular structure and reduces isotope fractionation [48]. Secondly, CI tends to generate molecular ions or adduct ions, simplifying the mass spectrum and making it easier to identify and quantify specific isotopic peaks. Thirdly, CI is considered a "soft" ionization technique, imparting less energy to the sample molecules during ionization, which reduces the chances of breaking chemical bonds within the sample.

6.7.5.3 *Field Ionization (FI)*

Field Ionization (FI) is an incredibly crucial ionization method used in mass spectrometry, particularly in Isotope Ratio Mass Spectrometry (IRMS). The process involves applying a high electric field to the sample, which exerts a force on the sample molecules, resulting in the formation of positively charged ions (cations) that are then analyzed. The advantages of Field Ionization in IRMS are impressive, especially its soft ionization technique, which maintains the molecular structure of the sample and reduces isotope fractionation [49]. Its high sensitivity and capacity to analyze small molecules and low molecular weight compounds are also noteworthy. Furthermore, it's astounding that Field Ionization can efficiently ionize and quantify rare stable isotopes, even when present in trace amounts. It's evident that Field Ionization is a potent ionization method that is ideal for high-sensitivity and high-precision Isotope Ratio Mass Spectrometry applications [50].

6.7.6 Mass Analyzer

Isotope Ratio Mass Spectrometry (IRMS) relies on a crucial component known as the mass analyzer, which separates ions based on their mass-to-charge ratio (m/z). The most widely used type of mass analyzer in IRMS is the magnetic sector analyzer. It works by deflecting ions using a strong magnetic field that is applied perpendicularly to their path [51]. As the ions travel through the magnetic field, the force they experience depends on their mass-to-charge ratio (m/z), which causes them to undergo circular motion with different radii. The detectors at the end of the analyzer measure the position of the ions and their corresponding m/z values, from which the isotopic ratios of the elements present in the sample can be calculated [39]. The magnetic sector analyzer is known for its high mass resolution and accuracy, making it an indispensable tool in a variety of fields, including geology, environmental science, archaeology, and forensic investigations.

6.7.7 Detector

In Isotope Ratio Mass Spectrometry (IRMS), the detector plays a crucial role in detecting the ions that pass through the mass analyzer and measuring their abundance. It is responsible for converting the ion signals into measurable quantities that are used to determine the isotopic ratios of the sample. The most used detector in IRMS is the Faraday cup. Once the ions are separated by the mass analyzer based on their mass-to-charge ratio (m/z), they enter the detector region, where they strike a metal plate in the Faraday cup. This transfer of charge creates an electric current, which is measured by an ammeter or electrometer [39]. The intensity of the current is directly proportional to the number of ions that struck the plate and represents the abundance of ions of a specific mass-to-charge ratio (m/z). This current measurement is related to the isotopic abundance of the corresponding isotope in the sample. The data recorded from the Faraday cup is processed to calculate the isotopic ratios of the sample, providing valuable information about its composition and origin. The Faraday cup detector is widely used in IRMS due to its high sensitivity and linearity, making it suitable for precise and accurate isotopic measurements. It is particularly useful for measuring the abundance of stable isotopes, such as carbon, nitrogen, oxygen, and sulphur [39].

6.7.8 Isotope Ratio Measurement System

The Isotope Ratio Measurement System (IRMS) is a critical component in Isotope Ratio Mass Spectrometry (IRMS) instruments. It calculates the isotopic ratios of the sample based on the data obtained from the detector. The IRMS system usually includes a computer and specialized software that process and analyzes the data generated by the mass spectrometer and detector [52]. The Faraday cup or other detectors detect the ions passing through the mass analyzer and measure the abundance of ions of specific mass-to-charge ratios (m/z) and convert them into electrical signals. These electrical signals are then turned into digital data, which is processed and converted into usable formats by the computer. The IRMS software analyzes the data and calculates the isotopic ratios of the sample by comparing the intensities or abundances of the isotopes present in the sample to a known standard or reference material [53]. Necessary corrections and calibrations are applied to the data to account for instrumental and sample-specific factors that may affect the accuracy and precision of the isotopic measurements. The calculated isotopic ratios are then presented in a readable format, such as a table or graph, allowing researchers to interpret and analyze the isotopic composition of the sample. The IRMS software often includes quality control features to assess the reliability and validity of the measurements, such as assessing precision, signal-to-noise ratio, and instrument stability [54].

6.7.9 Gas Handling System

The Gas Handling System is a crucial component in Isotope Ratio Mass Spectrometry (IRMS). Its main role is to prepare the sample for analysis and introduce it into the ion source [55]. Depending on the type of sample, different techniques are employed to convert it into a suitable form for analysis. For solid or liquid samples, a gas conversion system may be used, which converts the sample into a gaseous form. The Gas Handling System then carefully controls the flow rate and pressure of the sample gases to ensure stable ionization conditions and consistent ion production throughout the analysis [56]. Proper sample handling, isolation, and purification are also essential to minimize potential sources of contamination and ensure the highest quality data. In some cases, a carrier gas is used to aid in sample introduction and ionization, and purification units may be included to remove unwanted components or impurities from the sample before analysis [57].

6.8 Applications of Isotope Ratio Mass Spectroscopy in Forensics

The analysis of stable isotopes using IRMS has broad applications in various scientific disciplines. While a number of these disciplines utilize IRMS as a standard analytical technique, its application in other areas remains largely at an experimental stage. This section of the Chapter includes a summary of the applications of IRMS in various scientific fields, with the focus being on forensic applications and the analysis of illicit drugs, explosives, and ignitable liquids. This summary does not comprise an exhaustive list of all the research conducted in each of the scientific disciplines mentioned.

6.8.1 Environmental Forensic Applications

The use of IRMS can be extremely helpful in determining the origin of oil spills and other types of environmental contamination. Researchers conducted a thorough review of how CSIA can be used to analyze organic contaminants in the environment, while also discussing the identification and quantification of biodegradation processes and fractionation effects on a range of environmental samples [58]. Some researchers discussed the analysis of samples commonly found as contaminants in the environment, such as MTBE in petrol and TCE. The isotopic composition of these samples and their environmental effects were also evaluated. Research performed on the analysis of carbon and chlorine isotopes in chlorinated organic compounds in groundwater and the effect of various environmental processes on the isotopic composition of the samples was also evaluated. The Ignitable Liquid Applications section of this Chapter contains a summary of the application of IRMS for the analysis of petroleum products, which are common environmental contaminants [59]. IRMS is typically used to study manmade pollutants, which have a different isotope profile than natural sources of the same substance. Overall, a variety of analytical techniques are often necessary in environmental forensics to determine the origin of pollutants, and IRMS is a valuable tool in this process [60].

6.8.2 Wildlife Forensic Applications

IRMS has been a valuable tool for studying the migratory behavior of various animals such as the North American Monarch butterfly, Bowhead (baleen) whales, and birds. Additionally, it has been used to analyze the stable isotopic compositions in elephant bone tissue and ivory to determine whether elephant populations in Africa can be discriminated against [61]. Moreover, several studies have been conducted on the characterization of animal products using isotope ratio mass spectrometry according to geographic origin and feeding diet. In forensic science applications, the Forensic Isotope Ratio Mass Spectrometry (FIRMS) Network has been formed to raise awareness of the potential for IRMS in forensic science and to encourage collaboration between various scientific disciplines. The Network has also aimed to develop and validate methods for the analysis of trace elements and isotopes in forensic samples, including float glass, bullets, hair and nails, steel, tape, marble, and methylenedioxymethamphetamine (MDMA) [62]. Research showed the carbon and nitrogen isotope ratio values in paint and varnish samples using an EA/IRMS. Moreover, IRMS has been used to analyze samples relating to the investigation of terrorism offenses. The analysis of stable isotopes in bone and teeth has also assisted in the determination of the recent location of a person, i.e., geolocation. Some Researchers reported that stable isotope ratio data may be useful when trying to determine the origin of microbial cultures, and it should thus be possible to deduce information about the growth environment from samples of suspect pathogen culture [63].

6.8.3 Illicit Drug Applications

There have been several publications addressing the analysis of stable isotopes in illicit drugs to differentiate products and constituents from different geographical regions and different products from different manufacturing batches and processes. It has been demonstrated that illicit narcotics have stable isotope ratio values that characterize the region from whence a drug sample originated. An "isotopic fingerprint" has been found in marijuana, heroin, and cocaine, which is often a mixture of carbon and nitrogen isotope ratio values [64]. Previous research was hampered by a small number of genuine exhibits, but it demonstrated the comparative relevance of isotopic analysis in comparing different heroin samples. The carbon and nitrogen isotope ratios of heroin from the world's major poppy-growing regions aggregated into four separate groups, enabling the identification of the region of origin of different heroin exhibits, according to research. It should be remembered, however, that heroin is a manufactured chemical, as is cocaine. Hoping as it is the result of the acetylation of morphine with acetic anhydride. As a result, any isotopic fingerprint in morphine (biological product), which contributes 17 of the 21 carbon atoms and all the nitrogen atoms in heroin is recorded [65]. The carbon isotope ratios of acetic anhydride will vary depending on the carbon source utilized to manufacture the molecule (for example, fossil fuel, biogenic, and syngas sources) and illustrate the carbon isotope ratios of various DEA exhibits collected in one location of the world. Take note of the similarities in values between the various exhibitions. The stable isotope ratio information was significant in this case for further defining the acetic anhydride and allowing scientists to link multiple exhibits to identify a common source. Major coca-growing areas. Stable isotope analyses are now a major measurement in the United States Drug Enforcement Administration's Cocaine Signature Program, providing critical information regarding the provenance of confiscated samples [66]. According to a 2013 National Survey on Drug Use and Health report, around 24.6 million Americans aged 12 or older admitted to using illicit drugs in the previous year. One technique that has emerged as a potential tool for forensic purposes is isotope ratio mass spectrometry (IRMS), which can help infer the cultivation location of drugs of plant origin, establish trafficking routes, and determine the synthetic pathways and chemical lots used in clandestine laboratories. *Cannabis sativa* L., also known as marijuana or cannabis, is the most used plant-derived illicit drug in the US and across the world. With the legalization of medical and recreational marijuana in some US states, its use has increased significantly. IRMS has been mostly applied to infer cannabis source and distribution networks. Carbon and nitrogen stable isotopes are the most well-explored isotopes for the origin determination and growth conditions assessment of Cannabis seized in different countries. Cocaine's production and trafficking routes around the world are also of particular interest to law enforcement agencies, and SIA appears to be well-suited to the task because seized cocaine samples closely reflect the growth environment of coca plants. IRMS has also been used in combination with other profiling techniques to classify car fentanyl seizures [67].

6.8.4 Forensic Applications of Archaeology and Anthropology

Forensic archaeology and anthropology make use of stable isotopes to gain valuable insights into the diets, geographic origins, and migrations of individuals in the past. By studying the isotopic composition of human remains, researchers can reconstruct the dietary patterns of ancient populations and differentiate between various dietary preferences, such as marine and terrestrial diets or different types of plant-based diets [68]. Forensic archaeology and anthropology have found stable isotopes to be incredibly useful in gaining insights into the diets, geographic origins, and migrations of individuals from the past. By studying the isotopic composition of human remains, researchers can reconstruct the dietary patterns of ancient populations and differentiate between various dietary preferences, such as marine and terrestrial diets or different types of plant-based diets. When it comes to forensic archaeology, teeth, bones, and hair are essential sources of information. Analyzing the carbon and nitrogen isotope ratios in bone collagen allows investigators to create long-term records of dietary habits. This enables them to reconstruct the dietary histories of both recent and prehistoric individuals. In forensic anthropology, teeth are particularly valuable because they preserve trace elements such as lead, strontium, and carbonates, each with unique isotope variations. These elements provide information about the geographic origins or movements of individuals. Human hair and fingernails also play a significant role in forensic studies. Stable isotope ratios in hair and fingernails can be used to differentiate individuals with different geographic origins. Despite the trend towards globalized diets, distinct dietary preferences in different countries lead to differences in the isotope ratios of human hair and fingernails, allowing researchers to determine geographic origins. The isotopic composition of an organism reflects the food and water it consumes. Different plants have varying carbon isotope ratios, which lead to diverse dietary inputs. The dietary sources are stored in an organism's tissues like muscles, bones, teeth, and hair, creating a record of its diet. Carbon and nitrogen isotope analyses of collagen in bone offer insights into the dietary histories of both ancient and modern humans over several years. Stable isotope analyses have been used to study diet changes in various historical populations. The heavier element strontium shows geographic variation related to soil differences in regions and countries. Plants absorb strontium, which then enters the food chain and becomes incorporated into human diets. Strontium signals help trace the geographic origins or movements of individuals across different terrains, aiding in distinguishing migrants from locals in a population. Lead isotope ratios in human teeth have been used to differentiate individuals from different regions. Human hair and fingernails also record the dietary and water source information, providing geographic data for forensic studies. Stable isotopes provide valuable information about an individual's past diet and geographic origin, making them a valuable tool in forensic investigations [69]. Strontium signals reflect variations in soil composition across different regions and countries. The lead isotope composition in human teeth has also been used successfully to distinguish individuals from various parts of the world, including Eastern and Southern Europe, Australia, the Middle East, and Western Europe.

Human hair and fingernails also play a significant role in forensic studies. Stable isotope ratios in hair and fingernails can be used to differentiate individuals with different geographic origins, including citizens from different countries such as Europe, the United States, and Brazil. Despite the trend towards globalized diets, distinct dietary preferences in these countries lead to differences in the isotope ratios of human hair and fingernails, allowing researchers to determine geographic origins. The isotopic composition of an organism reflects the food and water it consumes [70]. Different plants have varying carbon isotope ratios, which lead to diverse dietary inputs. The dietary sources are stored in an organism's tissues like muscles, bones, teeth, and hair, creating a record of its diet. Hair can serve as a chronological record of an organism's diet, making it useful for studying traveling humans or migrating animals like elephants. Geographic variations in stable isotopes have been used to associate individuals with specific regions of the world. Hydrogen and oxygen isotope ratios in water form a geographic signal recorded in the organic matter of animals. Researchers can trace microbial spores using known variations in isotope ratios of water, which helps eliminate potential sources and guide investigations. Carbon and nitrogen isotope ratios of spores also provide insights into the nutrient media for microbial growth.

In humans, bones, hair, and teeth contain trace components like lead, strontium, and carbonates, each with isotope variations (C, O, Pb, Sr) that offer geographic and dietary information to forensic investigators. Carbon isotopes in teeth reveal dietary information from early life, reflecting the consumption of C3 and C4 plants. Oxygen isotopes in teeth reflect the oxygen of the drinking water, allowing researchers to study geographical variations. Carbon and nitrogen isotope analyses of collagen in bone offer insights into the dietary histories of both ancient and modern humans over several years. Collagen is preserved in bones, degrading slowly over time, making it suitable for dietary reconstructions. Stable isotope analyses have been used to study diet changes in various historical populations. The heavier element strontium shows geographic variation related to soil differences in regions and countries [71]. Plants absorb strontium, which then enters the food chain and becomes incorporated into human diets. Strontium signals help trace the geographic origins or movements of individuals across different terrains, aiding in distinguishing migrants from locals in a population. Lead isotope ratios in human teeth have been used to differentiate individuals from different regions. Human hair and fingernails also record the dietary and water source information, providing geographic data for forensic studies. Stable isotope ratios in hair can distinguish between individuals with different geographic origins, and recent studies have shown similar distinctions in fingernails. The stable isotope approach is valuable in forensic investigations and provides valuable information about an individual's past diet and geographic origin [72]. For instance, the case of the Ice Man discovered on the border between Austria and Italy was studied using stable isotopes to gain insights into his past.

6.8.5 Food Forensic Applications

When it comes to food authentication, the nitrogen isotope signature is often used to determine the organic authenticity of crops. However, there are several factors that can influence the nitrogen signature, including agricultural practices, atmospheric nitrogen deposition, and the plant's internal nitrogen balance. Therefore, $\delta 15N$ analysis alone may not be the most suitable parameter for organic authentication [73]. Instead, a combination of multiple isotopes, multivariate statistics, and other analytical techniques is preferred. IRMS with ICP-MS and IRMS with mid-infrared spectroscopy have both been successful in classifying organic vs. conventionally grown tomatoes. However, there are still limitations to IRMS in practical food applications, including the high costs of maintaining the instrument and the lack of an extensive reference database containing products from different diets, production conditions, locations, and seasons [74]. Despite these challenges, IRMS has demonstrated good discriminatory power between plants grown under different conditions.

6.8.6 Application of IRMS in Questioned Documents

Discrimination and source determination of documents are still major issues in forensic science. The process involves verifying documents, signatures, and dating, as well as analyzing threatening letters and other materials. The FBI's investigation of the Anthrax letters in 2001 brought attention to the analysis of paper products. However, little discrimination was found in that case [74]. In 2013, researchers found that 13C analysis could help distinguish the manufacturing source of document papers. They tested different brands of office papers from Australia and New Zealand and suggested a confidence interval to discriminate documents. Recently, they incorporated oxygen isotope values into their research, which showed the potential of IRMS to discriminate paper samples. A dual-isotope approach using carbon and oxygen was indicated as the next step to optimize and validate an operation protocol suitable for paper document casework analysis [75]. The combination of IRMS and XRF appeared to be even more effective at distinguishing between paper products. Regarding ink and toner analysis, Raman spectroscopy and Fourier transform infrared spectroscopy (FTIR) are the most frequent, reliable, and non-destructive methods to differentiate variations found in ballpoint pens. IRMS has only just begun to be explored for inks. Additional method development is still required before IRMS can be used in questioned-document casework [76].

6.8.7 Miscellaneous

Trace evidence studies involving clothing fibers, the implementation of IRMS is relatively understudied. However, isotope ratio analysis appears to be a promising method to determine the source of similar fibers when alternative analytical methods struggle to provide information beyond the polymer type and color of fibers. $\delta13C$, $\delta15N$, and $\delta18O$ values have been used to discriminate between valuable natural fibers and cheaper synthetic fibers used as a substitute for cashmere in the manufacturing process [77]. A pilot multi-element study using IRMS also showed differences in un-dyed spun cotton fabric fibers from different countries. However, a larger number of cotton fiber samples would be required to achieve more robust statistical results of within-region variability. To overcome this issue, hierarchical cluster analysis has been used to compare the isotopic compositions of cotton samples from different regions [78]. The δ2 H and δ18O values of cotton can also be used to identify counterfeit currency. Isotope ratio values of cable ties were significantly different between batches, and the δ2 H and δ13C values of cling wraps and resealable bags have been used to distinguish between samples. SIA of plastic wraps has also been demonstrated to contribute to the source elucidation of illicit materials [79].

6.9 Case Study

In 2016, a major scandal erupted in the UK when a well-known retailer confirmed that some of its own-brand 100% beef lasagna products contained horse meat. The incident prompted an investigation by the UK Food Standards Agency (FSA), which conducted a forensic analysis to determine the source of the horse meat and to identify whether it was intentionally added to the products. By collecting samples of 100% beef lasagna products from various retail outlets and subjecting them to IRMS analysis, the FSA was able to measure the ratio of carbon isotopes in the meat samples. The analysis revealed that the samples contained horse meat, which was likely to have originated from Romania. The carbon isotope ratios in the horse meat samples were consistent with those found in animals that had been raised in Romania, indicating that the horse meat had been intentionally added to the beef lasagna products and was not a result of accidental contamination. The FSA traced the source of the horse meat to a Romanian slaughterhouse, which had supplied beef to several European food processors that had then supplied it to various retailers. The investigation revealed that the horse meat had been fraudulently labeled as beef and added to the 100% beef lasagna products. In 2016, a large UK retailer reported that some of its own-brand 100% beef lasagna products contained horse meat. This resulted in a major scandal and prompted a nationwide investigation by the UK Food Standards Agency (FSA). The FSA conducted a forensic investigation to identify the source of the horse meat and determine whether it had been intentionally added to the products. The FSA collected samples of 100% beef lasagna products from various retail outlets and subjected them to IRMS analysis. IRMS measures the ratio of stable isotopes of carbon, nitrogen, oxygen, and hydrogen in a sample, which can be used to determine the geographical origin of the sample. In this case, the FSA used IRMS to measure the ratio of carbon isotopes in the meat samples. The IRMS analysis revealed that the samples of the 100% beef lasagna contained horse meat, which was likely to have originated from Romania.

The carbon isotope ratios in the horse meat samples were consistent with the ratios found in animals that had been raised in Romania. This suggested that the horse meat had been intentionally added to the 100% beef lasagna products and was not a result of accidental contamination. The FSA conducted further investigations and traced the source of the horse meat to a Romanian slaughterhouse. The slaughterhouse had supplied beef to several European food processors, who had then supplied it to various retailers. The investigation revealed that the horse meat had been fraudulently labeled as beef and added to the 100% beef lasagna products [80].

6.10 Challenges and Limitations of Mass Spectrometry in Forensics

Sample Contamination: One of the primary challenges in mass spectrometry is the potential for sample contamination. Forensic samples are often small and easily susceptible to contamination from various sources, such as the environment, handling, or previous analyses. Contaminants can introduce foreign isotopes and compromise the accuracy and reliability of the results. To mitigate this issue, strict protocols for sample collection, handling, and analysis must be followed, and laboratories need to implement rigorous quality control measures.

Analyzing Complex Mixtures: Forensic samples can be highly complex mixtures, containing a wide range of compounds and elements. This complexity can make it difficult to separate and identify individual components accurately. In mass spectrometry, complex mixtures may lead to overlapping mass spectra, resulting in challenges in peak assignment and accurate quantification. Advanced separation techniques like chromatography or multidimensional mass spectrometry are often employed to address this limitation.

Sensitivity and Detection Limits: Some forensic samples may contain trace amounts of analytes, making their detection challenging. Low analyte concentrations can lead to reduced signal intensity in mass spectra, affecting the sensitivity of the analysis. To overcome this limitation, researchers continually work on improving the sensitivity of mass spectrometers and developing more sensitive ionization techniques.

Isobaric Interferences: Isobaric interferences occur when two or more compounds have the same nominal mass but different chemical compositions, making it difficult to differentiate them based solely on mass measurements. Such interferences can lead to misidentification of compounds or elements, particularly in complex forensic samples. Isobaric interferences require careful consideration and additional techniques, such as tandem mass spectrometry (MS/MS), to distinguish between compounds accurately.

Calibration and Standardization: Accurate quantification in mass spectrometry relies on calibration using appropriate standards. However, obtaining suitable reference standards for all analytes of interest can be challenging, especially in the field of forensics where new drugs or compounds may constantly emerge. The lack of well-characterized standards can lead to uncertainties in quantification and limit the reliability of results.

Instrumentation Costs and Expertise: Mass spectrometry instruments can be expensive and require specialized training to operate and maintain. Smaller forensic laboratories may face budgetary constraints, limiting access to advanced mass spectrometers. Additionally, the complex data analysis and interpretation involved in mass spectrometry require skilled experts, which can be a limitation in some settings.

Despite these challenges and limitations, mass spectrometry remains a valuable tool in forensic science. Advances in technology and methodology continue to address these issues, improving the accuracy, sensitivity, and applicability of mass spectrometry in solving complex forensic cases and providing critical scientific evidence in legal proceedings.

6.11 Conclusion

In Conclusion, the use of mass spectrometry and isotope ratio mass spectrometry (IRMS) in forensic science has brought about a significant paradigm shift, revolutionizing the investigation and analysis of forensic evidence. These powerful analytical techniques have opened new avenues of understanding and unravelling complex forensic puzzles. Through mass spectrometry, forensic investigators can identify and quantify various compounds, drugs, and toxins in forensic samples with high sensitivity and specificity. This capability has played a crucial role in drug testing, toxicology, and identifying illicit substances in criminal cases. Moreover, the ability to analyze complex mixtures has facilitated the detection of trace elements, aiding in identifying geographic origins, reconstructing diets, and providing valuable information about the lifestyle and movement of individuals in the past. Isotope ratio mass spectrometry has emerged as a game-changer in the forensic world, offering unique insights into geographic origins, dietary habits, and migration patterns. This technology has significantly improved our understanding of ancient populations, helped solve historical mysteries, and supported efforts in wildlife conservation. Despite the remarkable advancements, these techniques do come with challenges and limitations. Sample contamination, the complexity of mixtures, and isobaric interferences necessitate careful handling, advanced separation techniques, and sophisticated data interpretation methods. The availability of appropriate standards for calibration remains an ongoing concern, requiring continuous efforts to develop and validate new reference materials. Nonetheless, the benefits of mass spectrometry and IRMS in forensics far outweigh the challenges. These methods have provided critical scientific evidence in legal proceedings, aiding in solving complex cases and ensuring justice is served. Additionally, the integration of these techniques with other forensic tools has significantly enhanced the capabilities of forensic investigations, leading to more accurate and reliable results. Looking ahead, further advancements in mass spectrometry instrumentation, method development, and data analysis will undoubtedly enhance the precision and efficiency of forensic analyses. Collaboration among researchers, forensic experts, and law enforcement agencies will continue to be pivotal in pushing the boundaries of forensic science and maximizing the potential of mass spectrometry in unravelling the mysteries of the past and addressing the challenges of the future. The profound impact of mass spectrometry and IRMS in the realm of forensic science is undeniable, paving the way for a deeper understanding of past civilizations, the dynamics of crime, and the advancement of justice.

References

1. *Forensic Analysis on the Cutting Edge*. Wiley, 2007. doi: 10.1002/9780470166932.
2. "Web Importer | Mendeley." Accessed: Jan. 03, 2024. [Online]. Available: https://www.mendeley.com/reference-management/web-importer?utm_source=science_direct&utm_campaign=web_importer_cross_sell
3. A. J. Folayan, A. Dosunmu, and B. Oriji, "Aerobic and anaerobic biodegradation of synthetic drilling fluids in marine deep-water offshore environments: Process variables and empirical investigations," *Energy Reports*, vol. 9, pp. 2153–2168, Dec. 2023, doi: 10.1016/j.egyr.2023.01.034.

4. B. d. A. Zellner, P. Dugo, G. Dugo, and L. Mondello, "Flavors and Odors," *Chemical Analysis of Food: Techniques and Applications*, pp. 599–663, Jan. 2012, doi: 10.1016/B978-0-12-384862-8.00019-4.
5. A. Barry, S. Thomson, I. Dimayuga, A. Chaudhuri, and T. Do, "Isotope ratio method: state-of-the-art of forensic applications to CBRNE materials," *Canadian Society of Forensic Science Journal*, vol. 55, no. 3, pp. 115–141, Jul. 2022, doi: 10.1080/00085030.2022.2054109.
6. M. Sun, C. Archer, and D. Vance, "New Methods for the Chemical Isolation and Stable Isotope Measurement of Multiple Transition Metals, with Application to the Earth Sciences," *Geostand. Geoanal. Res.*, vol. 45, no. 4, pp. 643–658, Dec. 2021, doi: 10.1111/ggr.12402.
7. C. Hillaire-Marcel *et al.*, "A stable isotope toolbox for water and inorganic carbon cycle studies," *Nat. Rev. Earth Environ.*, vol. 2, no. 10, pp. 699–719, Sep. 2021, doi: 10.1038/s43017-021-00209-0.
8. R. Sleeman and J. F. Carter, "Mass Spectrometry - Overview," *Encyclopedia of Analytical Science: Second Edition*, pp. 337–344, Jan. 2004, doi: 10.1016/B0-12-369397-7/00342-3.
9. J. Lisec, N. Schauer, J. Kopka, L. Willmitzer, and A. R. Fernie, "Gas chromatography mass spectrometry–based metabolite profiling in plants," *Nat. Protoc.*, vol. 1, no. 1, pp. 387–396, Jun. 2006, doi: 10.1038/nprot.2006.59.
10. T. O. Alves, C. T. S. D'Almeida, K. A. Scherf, and M. S. L. Ferreira, "Modern Approaches in the Identification and Quantification of Immunogenic Peptides in Cereals by LC-MS/MS," *Front. Plant Sci.*, vol. 10, Nov. 2019, doi: 10.3389/fpls.2019.01470.
11. A. P. Kafka, T. Kleffmann, T. Rades, and A. McDowell, "The application of MALDI TOF MS in biopharmaceutical research," *Int. J. Pharm.*, vol. 417, no. 1–2, pp. 70–82, Sep. 2011, doi: 10.1016/j.ijpharm.2010.12.010.
12. F. Taguchi *et al.*, "Mass spectrometry to classify non-small-cell lung cancer patients for clinical outcome after treatment with epidermal growth factor receptor tyrosine kinase inhibitors: a multicohort cross-institutional study.," *J. Natl. Cancer Inst.*, vol. 99, no. 11, pp. 838–846, 2007, doi: 10.1093/JNCI/DJK195.
13. J. Albrethsen, "The first decade of MALDI protein profiling: A lesson in translational biomarker research," *J. Proteomics*, vol. 74, no. 6, pp. 765–773, May 2011, doi: 10.1016/J.JPROT.2011.02.027.
14. S. Kumar, "Developments, advancements, and contributions of mass spectrometry in omics technologies," *Advances in Protein Molecular and Structural Biology Methods*, pp. 327–356, Jan. 2022, doi: 10.1016/B978-0-323-90264-9.00021-0.
15. G. Siuzdak, "An Introduction to Mass Spectrometry Ionization: An Excerpt from *The Expanding Role of Mass Spectrometry in Biotechnology*, 2nd ed.; MCC Press: San Diego, 2005," *JALA: Journal of the Association for Laboratory Automation*, vol. 9, no. 2, pp. 50–63, Apr. 2004, doi: 10.1016/j.jala.2004.01.004.

16. K. H. Cheong and A. Khursheed, "A parallel magnetic sector mass analyzer design," *Nucl. Instrum. Methods Phys. Res. A*, vol. 645, no. 1, pp. 221–226, Jul. 2011, doi: 10.1016/J.NIMA.2010.12.017.
17. B. Mindur, T. Fiutowski, S. Koperny, P. Wiącek, and W. Dąbrowski, "Investigation of Copper-Less Gas Electron Multiplier Detectors Responses to Soft X-rays," *Sensors*, vol. 20, no. 10, p. 2784, May 2020, doi: 10.3390/s20102784.
18. I. V. Chernushevich, A. V. Loboda, and B. A. Thomson, "An introduction to quadrupole-time-of-flight mass spectrometry," *J. Mass Spectrom.*, vol. 36, no. 8, pp. 849–865, Aug. 2001, doi: 10.1002/jms.207.
19. L. A. Malik, A. Bashir, A. Qureashi, and A. H. Pandith, "Detection and removal of heavy metal ions: a review," *Environ. Chem. Lett.*, vol. 17, no. 4, pp. 1495–1521, Dec. 2019, doi: 10.1007/s10311-019-00891-z.
20. G. Kaklamanos, E. Aprea, and G. Theodoridis, "Mass spectrometry: principles and instrumentation," *Chemical Analysis of Food*, pp. 525–552, Jan. 2020, doi: 10.1016/B978-0-12-813266-1.00011-5.
21. M. G. Alaimo and D. Varrica, "Global public health and toxicology," *Reference Module in Biomedical Sciences*, 2023, doi: 10.1016/B978-0-12-824315-2.00445-0.
22. O. H. Drummer, "Forensic toxicology," 2010, pp. 579–603. doi: 10.1007/978-3-7643-8338-1_18.
23. N. Vanderheyden, E. Verhoeven, S. Vermeulen, and B. Bekaert, "Survival of forensic trace evidence on improvised explosive devices: perspectives on individualisation," *Sci. Rep.*, vol. 10, no. 1, p. 12813, Jul. 2020, doi: 10.1038/s41598-020-69385-1.
24. P. Munjal, B. Sharma, J. R. Sethi, A. Dalal, and S. L. Gholap, "Identification and analysis of organic explosives from post-blast debris by nuclear magnetic resonance," *J. Hazard. Mater*, vol. 403, p. 124003, Feb. 2021, doi: 10.1016/J.JHAZMAT.2020.124003.
25. J. Yinon, "Chapter 17 Explosives," *Handbook of Analytical Separations*, vol. 2, pp. 603–616, Jan. 2000, doi: 10.1016/S1567-7192(00)80072-8.
26. E. B. Kujawinski, "Electrospray Ionization Fourier Transform Ion Cyclotron Resonance Mass Spectrometry (ESI FT-ICR MS): Characterization of Complex Environmental Mixtures," *Environ. Forensics*, vol. 3, no. 3–4, pp. 207–216, Sep. 2002, doi: 10.1006/ENFO.2002.0109.
27. A. O. Barakat, Y. Qian, M. Kim, and M. C. Kennicutt, "Compositional Changes of Aromatic Steroid Hydrocarbons in Naturally Weathered Oil Residues in the Egyptian Western Desert," *Environ. Forensics*, vol. 3, no. 3–4, pp. 219–225, Sep. 2002, doi: 10.1006/ENFO.2002.0095.
28. G. J. Parker, H. E. McKiernan, K. M. Legg, and Z. C. Goecker, "Forensic proteomics," *Forensic Sci. Int. Genet.*, vol. 54, p. 102529, Sep. 2021, doi: 10.1016/J.FSIGEN.2021.102529.

29. E. D. Merkley, D. S. Wunschel, K. L. Wahl, and K. H. Jarman, "Applications and challenges of forensic proteomics," *Forensic Sci. Int*, vol. 297, pp. 350–363, Apr. 2019, doi: 10.1016/J.FORSCIINT.2019.01.022.
30. W. Timp and G. Timp, "Beyond mass spectrometry, the next step in proteomics," *Sci. Adv.*, vol. 6, no. 2, Jan. 2020, doi: 10.1126/sciadv.aax8978.
31. I. R. Kaplan, Y. Galperin, S. T. Lu, and R. P. Lee, "Forensic Environmental Geochemistry: differentiation of fuel-types, their sources and release time," *Org. Geochem.*, vol. 27, no. 5–6, pp. 289–317, Nov. 1997, doi: 10.1016/S0146-6380(97)87941-7.
32. Z. Millbern, A. Trettin, R. Wu, M. Demmler, and N. R. Vinueza, "Synthetic dyes: A mass spectrometry approach and applications," *Mass Spectrom. Rev.*, Nov. 2022, doi: 10.1002/mas.21818.
33. N. Sugaya, M. Takahashi, K. Sakurai, N. Tanaka, I. Okubo, and T. Kawakami, "Mass Spectrometric Analysis of Synthetic Organic Pigments," *J. AOAC Int.*, vol. 101, no. 5, pp. 1328–1340, Sep. 2018, doi: 10.5740/jaoacint.18-0049.
34. K. Lech and E. Fornal, "A Mass Spectrometry-Based Approach for Characterization of Red, Blue, and Purple Natural Dyes," *Molecules*, vol. 25, no. 14, p. 3223, Jul. 2020, doi: 10.3390/molecules25143223.
35. Z. Muccio and G. P. Jackson, "Isotope ratio mass spectrometry," *Analyst*, vol. 134, no. 2, pp. 213–222, 2009, doi: 10.1039/B808232D.
36. G. Kaklamanos, E. Aprea, and G. Theodoridis, "Mass spectrometry: principles and instrumentation," *Chemical Analysis of Food*, pp. 525–552, 2020, doi: 10.1016/B978-0-12-813266-1.00011-5.
37. S. Kelly, C. Brodie, and A. Hilkert, "Isotopic-Spectroscopic Technique: Stable Isotope-Ratio Mass Spectrometry (IRMS)," *Modern Techniques for Food Authentication*, pp. 349–413, Jan. 2018, doi: 10.1016/B978-0-12-814264-6.00011-6.
38. Q. T. Birch, P. M. Potter, P. X. Pinto, D. D. Dionysiou, and S. R. Al-Abed, "Isotope ratio mass spectrometry and spectroscopic techniques for microplastics characterization," *Talanta*, vol. 224, p. 121743, Mar. 2021, doi: 10.1016/J.TALANTA.2020.121743.
39. G. Kaklamanos, E. Aprea, and G. Theodoridis, "Mass spectrometry: principles and instrumentation," *Chemical Analysis of Food*, pp. 525–552, 2020, doi: 10.1016/B978-0-12-813266-1.00011-5.
40. Q. T. Birch, P. M. Potter, P. X. Pinto, D. D. Dionysiou, and S. R. Al-Abed, "Isotope ratio mass spectrometry and spectroscopic techniques for microplastics characterization," *Talanta*, vol. 224, p. 121743, Mar. 2021, doi: 10.1016/J.TALANTA.2020.121743.
41. O. Abbas *et al.*, "Analytical methods used for the authentication of food of animal origin," *Food Chem.*, vol. 246, pp. 6–17, Apr. 2018, doi: 10.1016/J.FOODCHEM.2017.11.007.
42. G. P. Danezis, A. S. Tsagkaris, F. Camin, V. Brusic, and C. A. Georgiou, "Food authentication: Techniques, trends & emerging approaches," *TrAC Trends*

in Analytical Chemistry, vol. 85, pp. 123–132, Dec. 2016, doi: 10.1016/J.TRAC.2016.02.026.

43. B. A. Eckenrode, S. A. McLuckey, and G. L. Glish, "Comparison of electron ionization and chemical ionization sensitivities in an ion trap mass spectrometer," *Int. J. Mass Spectrom. Ion Process*, vol. 106, pp. 137–157, May 1991, doi: 10.1016/0168-1176(91)85015-E.
44. E. Sieniawska and T. Baj, "Tannins," *Pharmacognosy: Fundamentals, Applications and Strategy*, pp. 199–232, 2017, doi: 10.1016/B978-0-12-802104-0.00010-X.
45. R. Sleeman and J. F. Carter, "Mass Spectrometry - Overview," *Encyclopedia of Analytical Science: Second Edition*, pp. 337–344, Jan. 2004, doi: 10.1016/B0-12-369397-7/00342-3.
46. Y. Fang, D. Jia-hua, and L. Shu-li, "A Comparison Between Chemical Ionization And Electron Impact Techniques Of Mass Spectrometry For The Estimation Of N-Nitrosodimethylamine," *Anal. Lett.*, vol. 14, no. 14, pp. 1165–1175, Jan. 1981, doi: 10.1080/00032718108059813.
47. B. Munson, "Chemical Ionization Mass Spectrometry: Theory and Applications," in *Encyclopedia of Analytical Chemistry*, Chichester, UK: John Wiley & Sons, Ltd, 2000. doi: 10.1002/9780470027318.a6004.
48. A. Dasgupta and A. Wahed, "Instrumentation and Analytical Methods," *Clinical Chemistry, Immunology and Laboratory Quality Control*, pp. 1–18, 2014, doi: 10.1016/B978-0-12-407821-5.00001-2.
49. R. S. Lehrle, M. Rollinson, N. Dadvand, and I. W. Parsons, "Mass spectrometry detection versus flame ionisation detection in pyrolysis–gas chromatography: spurious pyrolysis peaks and possible errors in estimating relative product yields," *Polym. Degrad. Stab.*, vol. 66, no. 2, pp. 221–231, Nov. 1999, doi: 10.1016/S0141-3910(99)00069-5.
50. C. Hasse, "Models for Coal Kinetics," *Reference Module in Chemistry, Molecular Sciences and Chemical Engineering*, 2015, doi: 10.1016/B978-0-12-409547-2.11520-3.
51. Y. Picó and D. Barceló, "Isotopic Mass Spectrometry in Food and Environmental Chemistry," 2022, pp. 99–125. doi: 10.1007/698_2022_907.
52. A. J. Walder, I. D. Abell, I. Platzner, and P. A. Freedman, "Lead isotope ratio measurement of NIST 610 glass by laser ablation inductively coupled plasma mass spectrometry," *Spectrochim. Acta Part B At Spectrosc*, vol. 48, no. 3, pp. 397–402, Feb. 1993, doi: 10.1016/0584-8547(93)80044-U.
53. K. G. Heumann, S. M. Gallus, G. Rädlinger, and J. Vogl, "Precision and accuracy in isotope ratio measurements by plasma source mass spectrometry," *J. Anal. At Spectrom.*, vol. 13, no. 9, p. 1001, 1998, doi: 10.1039/a801965g.
54. H.-P. Sieper *et al.*, "A measuring system for the fast simultaneous isotope ratio and elemental analysis of carbon, hydrogen, nitrogen and sulfur in food commodities and other biological material," *Rapid Communications in Mass Spectrometry*, vol. 20, no. 17, pp. 2521–2527, Sep. 2006, doi: 10.1002/rcm.2619.

55. Y. Zhang, H. J. Tobias, G. L. Sacks, and J. Thomas Brenna, "Calibration and data processing in gas chromatography combustion isotope ratio mass spectrometry," *Drug Test. Anal.*, vol. 4, no. 12, pp. 912–922, Dec. 2012, doi: 10.1002/dta.394.
56. M. J. Zeeman *et al.*, "Optimization of automated gas sample collection and isotope ratio mass spectrometric analysis of δ^{13} C of CO_2 in air," *Rapid Communications in Mass Spectrometry*, vol. 22, no. 23, pp. 3883–3892, Dec. 2008, doi: 10.1002/rcm.3772.
57. K. A. van Leeuwen, P. D. Prenzler, D. Ryan, and F. Camin, "Gas Chromatography-Combustion-Isotope Ratio Mass Spectrometry for Traceability and Authenticity in Foods and Beverages," *Compr. Rev. Food Sci. Food Saf.*, vol. 13, no. 5, pp. 814–837, Sep. 2014, doi: 10.1111/1541-4337.12096.
58. B. A. Eckenrode, "Environmental and Forensic applications of field-portable GC-MS: An overview," *J. Am. Soc. Mass Spectrom.*, vol. 12, no. 6, pp. 683–693, Jun. 2001, doi: 10.1016/S1044-0305(01)00251-3.
59. B. Kasprzyk-Hordern, R. M. Dinsdale, and A. J. Guwy, "Illicit drugs and pharmaceuticals in the environment – Forensic applications of environmental data. Part 1: Estimation of the usage of drugs in local communities," *Environ. Pollut.*, vol. 157, no. 6, pp. 1773–1777, Jun. 2009, doi: 10.1016/J.ENVPOL.2009.03.017.
60. D. Megson, E. J. Reiner, K. J. Jobst, F. L. Dorman, M. Robson, and J. F. Focant, "A review of the determination of persistent organic pollutants for environmental forensics investigations," *Anal. Chim. Acta*, vol. 941, pp. 10–25, Oct. 2016, doi: 10.1016/J.ACA.2016.08.027.
61. G. J. Bowen, L. I. Wassenaar, and K. A. Hobson, "Global application of stable hydrogen and oxygen isotopes to wildlife forensics," *Oecologia*, vol. 143, no. 3, pp. 337–348, Apr. 2005, doi: 10.1007/s00442-004-1813-y.
62. V. Bourret, V. Albert, J. April, G. Côté, and O. Morissette, "Past, present and future contributions of evolutionary biology to wildlife forensics, management and conservation," *Evol. Appl.*, vol. 13, no. 6, pp. 1420–1434, Jul. 2020, doi: 10.1111/eva.12977.
63. S. K. Verma and L. Singh, "Novel universal primers establish identity of an enormous number of animal species for forensic application," *Mol. Ecol. Notes*, vol. 3, no. 1, pp. 28–31, Dec. 2002, doi: 10.1046/j.1471-8286.2003.00340.x.
64. C. G. Daughton, "Illicit Drugs: Contaminants in the Environment and Utility in Forensic Epidemiology," 2011, pp. 59–110. doi: 10.1007/978-1-4419-7615-4_3.
65. B. Kasprzyk-Hordern, R. M. Dinsdale, and A. J. Guwy, "Illicit drugs and pharmaceuticals in the environment – Forensic applications of environmental data. Part 1: Estimation of the usage of drugs in local communities," *Environmental Pollution*, vol. 157, no. 6, pp. 1773–1777, Jun. 2009, doi: 10.1016/J.ENVPOL.2009.03.017.

66. M. Morelato *et al.*, "Forensic intelligence framework—Part I: Induction of a transversal model by comparing illicit drugs and false identity documents monitoring," *Forensic Sci. Int.*, vol. 236, pp. 181–190, Mar. 2014, doi: 10.1016/J.FORSCIINT.2013.12.045.
67. C. Ribeiro, C. Santos, V. Gonçalves, A. Ramos, C. Afonso, and M. Tiritan, "Chiral Drug Analysis in Forensic Chemistry: An Overview," *Molecules*, vol. 23, no. 2, p. 262, Jan. 2018, doi: 10.3390/molecules23020262.
68. R. W. Mathewes, "Forensic palynology in Canada: An overview with emphasis on archaeology and anthropology," *Forensic Sci. Int.*, vol. 163, no. 3, pp. 198–203, Nov. 2006, doi: 10.1016/J.FORSCIINT.2006.06.069.
69. D. C. Dirkmaat, L. L. Cabo, S. D. Ousley, and S. A. Symes, "New perspectives in forensic anthropology," *Am. J. Phys. Anthropol.*, vol. 137, no. S47, pp. 33–52, 2008, doi: 10.1002/ajpa.20948.
70. D. H. Ubelaker, "A history of forensic anthropology," *Am. J. Phys. Anthropol.*, vol. 165, no. 4, pp. 915–923, Apr. 2018, doi: 10.1002/ajpa.23306.
71. R. W. Mathewes, "Forensic palynology in Canada: An overview with emphasis on archaeology and anthropology," *Forensic Sci. Int.*, vol. 163, no. 3, pp. 198–203, Nov. 2006, doi: 10.1016/J.FORSCIINT.2006.06.069.
72. R. Premathilake and T. S. Erandathee Kumari, "Palynological Evidence from Sediment Samples Associated with the Early Holocene Human Skeleton from Fa Hien-lena, Sri Lanka," *Ancient Lanka*, vol. 1, Nov. 2022, doi: 10.29173/anlk656.
73. F. Da Silva Santos, L. Vitor da Silva, P. V. S. Campos, C. de Medeiros Strunkis, C. M. G. Ribeiro, and M. O. Salles, "Review—Recent Advances of Electrochemical Techniques in Food, Energy, Environment, and Forensic Applications," *ECS Sensors Plus*, vol. 1, no. 1, p. 013603, Mar. 2022, doi: 10.1149/2754-2726/ac5cdf.
74. F. Teletchea, C. Maudet, and C. Hänni, "Food and forensic molecular identification: update and challenges," *Trends Biotechnol.*, vol. 23, no. 7, pp. 359–366, Jul. 2005, doi: 10.1016/j.tibtech.2005.05.006.
75. C. M. Deviterne-Lapeyre, "Interpol review of questioned documents 2016–2019," *Forensic Sci. Int.*, vol. 2, pp. 429–441, Jan. 2020, doi: 10.1016/J.FSISYN.2020.01.012.
76. M. Calcerrada and C. García-Ruiz, "Analysis of questioned documents: A review," *Anal. Chim. Acta*, vol. 853, no. 1, pp. 143–166, Jan. 2015, doi: 10.1016/J.ACA.2014.10.057.
77. E. Mistek, M. A. Fikiet, S. R. Khandasammy, and I. K. Lednev, "Toward Locard's Exchange Principle: Recent Developments in Forensic Trace Evidence Analysis," *Anal. Chem.*, vol. 91, no. 1, pp. 637–654, Jan. 2019, doi: 10.1021/acs.analchem.8b04704.

78. M. P. V. Matos and G. P. Jackson, "Isotope ratio mass spectrometry in forensic science applications," *Forensic Chem.*, vol. 13, p. 100154, May 2019, doi: 10.1016/J.FORC.2019.100154.
79. T. A. Brettell, J. M. Butler, and R. Saferstein, "Forensic Science," *Anal. Chem.*, vol. 77, no. 12, pp. 3839–3860, Jun. 2005, doi: 10.1021/ac050682e.
80. A. Lianou, M. Papakonstantinou, G.-J. E. Nychas, and J. Stoitsis, "Fraud in meat and poultry products," in *Food Fraud*, Elsevier, 2021, pp. 85–108. doi: 10.1016/B978-0-12-817242-1.00012-9.

7

Application of Plasma and Atomic Absorption Spectroscopy in Sample Analysis

Jyoti Singh* and Shrutika Singla

Amity Institute of Forensic Science, Amity University, Noida, Uttar Pradesh, India

Abstract
Atomic Absorption Spectroscopy (AAS) and Inductively Coupled Plasma Optical Emission Spectroscopy (ICP-OES) serves as a valuable analytical technique for quickly assessing trace metallic elements and quantifying the concentrations of unknown sample constituents. Both these techniques are applicable to discern heavy metals, trace elements, impurities, and contaminants within various biological matrices and offer advantages over traditional gravimetric approaches in terms of speed, sensitivity, and clarity. Due to their exceptional accuracy and regulatory compliance and ability to quantitatively estimate and map the elements present in the sample, AAS and ICP-OES have gained widespread use in forensic evidence analysis to investigate explosives, gunshot residue (GSR) particles, and other ammunition components.. This chapter provides a concise overview of the principles and theories behind AAS and ICP-OES techniques, their instrumental setups, and forensic application applications.

Keywords: Atomic absorption spectroscopy, plasma spectroscopy, spectroscopy, analytical approach, detection, trace elements, forensic evidence

7.1 Introduction

Spectroscopy is a technique of the fragmentation of a single white light into its color components. It is the study of light absorbed or emitted by

**Corresponding author*: jsingh4@amity.edu.in

Priyanka Chhabra, Divya Bajpai Tripathy, Anjali Gupta, Rajeev Kumar, Kajol Bhati and Shruti Shukla (eds.) Advances in Analytical Techniques for Forensic Investigation, (189–214) © 2024 Scrivener Publishing LLC

a substance when a light of particular wavelength strikes on it. Light is composed of electromagnetic radiation of varying wavelength and frequency. Spectroscopy mainly studies the interaction of electromagnetic radiations with the substance. The use of spectroscopy is wide due to its property of interaction with different matter as a function of wavelength and frequency. Electromagnetic radiation has both electric and magnetic fields, and includes radio waves, microwaves, infrared, visible, ultraviolet, X-rays and gamma rays (with shortest wavelength and longest frequency) (Figure 7.1).

Depending on the inter-action of electromagnetic radiation with the target substance, spectroscopy can be of different types such as absorption spectroscopy, emission spectroscopy, resonance spectroscopy and many more [5].

Atomic spectroscopy has led to the advancement of three analytical techniques: atomic emission, atomic absorption, and atomic fluorescence. All these methods involve an atomic process which relates all the techniques with each other. AAS has many uses, such as detection of trace metals in different samples including drinking water, pharmaceuticals, beverages, petroleum samples, and forensic analysis. Also, it has its applications in geological and mineralogical samples, food testing and industrial applications.

Atomic Absorption Spectroscopy offers applied and reasonable options for the investigation of trace amounts of metals in a variety of things, including geographical samples, environmental samples, biological specimens, agricultural products and soils, pharmaceuticals, foods, and drinking water.

Robert Wilhelm Bunsen and Gustav Robert Kirchhoff, Professors at the University of Heidelberg in Germany, created the fundamental concepts of atomic emission spectroscopy in the latter half of the nineteenth century. Initial applications of atomic emission spectroscopy were as analytical tools. A group of Australian chemists spent the 1950s substantially developing the contemporary version of AAS. They were led by Sir Alan Walsh at the Chemical Physics Division of the Commonwealth Scientific and Industrial Research Organization (CSIRO) in Melbourne, Australia [1].

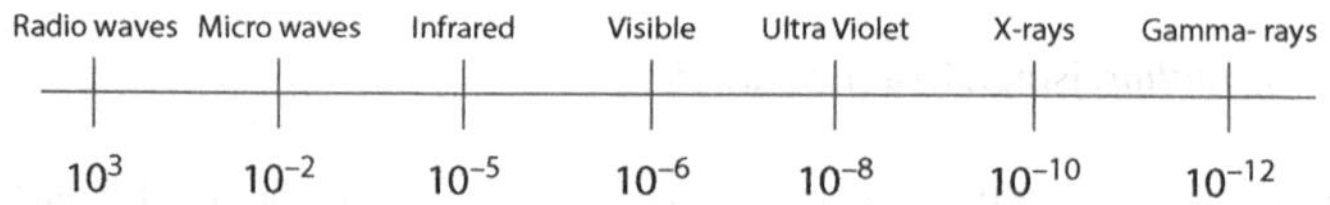

Figure 7.1 Diagram of electromagnetic radiation.

The atom is composed of an electron-encircled nucleus. A specified number of electrons are present in each element that depends on the atomic number of the element which is specific for each element. The orbital locations of the electrons are filled in a systematic and predictable manner. The typical orbital arrangement for an atom is that of its "ground state," which is the lowest energy and most stable electronic form. If enough photons are delivered to the atoms, the electrons in the atom absorb the energy due to which it gets excited from a highly stable or ground state to a less stable or excited state. Due to the un-stability of the electron at the excited state, it comes back to the ground state. The energy that was initially absorbed during the excitation process will be released as radiant energy as the electron moves back to its original, and stable orbital location [2].

The electronic transition that has taken place is closely related to the wavelength of the radiant energy that has been emitted. As we know, each element has a distinct electrical structure, thus the wavelength of light it emits is a characteristic that is exclusive to that element. A complex atom have complicated orbital arrangement due to which it is possible that numerous electronic transitions take place, each of which results in the emission of a distinct wavelength of light [3].

All three of the domains of atomic spectroscopy entail the excitation and decay to the ground state. For AAS to be used for the analytical purpose, there can be 2 ways – first, energy absorbed during the excitation process and second, energy released during the decay process. In both cases, energy is measured. In case of atomic emission, high energy is supplied to the sample, creating a thermal environment which then excites electrons to the excited state, which then emits energy in the form of light. There are many sources of energy, also termed radiation sources such as electric arcs, plasma, flame and many more. The emitted energy can be seen in the form of an emission spectrum which contains discrete lines corresponding to the wavelength emitted, known as emission lines. As each element gives different emission lines, due to this reason it can be used for the qualitative identification of the element [4].

When a beam of electromagnetic radiation is imparted on a ground state atom, the electrons absorb energy due to which they get excited to excited state. The process of absorbing energy is known as atomic absorption. These atoms absorb at specific wavelength and this property of absorption is used in AAS.

In this chapter we mainly focus on absorption spectroscopy.

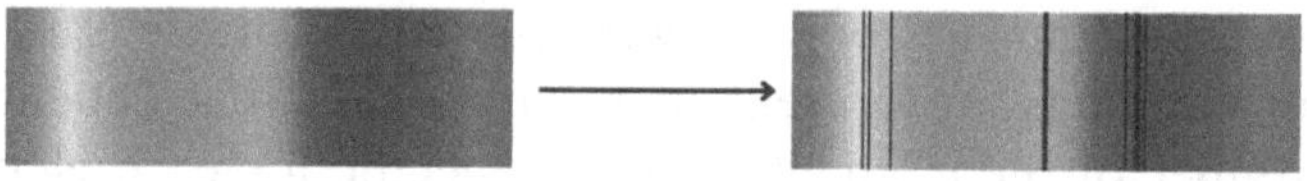

Figure 7.2 Electromagnetic radiation converting into Black line of electromagnetic spectrum.

7.2 Absorption Spectroscopy

Absorption spectroscopy, as the name indicates, is the type of spectroscopy in which there is absorption of radiation of particular wavelength when electromagnetic radiation interacts with some material. As we all know, white light contains electromagnetic radiation with different frequency and wavelength. Whenever this bunch of different radiation passes through a sample, it leads to absorption of a particular wavelength by the sample. Due to absorption of particular wavelength, a black line is seen on electromagnetic spectrum (Figure 7.2). The absorption of electromagnetic radiation is different for different substances. Absorption depends on the composition of that substance [5].

Now, the main thing is, why is absorption happening? We all know that a substance is composed of compounds and molecules. Atoms are the basic unit of these molecules and substances. Atoms contain electrons, protons and neutrons. Whenever light is passed through a substance, electrons when gets their sufficient amount of energy to jump to a higher level, absorb some energy from electromagnetic radiation or light and get excited. When that wavelength of light is absorbed by electrons, then it is known as absorption spectroscopy. At that wavelength, the transmittance becomes low and black bands are seen in the radiation spectrum [6].

There are different types of absorption spectroscopy. In this chapter, we will be studying plasma absorption spectroscopy and atomic absorption spectroscopy.

7.3 Atomic Absorption Spectroscopy (AAS)

Atomic absorption spectrometry is a technique for identifying elements in either liquid or solid samples by using certain wavelengths of electromagnetic radiation from a radiation source. All these elements absorb at specific wavelengths, and these absorbances are compared with the known absorbance for identification of the element. AAS basically uses the different light wavelengths that are absorbed by different atoms [7]. In AAS, the foremost step is atomization of the element followed by absorption of energy at specific wavelengths due to which discrete black lines are observed in the absorption spectrum.

There are different categories of AAS-

Flame Atomic Absorption Spectroscopy - This technique was first developed by Sir Alan Walsh and since then it has proved to be a powerful technique for the purpose of identifying and measuring trace components in the sample. It is a highly sensitive tool that can detect concentration up to 1 ppm. The main drawback of this method is that simultaneous detection is not possible for more than 1 metal [8]. In FAAS, atoms get atomized by flame atomizer. The atomized elements absorb energy at specific wavelengths and gives spectra with black lines at discrete sites due to absorption of desired wavelengths. There are many advantages of this technique such as it is less costly, highly sensitive, less complex and due to these reasons, it has become the first choice of researchers for the analysis of trace elements [2].

Cold Vapor Atomic Absorption Spectroscopy - Cold Vapour Atomic Absorption Spectroscopy (CVAAS) does not require the step of vaporization as it is done for volatile elements such as Hg, which is already in vapor form at room temperature. It was first introduced by Hatch and Ott when they attached an additional instrument that reduces Hg^{2+} (stable form) to Hg^0 (excited form) for the monitoring of drinking water [9]. The market was then opened up to CV-AAS for the purpose of identifying dangerous substances obtained from the environment. Afterwards, it was also used for the detection of Hg in soil and aquatic animals like fish and prawns. CV-AAS can be used to determine the amount of element up to 10^{-3} ng/L. It is one of the most efficient, sensitive and fast techniques that can determine Hg [10]. Hydride Generation Atomic Absorption Spectroscopy (HGAAS) - As the name indicates, hydrides are generated for some of the metals such as As, Pb, Te, Sb and many more for their detection by AAS. The working of HGAAS is very similar to AAS. In addition, it includes Hydride generation apparatus [11]. Hydride generation setup is responsible for producing volatile hydrides by the reaction of oxyanions of metalloids with sodium borohydride and HCl. The hydrides thus produced for certain elements such as H2Te, H3Sb, etc. are thus transferred to the flame atomizer as it allows efficient nebulization than metals as such. The atoms thus formed absorb energy at specific wavelength which is then detected by optical cells and other detectors including Photomultiplier tube.

This technique can be used for the detection of above-mentioned metals in the small concentration with high specificity and efficiency [12].

Graphite Furnace Atomic Absorption Spectroscopy (GFAAS) – Graphite Furnace Atomic Absorption Spectroscopy is also known as Electrothermal Atomic absorption Spectroscopy, and it is a more sophisticated sort of Atomic Absorption Spectroscopy. It uses a graphite – or pyrolytic coated graphite furnace for the vaporization of the sample [13].

In GFAAS, a specific amount of known sample is injected into a graphite-coated furnace in which high temperature is regulated up to 3000°C electrically. Vaporization and atomization of elements takes place in the furnace [14]. It can detect elements up to the range of 10^{-2} μL, less expensive, easy to use and highly precise. Major disadvantage with Graphite Furnace Atomic Absorption Spectroscopy is, it is less sensitive, and for the analysis a large amount of sample is required [15]. Improvements in the suppression of matrix interferences, flow injection analysis, and the introduction of accessories like graphite furnaces have all helped to increase the susceptibility and choosability of analytes in complex matrices. When utilizing graphite furnace atomization, it is typical to obtain findings at ppm levels as well as in ppb levels of higher sensitivity. Atomic absorption spectroscopy is used to estimate the concentration of any element, especially metals, in a sample. It is an instrument which uses the ionic state of an element for their detection. This instrument is highly specific as it produces narrow spectra.

7.3.1 Principle

AAS atomizes an element to its ionic form. When a beam of radiation falls on the ion, the ion absorbs energy and gets excited to a higher ionic level. This absorbed energy of the ion can be directly related to the element as it is a unique feature of all the elements and the corresponding wavelength is measured for the analysis purpose [16].

7.3.2 Instrumentation

Instrumentation of AAS consists of following parts (Figure 7.3):

Radiation Source: The hollow cathode lamp (HCL) is the primary radiation source in AAS. It is a hollow tube filled with noble gas, mainly argon or neon. It consists of an anode made of tungsten and cathode made up of

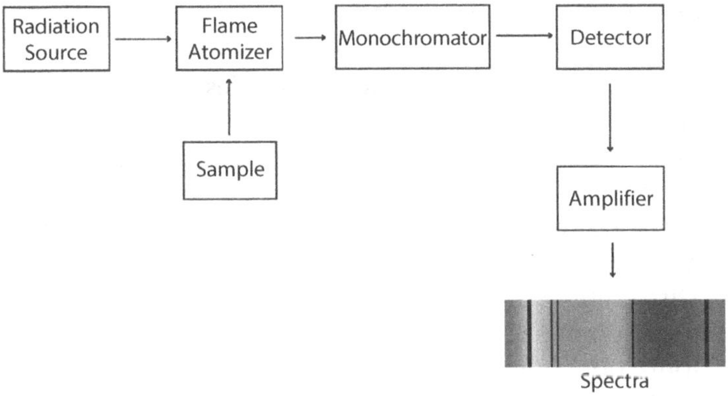

Figure 7.3 Basic instrumentation of atomic absorption spectroscopy.

the desired element. The complete apparatus is kept at a pressure of 1–5 torr. Potential is provided from the outside of the outside of the setup of about 300V.

Flame Atomizer: For any element to be detected by AAS, it is first necessary to have those in their atomic form. For this purpose, we use an atomizer in AAS. An atomizer is a setup that converts an element into its atomic form, and the process of converting into an atom is known as atomization. In AAS, we mainly have different types of atomization – Flame atomization, Electrothermal Atomization, Glow-Discharge Atomization, Hydride Atomization and many more.

Most commonly, flame atomization is used in AAS. The complete process of atomization is given in Figure 7.4.

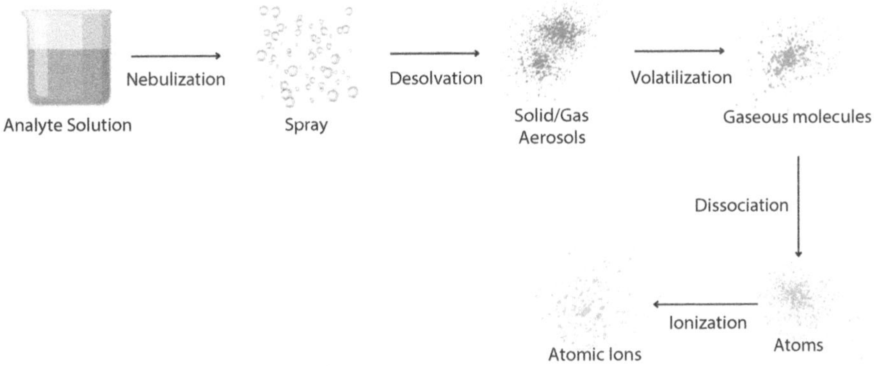

Figure 7.4 Process of atomization.

In the process of atomization, following steps are included:

a) Nebulization: In this step, larger particles get converted into smaller ones.
b) Desolvation: In this process solvent further evaporates and forms solid molecular aerosols.
c) Volatilization: In the step of volatilization, aerosols get volatilized to gaseous molecules.
d) Dissociation: In this process, molecules get dissociated into their component atoms.
e) Ionization: It is the last step of atomization in which atoms get ionized to form their respective cations and anions.

For the process of atomization, fuel, oxidants and high temperature is a necessity. Fuel can be natural gas, hydrogen and acetylene. Oxidant used for the AAS is mainly air and oxygen, but nitrous oxide is also used. Depending on the fuel and oxidant being utilized, temperature ranges from 1700°C to 2800°C [17]. The primary combustion zone, the interzone region, and the secondary combustion zone are the three main zones of flame. The region where the atomization process is accomplished is termed as the interzonal region. The primary combustion region mainly contains pure hydrocarbons with blue flame and the secondary combustion region gives stable oxides of elements.

After atomization, ions formed are moved on the monochromator [18].

Monochromator: Monochromator is a device used to separate a single wavelength band from a mixture of wavelengths. Monochromator consists of mainly 5 parts (Figure 7.5):

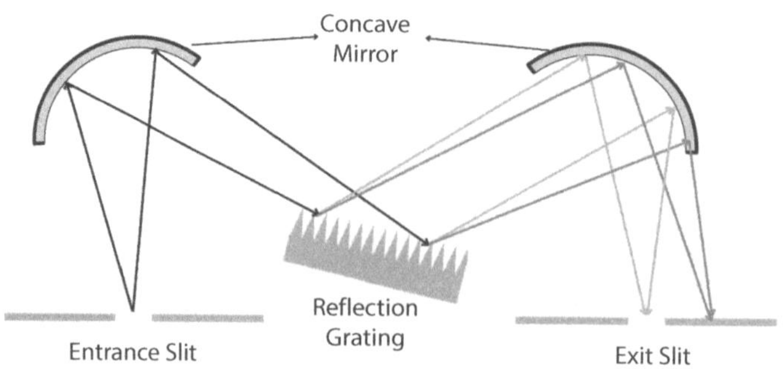

Figure 7.5 Diagram of monochromator.

a) Entrance Slit - An entry to the beam of wavelength.
b) Collimator - Collimator mirror or lens produces a parallel beam of radiation.
c) Grating - Grating or prism is used to separate components of a wavelength from radiation.
d) Focusing Mirror - Focusing mirror focuses the separated components of wavelength to planer surface, also known as focal plane.
e) Exit Slit - It is a focal plane through which an isolated beam of light takes exit from a device.

Detector: Detector is a mechanical, electrical, or chemical device which is used to measure the change in one or other variables and give results in readable form. Different detectors can be used such as Photomultiplier tube, photodiodes, charged coupled devices and many more.
Amplifier: Amplifier is an electronic device which is used to enhance the magnitude of signal reached at the detector.

7.3.3 Working

All the parts of the instrument have been explained in the above section. The process starts from the radiation source which is a hollow cathode lamp which emits a beam of radiation toward the flame atomizer where atomization and ionization of elements takes place. Atoms and ions thus formed absorb at particular wavelength and the remaining wavelengths are passed on to monochromator [19]. Monochromator isolates desired wavelength from a mixture of wavelengths. That specific wavelength is detected by the detector and amplified by the amplifier. The results are then shown on the screen in the form of spectrum [20].

7.4 Plasma Absorption Spectroscopy (PAS)

Plasma is a mixture of ionized gases that consists of electrons, ions (anions and cations) and also neutral species [21]. In plasma, mainly Argon gas is carried which is ionized by electrical discharge. The resultant plasma can be of 2 types depending on the source of electric field - Inductively Coupled Plasma (ICP) and Direct Current Plasma (DCP) [26]. In DCP, 2-3 electrodes made of argon combining into a discharge tube is used for the ionization purpose. On the other hand, in ICP, Argon gas is passed to the sample in the form of aerosols through 3 concentric silica quartz tubes.

Plasma is mainly formed by ionization of Argon gas by a spark generated from the Tesla coil. Plasma absorbs the majority of electromagnetic radiation in the UV range [22].

Plasma is mainly a source belonging to the high-temperature category of a source gas, which in most of the cases, is argon. Inductive coupling from electrical coils at megahertz frequencies sustains and maintains the plasma. The temperature of the available source is mainly from 5700°C to 9700°C. Elemental composition of the sample is directly related to the strength of emitted radiation.

PAS is a type of instrument where absorption of a definite wavelength of electromagnetic radiation takes place as a function of frequency or wavelength. For absorption, it is very important for the substance to get atomized, and for the same purpose, plasma is used. It is an effective atomization technique consisting of ions of mainly Argon which strikes with the matter, making those atomized. Plasma is also used in emission spectroscopy, also known as, Plasma Emission Spectroscopy (PES) [23]. Numerous industrial and academic contexts have used AA or AE spectrometers. A medical laboratory, for instance, might identify the kinds and quantities of dangerous metals that might be present in a patient's urine or blood. Metal contaminants in soil and water could be monitored by environmental experts. These devices are used by the pharmaceutical industry to check whether a metal catalyst is present after a medication has been purified. Finally, these tools would be used by the mining sector to gauge the quantity and existence of valuable metals like gold and silver.

Plasma spectroscopy can be further classified into:

a) Emission spectroscopy (Passive method)
b) Absorption Spectroscopy (Active method)

In plasma emission spectroscopy, radiation emitted by the electrons after passing from the plasma is recorded. The absorption of energy excites electrons from lower energy to higher energy state. And these electrons then come back to their ground state or lower energy state emitting some wavelength which is termed as decay process. When analytical samples are introduced into plasma, light and ions are produced. Trace amounts of the elements in the samples can be evaluated by detecting these ions and light. In addition to the plasma's tremendous temperature, the intricate atomic/molecular processes within the plasma also produce light and ions. A thorough comprehension of phenomena like the matrix effect can be attained by comprehending this process, the properties of plasma, and the effect on materials other than analytes. In absorption plasma spectroscopy, electrons are stimulated to higher energy levels after absorbing energy from lower energy state. This absorption of energy or photons is then noted down by the detector and it is given in the form absorption spectrum [24].

7.4.1 Principle

Plasma is used for the ionization of compounds. Ionized products then absorb electromagnetic radiation of particular wavelength depending on the type of atom present to get excited to higher level [25].

7.4.2 Instrumentation

Instrument of PAS consist of the following components (Figure 7.6):

Radiation Source: PAS uses a Hollow Cathode Lamp (HCL) as its radiation source. It is the most common radiation source used for absorption spectroscopy. It is composed of a tungsten anode and a metal cathode that is intended to be detected and this complete setup is filled by argon or neon gas (Figure 7.6).
Ionization Source: Ionization source is used for the ionization of samples to be detected. In PAS, plasma is used as an ionization source because it contains ionized gas, cations and anion species. Mainly Inductively Coupled Plasma (ICP) is used as the ionization source as shown in Figure 7.7.

Inductively coupled Plasma consists of three concentric quartz tubes from argon gas flow. In the inner tube, the sample is allowed to flow and

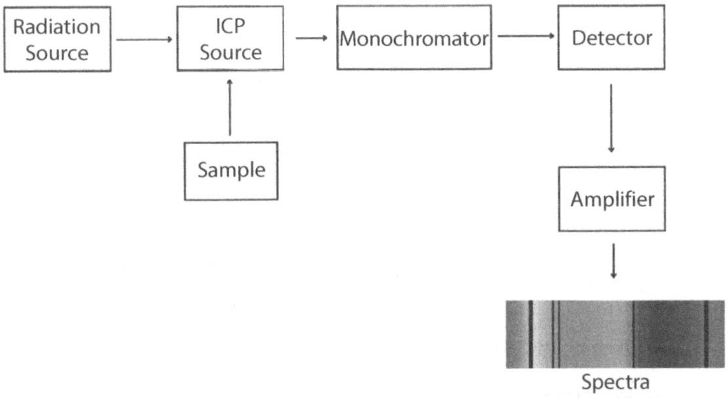

Figure 7.6 Instrumentation of plasma absorption spectroscopy (PAS).

in the outermost tube, argon gas flows in tangential manner. There is a radio frequency coil at the top of the setup which induces a magnetic field. The ionization of flowing argon gas occurs by spark produced from Tesla coil, ions that interact with the magnetic field produced by frequency coil. These ions then interact with the sample causing their ionization. The radiation produced by the ICP is then transferred to the monochromator for further process.

Monochromator: Monochromator is a device used to separate a single wavelength band from a mixture of wavelengths. Monochromator consists of mainly 5 parts (Figure 7.7):

a) Entrance Slit – An entry to the beam of wavelength.
b) Collimator – Collimator mirror or lens produces parallel beam of radiation.
c) Grating – Grating or prism is used to separate components of a wavelength from radiation.
d) Focusing Mirror – Focusing mirror focuses the separated components of wavelength to planer surface, also known as focal plane.
e) Exit Slit – It is a focal plane to through which isolated beam of light takes exit from device.

Detector: Detector is a mechanical, electrical, or chemical device which is used to measure the change in one or other variables and give results in readable form. Different detectors can be used such as Photomultiplier tubes, photodiodes, charged coupled devices and many more.

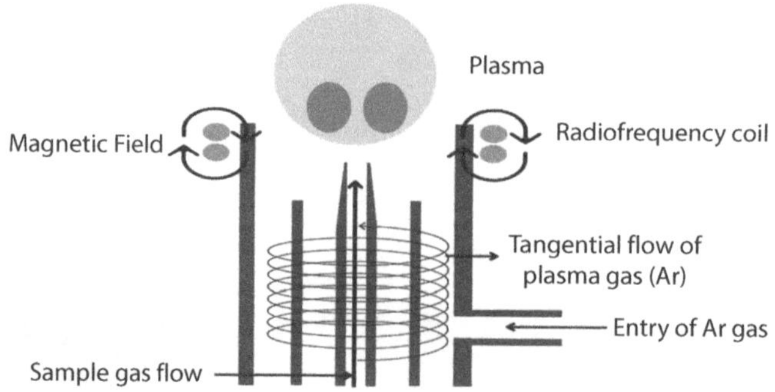

Figure 7.7 Diagram of ICP.

Amplifier: Amplifier is an electronic device which is used to enhance the magnitude of signal reached at the detector.

7.4.3 Working

Complete instrumentation of Plasma Absorption Spectroscopy has been explained in the previous section. The radiation comes from a hollow cathode bulb in the form of a beam of light towards the ICP ionization source where ionization of the sample takes place. After ionization of a sample, radiation of a certain wavelength is absorbed by the sample ions to get excited to higher energy levels. The radiation then passes through the monochromator to isolate desired wavelength at which absorption takes place. Desired wavelength is then detected by the detector. Amplifiers amplify the signal from the detector and the result is shown in the form of spectrum [26].

7.5 Analysis of Forensic Samples Using AAS and PAS

AAS has several applications and is still a well-liked choice for simple trace element research. Flame atomic absorption spectrometry (FAAS), which has obtained universal popularity in various areas, continues to be used in a number of industries due to its distinctive and specific advantages. Graphite furnace atomic absorption spectrometry is a well-known, deep rooted method for deciding the concentration of elements in parts per billion (ppb) with incredibly small sample sizes [27].

Inductively coupled plasma (ICP) and graphite furnace (GFAA) are other alternatives to flame-based AA/AE (ICP-AE or ICP-OES). The metallic sample is excited using the GFAA method in a furnace. This method has a lower threshold for metal detection than a flame AA/AE. Moreover, less sample volume is required for a GFAA. Plasma (a gas with charged ions) is used by ICP devices for the excitation procedure. Several of these tools can examine solid samples directly. ICP-AE instruments, sadly, produce data more slowly. Apart from these applications, there are various applications of AAS and ICP in forensic science which have been explained below:

7.5.1 Biological Samples and Matrices

Biological matrices and samples are very common in forensic science including blood, saliva, semen, urine, hairs and many more. AAS and PAS play a very important role in detection of various external constituents in these samples that can infer the reason of death of that individual.

ICP-OES is a useful method for detection of potential toxic metals, non-metals and trace elements such as Zn, Mn, Cu, B, Ba, Sr, Al, etc. in biological fluid and tissues obtained after autopsy [28].

Hairs are important evidence at crime scenes that can talk about drugs, heavy metals and medicine being taken a long time ago. It is very beneficial as compared to other biological samples like blood and urine as hairs open the gate for analysis after many years [29]. Lech *et al.*, conducted Thermal decomposition, amalgamation and AAS for detecting Hg in biological samples – blood, urine, hairs, bile, and vitreous humor. The LOD obtained for mercury found to be in the range of 0.10–0.20 μg/L [30]. Postuszny *et al.*, used electrothermal atomization – AAS for determination of Se in postmortem biological material obtained in case of acute Se poisoning. This method was easy to perform and time-efficient with a LOD value of Se-4.0 μg/L [31]. Ba is a toxic metal causing severe toxicity when found in concentration more than toxic level. It can be taken from drinking water, sometimes taken accidentally or even intentionally. Lech in her study utilized ICP-OES for detecting Ba in biological matrices including urine and blood. LOD and LOQ obtained for Ba were 0.11 and 0.4 μg/L [32]. Human bones and teeth are the evidence found in dangerous crime scenes and mass burial sites. Isotopic as well as elemental components of these materials helps in identification of individuals on the basis of their environmental exposure. ICP-SF-MS was used for elemental analysis of humerus and femur bones obtained from 12 different samples that can clearly discriminate between the samples [33]. In another study by Tofanelli *et al.*, Elemental analysis of bones was conducted by Laser-Induced Breakdown Spectroscopy (LIBS), followed by validation using ICP-OES [34]. In one of the studies, elemental composition of decomposing bone was done by measuring the concentration of a few elements such as Zn, P, Mg, K, Ba, Fe and Ca. This analysis helped in determining the time since death and the time since the bones have been present in soil [35].

ICP-MS is an important instrumentation technique used in clinical and forensic toxicology giving good reproducibility, accurate results with high sensitivity [36]. It can be used for analysis of multi-elementary metals and metalloids from biological matrices including blood, hair, urine and plasma. Single method was used as pre-treatment followed by determination using ICP-MS. This method leads to the identification of 27 elements in plasma and blood, 30 in urine and 32 in hair. LOQ of these methods depend on the element and ranged from 0.002 ng/mL to

8.1 ng/mL in blood, 0.2 pg/mg to 0.5 ng/mg for hair, 0.002 ng/mL to 7.7 ng/mL for plasma and 0.001 ng/mL to 2.2 ng/mL for urine [37].

Vitreous humor is the clear liquid that fills the space in our eyes. Vitreous humor is analyzed for trace elements and metals in forensic science for finding the cause of death and also to know the condition before death of an individual. Vazquez in his study analyzed vitreous humor in drowning cases using ICP-MS and ICP-OES for the detection of 14 elements. They conducted a comparative study for determination of elements using ICP-MS and ICP-OES and found that ICP-OES gives better results when liquid with high elemental concentration is analyzed whereas ICP-MS is more sensitive and can identify elements in low concentrations [38].

ICP-OES is also used to compare heavy metals concentration in body fluids. In one study done by Ahmed and others, ICP-OES was used to compare the occurrence of Cd and Pb in blood. The samples were first pretreated followed by their analysis. Validation of method was done after obtaining recovery, LOD, LOQ and linearity in acceptable range [39]. In another study, recovery of Pb and Cd from blood was compared using two extraction methods - Microwave digestion and Simple dilution digestion [40].

7.5.2 Drugs and Pharmaceutical Industry

Contamination and toxic substances might be present in drugs and pharmaceutical products including herbal medicine, medication drugs, infant formulas and many more. In one of the studies conducted by Gomez and others, leaves of plant *Hypericum perforatum*, used for treating depression, was analyzed for presence of trace elements using Electrothermal AAS and Ultrasonic Nebulization System-ICP-OES. Cr and Co were found to be above acceptable range whereas Al, Cd, Pb, and Fe were in acceptable range [41]. In another research, an anti-cancerous and anti-bacterial medicinal plant, *Tinnevelly Senna*, underwent spectrochemical analysis using LIBS followed by ICP-OES [42].

ICP-OES and AAS have been used for detection of purity in various pharmaceuticals preparation and generating impurity profiling [43].

ICP-OES was also used to determine elemental impurities in pharmaceutical tablets. In one research, a sample was prepared using Microwave-assisted acid digestion followed by instrumentation analysis using ICP-MS. The tablets were detected for the presence of many elements such as As, Cd, Fe, Mn, Mo and many more. LOD and LOQ obtained from this analysis was less than as mentioned in USP guidelines [44].

7.5.3 Forensic Medicine

Forensic medicine is the branch of forensic science that deals with the mode and manner of death of an individual. It also deals with injury caused by different ways including physical injury, burns, electrocution, drowning, etc. In one of the research projects conducted by Jakubeniene *et al.*, AAS was used to determine metals deposited in the electrical marks or injury caused by electrocution. Identification of traces of metal in electrocution injury using AAS has been a reliable method and the amount and type of metal depends on the impact of current duration and the type of wire coming in contact [45].

Hypothermia is a condition when a human body is exposed to low temperature for a longer period of time. Forensic medicine has always faced problems in identifying the cause of death in hypothermia cases. Jakubeniene *et al.*, in their study determined the concentration of Ca in post-mortem samples of liver, heart and skeletal muscles using Flame AAS [46].

In one of the researches conducted by Lech, a 14-year-old girl died suddenly in hospital while being treated for pains in hypogastrium. Blood and internal organs were analyzed for various trace elements using ICP-OES and Cold Vapour (CV)-AAS. A high level of mercury was found in the kidney and liver using ICP-OES and in blood and hair using CV AAS. From this study, it was concluded that ICP-OES can be used for screening of heavy metals in post-mortem samples and CV-AAS can be used for confirmation of heavy metals in blood [47].

7.5.4 Soil

Soil is important evidence in forensic science found in many cases including homicide, hit and run cases, sexual assault cases and many more. The presence of soil as evidence in most cases makes it important for its identification as constituents of soil act as a fingerprint for it. There are several constituents in soil that are similar in a given area and differ from the soil sample present in another area. Costley *et al.*, established the intensity of mercury in the soil samples utilizing Pyrolysis AAS with gold amalgamation with pyrolysis temperature of 750°C. This method did not require any treatment of the sample. It has an advantage of having no matrix interference with high accuracy and rapidity. The concentration of Hg obtained from this method was in the range of 0.035–7.06 mg/kg [48].

Maurya *et al.*, used AAS for relating the soil from a particular area with the heavy metals for the purpose of identification [49]. Moorthy in his research paper utilized AAS for soil profiling at Lamae district municipality ground, Chumphan city, Thailand to check the concentration of metallic ions like K, Na, Ca, Fe, Pb, Cu, Cr and Ca from varying depths and locations. This analysis concluded that the amount of ions vary from place to place and no two locations had similar amounts of ions [50]. In his other study, he used AAS for comparative study of subsoil profile at Golf ground of University, Malaysia for its application in forensic crime scene investigation [51].

In one of the studies, students identified the location of crime by collecting soil from the car of the suspect. They then picked up 7 soil samples from distances located near and far away from the crime scene. They found similarity in concentration of 22 elements (Co, Mg, Al, Fe, etc.) utilizing ICP-MS [52]. Soil contamination by heavy metals is an important aspect in forensic science. In one of the studies conducted by Brown *et al.*, soil samples from 3 locations – industrial, cemetery and control samples were collected from Windsor and Toronto, Ontario. Elemental composition of the soil was compared between these samples for the presence of As, Cd, Cu, Hg, Zn and other heavy metals using ICP-OES. The results showed that each location has its history and there was no relation of concentration of heavy metals with the type of land [53].

7.5.5 Explosives, Gunshot Residues, and Ammunition

Firearms and ammunition are other important forensic evidence found in crime scenes. This evidence are found in shooting cases, suicide and homicide cases. Krishnan in his research on investigation of Shooting cases analyzed 6 metals including Pb, Sn, As, Ba, Cu and Ag. This analysis helped in identification of hole of the bullet, the distance of shooter from the target, gunshot residue analysis and analysis of alloys and metals of ammunition [54]. Seltenhammer *et al.*, used AAS for analysis of Pb and Sb from GSR from 12 shots fired from 3 different firearms at varying distances on 3 surfaces including skin, cloth material and wood to check application of BTK3 [55]. The detection of GSR is becoming challenging due to varying composition of primers. Yuksel and others in their study generated elemental profiles of toxic as well as Pb-free primers that are commercially available in the Turkish ammunition market [56]. In another study conducted by Shrivastava *et al.*, a handheld device was developed for detection of Sb from GSR obtained in forensic cases. AAS was used for confirmation of presence of Antimony [57].

ICP-MS is a convincing tool in forensic science for determination of trace metals in very low concentrations up to ppm and ppb levels [58].

It is used for determination of GSR residues in shooting cases. In one of the studies, shooting was done on bare pork skin from varying distances. The swabbing of GSR was then taken for analysis using ICP-OES and ICP-MS resulting in maximum GSR was found in the case of firing range of 3 cm and then it decreased from 20 to 60 cm range [59].

7.5.6 Glass

Glass is a non-crystalline solid which is found in many forensic cases including robbery cases, burglary cases, hit and run cases, homicide cases, suicide cases and many more. Glass evidence from the crime scene is usually picked up for comparison purposes. For instance, broken glass pieces found at the crime scene can be compared with the known glass fragments obtained from the crime scene [60]. Elemental analysis of glass evidence provides details of constituents of the matter including trace metals, coloring reagents, binding reagents and many more. Buscaglia used many instrumental techniques such as X-ray fluorescence (XRF), ICP-AES, Flameless AAS and Energy Dispersive XRF for determination of elemental analysis of small glass fragments [61].

Laser ablation-ICP-MS has now become a mostly accepted method for examination of evidence in forensic science and its legal application [62]. In another study conducted by Trejos *et al.*, homogeneity in the elemental composition was analyzed in glass samples collected from various locations at crime scenes including containers, windows and windshields using ICP-MS [63].

7.5.7 Heavy Metals

There are various heavy metals that are present in the natural environment. The presence of these heavy metals can be detected in the body as well. The increase in concentration of these metals from a specific value causes toxicity in an individual causing rigorous symptoms and death of an individual.

AAS and PAS have been playing a valuable role in identification of these highly toxic metals in body, soil, water and food. Copper is one of the most commonly occurring heavy metals and its identification is important to know its toxicity. There are various methods available for detection of Cu but FAAS and ETAAS (Electrothermal AAS) have been efficient instruments for Cu detection in biological matrices. This method is less expensive, time efficient and more sensitive [64]. Tuzen *et al.*, used Furnace AAS for determination of heavy metals (Zn, Mn, Cu, etc.) in fish samples in the middle Black Sea (Turkey). They found good accuracy of the method and recovery of more than 95%. The level of heavy metals was less than the toxic level of these heavy metallic elements [65]. Heavy metals such as Zn, Cu, Mn, and many more catalyze various biological reactions inside a body cell that makes it important to determine the concentration of these metals to identify their roles in disease, human nutrition and regulatory functioning of the body. Falchuk, *et al.*, used AAS for determination of Zn in biological samples with ease of use, cost-efficiency and sensitivity [66]. Study conducted by Singhal, S.P., alloys were detected using AAS. Material of the bullet jacket was also identified using the instrument [67].

7.5.8 Environmental Samples

Geochemical analysis of samples helps forensic scientists to get data about the origin which helps in forensic crime scene investigation. In a study conducted by Carvalho *et al.*, geochemical data was obtained from 2 river beaches in Douro River, Portugal for elements including As, Cd, Cr, Mn, Zn, etc. using ICP-MS and ICP-OES. This geochemical study was useful in discriminating samples obtained from different areas but the elemental analysis in the same river does not show any significant changes over years [73].

7.5.9 Miscellaneous Samples

Trace elements are the material present in very small quantities. AAS and PAS are being used for their effective detection [68]. These instruments are rapid, sensitive, versatile and advanced [69]. Steel wires were forensically discriminated to detect the concentrations of trace elements using ICP-MS. The trace metal analysis can differentiate the origin of wires by comparing the elemental compositions. The samples were first extracted and then analyzed using ICP-MS for the presence of Cu, Cr, Mn, and Ni [70]. Cremains or cremated remains of humans are being contaminated. Due to this reason, these cremates are being analyzed for the presence of contamination. Brooks and others in their study took 88 known samples of concrete, cremains and its mixture and analyzed it using ICP-OES and identified 7 standard elements (V, Mn, Sr, Sb, Tl, Li, and B) [71]. AAS and ICP techniques play a huge role in determination of contamination and trace elements in agriculture crops and soil. In one of the studies, Rice grains were analyzed for determination of Zn concentration using ICP-OES and XRF. The results thus obtained were accurate, reliable and reproducible [72].

Consent for Publication

Consent of all authors

Conflict of Interest

No conflicts

Acknowledgement

All the authors have contributed to the chapter with interest.

References

1. J.W. Robinson, Atomic Absorption Spectroscopy. *Anal. Chem.*, 32 (1960) 17A-29A. https://doi.org/10.1021/ac60164a712.
2. N.R. Bader, Sample preparation for Flame Atomic Absorption Spectroscopy: An overview. *Rasayan J. Chem.*, 4 (2011) 49–55.
3. J.B. Willis, The determination of metals in blood serum by atomic absorption spectroscopy-I. *Spectrochim. Acta*, 16 (1960) 259–272. https://www.ufjf.br/baccan/files/2011/05/Willis-calcio.pdf.
4. J.B. Willis, Determination of Calcium and Magnesium in Urine by Atomic Absorption Spectroscopy. *Anal. Chem.*, 33 (1961) 556–559. https://doi.org/10.1021/ac60172a021.
5. W. Slavin, Atomic-Absortion Spectroscopy- a Critical Review. *Appl. Spectrosc.*, 20 (1996) 281–288. https://doi.org/https://opg.optica.org/as/abstract.cfm?URI=as-20-5-281.
6. S.R. Koirtyohann, A history of atomic absorption spectroscopy from an academic perspective. *Anal. Chem.*, 63 (1991) 1024A-1031A. https://doi.org/10.1021/ac00021a001.
7. W. Slavin, Atomic Absorption Spectroscopy- The present and Future. *Anal. Chem.*, 54 (1982) 685A-694A. https://doi.org/10.1021/ac00243a718.
8. B.V. L'vov, D.A. Katskov, L.P. Kruglikova, L.K. Polzik, Absolute analysis by flame atomic absorption spectroscopy: Present status and some problems. *Spectrochim Acta Part B At Spectrosc.*, 31 (1976) 49–80. https://doi.org/10.1016/0584-8547(76)80005-5.
9. S.C. Hight, J. Cheng, Determination of total mercury in seafood by cold vapor-atomic absorption spectroscopy (CVAAS) after microwave decomposition. *Food Chem.*, 91 (2005) 557–570. https://doi.org/10.1016/j.foodchem.2004.10.004.

10. M. Ghaedi, M.R. Fathi, A. Shokrollahi, F. Shajarat, Highly selective and Sensitive Preconcentration of Mercury Ion and Determination by Cold Vapor Atomic Absorption Spectroscopy. *Anal Lett.*, 39 (2006) 1171–1185. https://doi.org/https://doi.org/10.1080/00032710600622167.
11. A.R. Kumar, P. Riyazuddin, Mechanism of Volatile Hydride Formation and Their atomization in Hydride Generation Atomic Absorption Spectroscopy. *Anal. Sci.*, 21 (2005). https://www.jstage.jst.go.jp/article/analsci/21/12/21_12_1401/_pdf.
12. H.M. Anawar, Arsenic speciation in environmental samples by hydride generation and electrothermal atomic absorption spectrometry. *Talanta*, 88 (2012) 30–42. https://doi.org/10.1016/j.talanta.2011.11.068.
13. D.I. Bannon, C. Murashchik, C.R. Zapf, M.R. Farfel, J.J. Chisolm, Graphite Furnace Atomic Absorption Spectroscopic Measurement of Blood lead in Matrix-Matched Standards. *Clin. Chem*, 40 (1994) 1730–1734.
14. G.R. Carnrick, D.C. Manning, W. Slavin, Determination of selenium in biological materials with platform furnace atomic-absorption spectroscopy and Zeeman background correction. *Analyst*, 108 (1983) 1297. https://doi.org/10.1039/an9830801297.
15. W. Slavin, G.R. Carnrick, The possibility of standardless furnace atomic absorption spectroscopy. *Spectrochim. Acta Part B At Spectrosc.*, 39 (1984) 271–282. https://doi.org/10.1016/0584-8547(84)80035-X.
16. G.D. Christian, Meidicine, Trace Elements, and Atomic Absorption Spectroscopy. *Anal. Chem.*, 41 (1969) 24A-40A. https://doi.org/https://doi.org/10.1021/ac60270a719.
17. M.D. Amos, J.B. Willis, Use of high-temperature pre-mixed flames in atomic absorption spectroscopy. *Spectrochimica Acta*, 22 (1966) 1325–1343.
18. A.F. Lagalante, Atomic Absorption Spectroscopy: A Tutorial review, *Appl. Spectrosc. Rev.*, 34 (1999) 173–189. https://www.researchgate.net/profile/Anthony-Lagalante-2/publication/232974829_Atomic_Emission_Spectroscopy_A_Tutorial_Review/links/60b8d8f1458515218f87c828/Atomic-Emission-Spectroscopy-A-Tutorial-Review.pdf.
19. V.A. Fassel, V.G. Mossotti, W.L. Grossman, R.N. Kniseley, Evaluation of spectral continua as primary sources in atomic absorption spectroscopy. *Spectrochim. Acta*, 22 (1966) 347–357. https://doi.org/10.1016/0371-1951(66)80244-8.
20. W.W. Harrison, J.P. Yurachek, C.A. Benson, The determination of trace elements in human hair by atomic absorption spectroscopy. *Clin. Chim. Acta.*, 23 (1969) 83–91. https://doi.org/10.1016/0009-8981(69)90014-X.
21. S.A. Ruffolo, D. Barca, M. Alvarez de Buergo, M.F. La Russa, ICP-MS – Fundamentals and Application to Forensic Science, in: 2023: pp. 171–192. https://doi.org/10.1007/978-3-031-08834-6_6.
22. U. Fantz, Basics of plasma spectroscopy. *Plasma Sources Sci. Technol.*, 15 (2006) 137–147.

23. T. Fujimoto, Plasma Spectroscopy, in: Plasma Polarization Spectroscopy, Springer Berlin Heidelberg, Berlin, Heidelberg, n.d.: pp. 29–49. https://doi.org/10.1007/978-3-540-73587-8_3.
24. K.E. Jarvis, Handbook of Inductively Coupled Plasma Mass Spectrometry, 1991.
25. M.-H. Lee, C.-W. Chung, On the E to H and H to E transition mechanisms in inductively coupled plasma. *Phys. Plasmas.*, 13 (2006) 063510. https://doi.org/10.1063/1.2212387.
26. T. Okumura, Inductively Coupled Plasma Sources and Applications. *Physics Research International*, 2010 (2010) 1–14. https://doi.org/10.1155/2010/164249.
27. J.W. Robinson, Observations in atomic absorption spectroscopy. *Anal. Chim. Acta.*, 27 (1962) 465–469. https://doi.org/10.1016/S0003-2670(00)88539-6.
28. T. Lech, T. Lachowicz, APPLICATION OF ICP-OES TO MULTIELEMENT ANALYSIS OF BIOLOGICAL MATERIAL IN FORENSIC INORGANIC TOXICOLOGY. *Problems of Forensic Sciences*, (2009) 64–78.
29. M. Usman, A. Naseer, Y. Baig, T. Jamshaid, M. Shahwar, S. Khurshuid, Forensic toxicological analysis of hair: a review. *Egypt J. Forensic Sci.*, 9 (2019) 17. https://doi.org/10.1186/s41935-019-0119-5.
30. T. Lech, W. Turek, Application of TDA AAS to Direct Mercury Determination in Postmortem Material in Forensic Toxicology Examinations. *J. Anal. Toxicol.*, 43 (2019) 385–391. https://doi.org/10.1093/jat/bky107.
31. R. Wietecha-Posłuszny, T. Lech, P. Kościelniak, Application of Three Spectrometric Methods to Total Selenium Determination in Postmortem Material in a Case of Acute Selenium Compound Poisoning. *J. Forensic. Sci.*, 56 (2011) 518–521. https://doi.org/10.1111/j.1556-4029.2010.01660.x.
32. T. Lech, Application of ICP-OES to the Determination of Barium in Blood and Urine in Clinical and Forensic Analysis. *J. Anal. Toxicol.*, 37 (2013) 222–226. https://doi.org/10.1093/jat/bkt015.
33. W. Castro, J. Hoogewerff, C. Latkoczy, J.R. Almirall, Application of laser ablation (LA-ICP-SF-MS) for the elemental analysis of bone and teeth samples for discrimination purposes. *Forensic Sci. Int.*, 195 (2010) 17–27. https://doi.org/10.1016/j.forsciint.2009.10.029.
34. M. Tofanelli, L. Pardini, M. Borrini, F. Bartoli, A. Bacci, A. D'Ulivo, E. Pitzalis, M.C. Mascherpa, S. Legnaioli, G. Lorenzetti, S. Pagnotta, G. de Holanda Cavalcanti, M. Lezzerini, V. Palleschi, Spectroscopic analysis of bones for forensic studies. *Spectrochim. Acta Part B At Spectrosc.*, 99 (2014) 70–75. https://doi.org/10.1016/j.sab.2014.06.006.
35. S.J. Walden, J. Mulville, J.P. Rowlands, S.L. Evans, An Analysis of Systematic Elemental Changes in Decomposing Bone. *J. Forensic. Sci.*, 63 (2018) 207–213. https://doi.org/10.1111/1556-4029.13480.
36. J.-P. Goullé, E. Saussereau, L. Mahieu, M. Guerbet, Current role of ICP–MS in clinical toxicology and forensic toxicology: a metallic profile. *Bioanalysis*, 6 (2014) 2245–2259. https://doi.org/10.4155/bio.14.190.

37. J.-P. Goullé, L. Mahieu, J. Castermant, N. Neveu, L. Bonneau, G. Lainé, D. Bouige, C. Lacroix, Metal and metalloid multi-elementary ICP-MS validation in whole blood, plasma, urine and hair. *Forensic Sci. Int.*, 153 (2005) 39–44. https://doi.org/10.1016/j.forsciint.2005.04.020.
38. M. Vázquez, I. Ibarra, A. Sibón, M.D. Pérez-Cárceles, Multi-element Analysis of Vitreous Humor Samples by ICP-MS and ICP-OES. *At Spectrosc.*, 38 (2017) 124–132. https://doi.org/10.46770/AS.2017.05.002.
39. H.A.M. Ahmed, A.O. Alatawi, Comparison of the ICP OES viewing modes efficiency in the estimation of cadmium (Cd) and lead (Pb) in whole blood samples. *Arab J. Basic Appl. Sci.*, 29 (2022) 208–214. https://doi.org/10.1080/25765299.2022.2090148.
40. H. Ahmed, K.M.S. Almohammed, M.N. Janjua, N. Alhafez, Metals determination in the whole blood by ICP-OES: a comparison of two digestion procedures. *Int. J. Environ. Anal. Chem.*, (2022) 1–14. https://doi.org/10.1080/03067319.2022.2070011.
41. M.R. Gomez, S. Cerutti, L.L. Sombra, M.F. Silva, L.D. Martínez, Determination of heavy metals for the quality control in argentinian herbal medicines by ETAAS and ICP-OES. *Food Chem. Toxicol.*, 45 (2007) 1060–1064. https://doi.org/10.1016/j.fct.2006.12.013.
42. R.K. Aldakheel, M.A. Gondal, M.A. Almessiere, S. Rehman, M.M. Nasr, Z. Alsalem, F.A. Khan, Spectrochemical analysis using LIBS and ICP-OES techniques of herbal medicine (Tinnevelly Senna leaves) and its anti-cancerous/antibacterial applications. *Arab. J. Chem.*, 14 (2021) 103451. https://doi.org/10.1016/j.arabjc.2021.103451.
43. A.J. Majumdar, N. Dubey, Applications of inductively coupled plasma-atomic emission spectrometry (ICP-OES) in impurity profiling of Pharmaceuticals. *Int. J. Pharm. Life Sci.*, 8 (2017) 5420–5425.
44. C. Støving, H. Jensen, B. Gammelgaard, S. Stürup, Development and validation of an ICP-OES method for quantitation of elemental impurities in tablets according to coming US pharmacopeia chapters, *J. Pharm. Biomed. Anal.*, 84 (2013) 209–214. https://doi.org/10.1016/j.jpba.2013.06.007.
45. M. Jakubeniene, A. Zakaras, Z.N. Minkuviene, A. Benoshys, Application of atomic absorption spectroscopy for detection of multimetal traces in low-voltage electrical marks. *Forensic Sci. Int.*, 161 (2006) 36–40. https://doi.org/10.1016/j.forsciint.2005.10.019.
46. M. Jakubeniene, A. Irnius, G.A. Chaker, J.M. Paliulis, A. Bechelis, Post-mortem investigation of calcium content in liver, heart, and skeletal muscle in accidental hypothermia cases. *Forensic Sci. Int.*, 190 (2009) 87–90. https://doi.org/10.1016/j.forsciint.2009.05.017.
47. T. Lech, ICP OES and CV AAS in determination of mercury in an unusual fatal case of long-term exposure to elemental mercury in a teenager. *Forensic Sci. Int.*, 237 (2014) e1–e5. https://doi.org/10.1016/j.forsciint.2014.02.015.

48. C.T. Costley, K.F. Mossop, J.R. Dean, L.M. Garden, J. Marshall, J. Carroll, Determination of mercury in environmental and biological samples using pyrolysis atomic absorption spectrometry with gold amalgamation. *Anal. Chim. Acta.*, 405 (2000) 179–183. https://doi.org/10.1016/S0003-2670(99)00742-4.
49. A. Maurya, L. Kesharwani, M.K. Mishra, Analysis of Heavy Metal in Soil through Atomic Absorption Spectroscopy for Forensic Consideration. *International Journal for Research in Applied Science & Engineering Technology (IJRASET)*, 6 (2018).
50. T.N. Moorthy, Study on subsoil profile analysis at Lamae district municipality ground, Chumphon city, Thailand by atomic absorption spectroscopy for forensic application. *International Research Symposium on Pure and Applied Sciences* (IRSPAS), (2018).
51. N.T. Moorthy, A Comparative study of subsoil profile at the Southern end of the golf ground of university Sains Malaysia, Health Campus, Kubang Kerian by Atomic Absorption Spectroscopy- Potential application in Forensic Crime Investigation. *Buletin Penyelidikan Pusat Pengajian Sains Perubatan*, 7 (2007).
52. L. Reidy, K. Bu, M. Godfrey, J. V. Cizdziel, Elemental fingerprinting of soils using ICP-MS and multivariate statistics: A study for and by forensic chemistry majors. *Forensic Sci. Int.*, 233 (2013) 37–44. https://doi.org/10.1016/j.forsciint.2013.08.019.
53. E. Brown, P. Jasra, Estimation of Heavy Metal concentrations in soil for use in Forensic Investigations. *Journal of Emerging Forensic Sciences Research*, 1 (2016).
54. S.S. Krishnan, Trace Element Analysis by Atomic Absorption Spectrometry and Neutron Activation Analysis in the Investigation of Shooting Cases. *Can. Soc. Forensic Sci. J.*, 6 (1973) 55–77. https://doi.org/10.1080/00085030.1973.10757303.
55. M.H. Seltenhammer, C. Fitzl, I. Wieser, R. Binder, P. Paula, D.U. Risser, Does the Prior Application of the Field Kit Bullet Hole Testing Kit 3 on a Suspected Bullet Hole Bias the Analysis of Atomic Absorption Spectrophotometry?. *J. Forensic. Sci.*, 59 (2014) 1364–1367. https://doi.org/10.1111/1556-4029.12530.
56. B. Yüksel, N. Şen, G.I. Ögünç, A. Erdoğan, Elemental profiling of toxic and modern primers using ICP-MS, SEM-EDS, and XPS: an application in firearm discharge residue investigation. *Aust. J. Forensic Sci.*, 55 (2023) 529–546. https://doi.org/10.1080/00450618.2022.2043436.
57. P. Shrivastava, B.P. Singh, S.K. Jain, V.K. Jain, S. Nagpal, Novel Hand-Held Device for Detecting Antimony (Sb3+) in Gunshot Residue for Forensic Application. *SSRN Electronic Journal*, (2022). https://doi.org/10.2139/ssrn.4118358.
58. S.A. Ruffolo, D. Barca, M. Alvarez de Buergo, M.F. La Russa, ICP-MS – Fundamentals and Application to Forensic Science, in: 2023: pp. 171–192. https://doi.org/10.1007/978-3-031-08834-6_6.

59. D. Merli, A. Amadasi, D. Mazzarelli, A. Cappella, E. Castoldi, S. Ripa, L. Cucca, C. Cattaneo, A. Profumo, Comparison of Different Swabs for Sampling Inorganic Gunshot Residue from Gunshot Wounds: Applicability and Reliability for the Determination of Firing Distance. *J. Forensic. Sci.*, 64 (2019) 558–564. https://doi.org/10.1111/1556-4029.13870.
60. B.W. Kammrath, A.C. Koutrakos, M.E. McMahon, J.A. Reffner, The Forensic Analysis of Glass Evidence: Past, Present, and Future, in: *Forensic Sci*, Wiley-VCH Verlag GmbH & Co. KGaA, Weinheim, Germany, 2016: pp. 299–336. https://doi.org/10.1002/9783527693535.ch14.
61. J.A. Buscaglia, Elemental analysis of small glass fragments in forensic science. *Anal. Chim. Acta.*, 288 (1994) 17–24. https://doi.org/10.1016/0003-2670(94)85112-3.
62. J.R. Almirall, T. Trejos, Applications of LA–ICP–MS to Forensic Science. *Elements*, 12 (2016) 335–340. https://doi.org/10.2113/gselements.12.5.335.
63. T. TREJOS, J. ALMIRALL, Sampling strategies for the analysis of glass fragments by LA-ICP-MSPart I. Micro-homogeneity study of glass and its application to the interpretation of forensic evidence. *Talanta*, 67 (2005) 388–395. https://doi.org/10.1016/j.talanta.2005.01.042.
64. M.A. Sevenson, 26. Measurement of copper in biological samples by flame or electrothermal atomic absorption spectrometry, in: 1988: pp. 351–357. https://doi.org/10.1016/0076-6879(88)58066-7.
65. M. Tüzen, Determination of heavy metals in fish samples of the middle Black Sea (Turkey) by graphite furnace atomic absorption spectrometry. *Food Chem.*, 80 (2003) 119–123. https://doi.org/10.1016/S0308-8146(02)00264-9.
66. K.H. Falchuk, K.L. Hilt, B.L. Vallee, 33. Determination of zinc in biological samples by atomic absorption spectrometry, in: 1988: pp. 422–434. https://doi.org/10.1016/0076-6879(88)58073-4.
67. S.P. Singhal, Atomic Absorption Spectroscopy in Forensic Chemistry. *Can. Soc. Forensic Sci. J.*, 7 (1974) 7–17. https://doi.org/10.1080/00085030.1974.10757203.
68. G.H. Morrison, T.H. Risby, Elemental Trace Analysis of Biological Materials. *C R C Critical Reviews in Analytical Chemistry*, 8 (1979) 287–320. https://doi.org/10.1080/10408347908542713.
69. S.R. Khan, B. Sharma, P.A. Chawla, R. Bhatia, Inductively Coupled Plasma Optical Emission Spectrometry (ICP-OES): a Powerful Analytical Technique for Elemental Analysis. *Food Anal. Methods*, 15 (2022) 666–688. https://doi.org/10.1007/s12161-021-02148-4.
70. H. Ohsaki, K. Murakami, M. Kasamatsu, Y. Suzuki, S. Suzuki, Forensic Discrimination of Steel Wires by Quantitative Elemental Analysis with ICP-MS. *Japanese Journal of Forensic Science and Technology*, 14 (2009) 71–75. https://doi.org/10.3408/jafst.14.71.
71. T.R. Brooks, T.E. Bodkin, G.E. Potts, S.A. Smullen, Elemental Analysis of Human Cremains Using ICP-OES to Classify Legitimate and

Contaminated Cremains. *J. Forensic. Sci.,* 51 (2006) 967–973. https://doi.org/10.1111/j.1556-4029.2006.00209.x.

72. S. Sultana, H.A. Khatun, M. Faruquee, M.M.U. Islam, H.J. Tonny, M.R. Islam, Comparison between Acid Digestion (ICP-OES) and X-ray Fluorescence (XRF) Spectrometry for Zinc Concentration Determination in Rice (Oryza sativa L.). *Foods,* 12 (2023) 1044. https://doi.org/10.3390/foods12051044.
73. Áurea Madureira-Carvalho, Helena Ribeiro, Gareth Newman, Mark J. Brewer, Alexandra Guedes, Ilda Abreu, Fernando Noronha, Lorna Dawson, Geochemical analysis of sediment samples for forensic purposes: characterisation of two river beaches from the Douro River, Portugal. https://doi.org/10.1080/00450618.2018.1533037

8

Application of Gas Chromatography in Criminalistics

Ankit Singh[1*] **and Namrata Singh**[2]

[1]*Division of Forensic Science, School of Basic & Applied Sciences, Galgotias University, Greater Noida, U.P., India*
[2]*Department of Paramedical Sciences, IIAHSR, Integral University, Lucknow, U.P., India*

Abstract

Gas chromatography (GC) is a widely employed analytical method in the field of forensic science, serving various purposes. It finds application in the analysis of drugs, investigations related to arson, the examination of explosives, and the scrutiny of minute pieces of evidence like fibers, paint, and glass. Gas Chromatography proves to be a potent instrument for both identifying and quantifying drugs present in biological samples, and when combined with mass spectrometry (MS), it offers exceptionally precise and sensitive drug detection capabilities. Furthermore, this technique is instrumental in the scrutiny of trace evidence such as fibers, paint, and glass, providing valuable insights for criminal investigations, including details about the material's composition, its origin, and potential connections between suspects and crime scenes. GC coupled with MS, FID, or IR provides highly specific and sensitive detection of drugs, accelerants, explosives, and trace evidence, making it a critical tool in criminal investigations. The applications of GC in forensic science continue to evolve, and the use of this technique is likely to increase in the future.

Keywords: Chromatography, GC, criminalistics, trace-evidence analysis, HRGC, fast GC, GCxGC

**Corresponding author*: ankitsingh@galgotiasuniversity.edu.in

Priyanka Chhabra, Divya Bajpai Tripathy, Anjali Gupta, Rajeev Kumar, Kajol Bhati and Shruti Shukla (eds.) Advances in Analytical Techniques for Forensic Investigation, (215–240) © 2024 Scrivener Publishing LLC

8.1 Introduction

Separation techniques play a critical role in forensic investigations as they are used to separate and identify individual components within complex mixtures. Chromatography, Electrophoresis, Spectroscopy, Mass spectrometry, and Microscopy are some of the specific applications of separation techniques in forensic investigations. Overall, separation techniques are essential in forensic investigations as they provide valuable information about the composition and source of different types of evidence. By using a combination of separation techniques, forensic investigators can obtain a more complete picture of the evidence and use this information to identify suspects and solve crimes.

Gas chromatography has emerged as an indispensable tool in forensic science, aiding investigators in solving crimes and unravelling complex chemical compositions of various substances. One of the most effective chromatographic methods is Gas Chromatography, which is widely used in the fields of forensics and criminalistics to separate and analyze complex mixtures such as drugs, explosives and biological fluids in forensic investigations. Drug analysis, Explosive analysis, Forensic Toxicology Arson Investigation, and Food & Beverage Analysis are some of the specific applications of chromatography techniques in forensic investigations [1].

8.1.1 Evolution of Gas Chromatography

Chromatography originated in the early 20th century when the Russian botanist Mikhail S. Tswett used glass columns filled with calcium carbonate to separate plant pigments. It was not until the middle of the century that the technique was applied to the development of paper chromatography, high-performance liquid chromatography, and gas chromatography [2].

Gas Chromatography (GC) has a long history dating back to 1903 when Mikhail Semenovich Tswett developed the first chromatography method using a glass tube packed with calcium carbonate. In the 1940s and 1950s, advancements in column technology led to the development of new chromatographic methods. The introduction of paper chromatography and thin-layer chromatography allowed for the separation of a wider range of compounds, including amino acids, sugars, and steroids. Archer John Porter Martin and Richard Laurence Millington Synge developed the first gas-liquid chromatography (GLC) method in 1941. Erika Cremer invented the first capillary column in 1952, and James Lovelock and Albert

J. Seymour developed the most widely used flame ionization detector in 1953. Anthony T. James and A.T. G. James developed the first packed capillary column in 1957. In the 1960s, the development of gas chromatography (GC) and high-performance liquid chromatography (HPLC) revolutionized chromatography. GC uses a gas as the mobile phase, while HPLC uses a liquid. Both techniques allow for the separation and analysis of a wide range of compounds and have become critical tools in many areas of research and industry [2].

However, the development of high-performance liquid chromatography (HPLC) and other separation techniques led to a decline in GC use. Advances in technology, such as fused silica capillary columns and mass spectrometry detectors, have revived interest in GC in recent decades. Thus, the history of chromatography has been characterized by continual advancements in column technology, detection, and automation. These advancements have led to the development of new chromatographic methods, and have allowed for the separation and analysis of a wider range of compounds with greater accuracy and precision. Today, chromatography is a critical tool in many areas of research and industry, including pharmaceuticals, food science, and environmental science.

8.2 Gas Chromatography

Gas chromatography (GC) is an analytical separation technique that is used to separate and identify the components of a mixture. GC is based on the principle that different compounds have different affinities for a stationary phase and a mobile phase. In GC, a sample is vaporized and injected into a column packed with a stationary phase, which separates the components of the sample based on their affinity for the stationary phase. The separated components are then detected and quantified using a detector, such as a flame ionization detector (FID) or a mass spectrometer (MS) [3].

Gas Chromatography is a leading technique for organic analytical separations, with a broad range of applications spanning from natural compounds, environmental studies, and forensics to the petroleum/petrochemical industry. GC has enabled the rapid detection of previously unidentified components in complex mixtures, as well as the identification of trace chemicals that were previously unknown [4]. The emergence of hyphenated methods such as GC-MS, GC-MS-MS, GC-HS, GC-FT-IR, and GC-TGA-FT-IR, which have significantly enlarged the applications range of GC, has provided the biggest impetus to the evolution of gas chromatography. Today, GC is a widely used technique in many fields, including chemistry, biology, environmental science, and forensics. It is used to separate and analyze a wide range of compounds, from small molecules like gases and volatile organic compounds (VOCs) to complex biomolecules like proteins and peptides [5].

8.3 Principle of Gas Chromatography

The principle of Gas Chromatography (GC) is based on the separation of the individual components of a mixture based on their differences in partitioning between a stationary phase and a mobile phase. In GC, a sample is vaporized and introduced into the instrument's inlet, where it is mixed with a carrier gas such as helium or nitrogen. The sample is then injected into a long, thin, and coiled column that is packed with a stationary phase, typically a liquid or a polymer, which is coated onto the surface of the column. The mobile phase (carrier gas) carries the sample through the column, where the different components of the mixture interact differently with the stationary phase, resulting in their separation [4].

The separation of the mixture occurs due to two different processes: adsorption and partition. In adsorption, the stationary phase is typically a solid material, and the sample components adhere to its surface through intermolecular forces. In partition, the stationary phase is typically a liquid that coats the surface of the column packing material. The sample components partition between the stationary phase and the mobile phase based on their solubility in each phase. Components that are more soluble polar in the stationary phase will spend more time interacting with it and will take longer to travel through the column. Components that are insoluble in the mobile phase or non-polar components will travel through the column more quickly [5]. The separation process occurs as the sample components travel through the column at different rates, based on their interactions with the stationary and mobile phases. As the components pass through the column, they are detected by a detector, such as a flame ionization detector (FID), a thermal conductivity detector (TCD), or a mass spectrometer (MS), which produces a signal proportional to the amount of each component present. The output of the detector is recorded and analyzed to determine the identity and quantity of the individual components in the sample [6].

GC is a really good chemical analyzer that is great for looking at volatile and semi-vaporized compounds, like organic compounds and gasses. GC can be used to separate and identify a wide range of compounds, including small molecules, large biomolecules, and complex mixtures of organic compounds [7].

8.4 Instrumentation of Gas Chromatography

The instrumentation of Gas Chromatography (GC) typically consists of the following components (Figure 8.1)

Injection port: The injection port is where the sample is introduced into the GC system. The sample is typically injected using a syringe or an autosampler. Injectors are used to inject samples into the carrier gas stream at a consistent volume. In order to maintain a high degree of precision, injection must be inert and reproducible. Injectors must be able to handle tiny amounts on the order of microliters with the greatest accuracy [8].

Column: The column is a long, thin, and coiled tube that is packed with a stationary phase, typically a liquid or a polymer, which is coated onto the surface of the column. The mobile phase (carrier gas) carries the sample through the column, where the different components of the mixture interact differently with the stationary phase, resulting in their separation. Gas Chromatography columns can be categorized as short-length (1.5-2m) stainless steel or long-length (30m or greater) glass columns. Capillary columns are made up of flexible fused silica tubing and are coated with an absorbent phase layer on the interior wall of the capillary tube, whereas packed columns are filled with the stationary phase. It is essential to carefully maintain the column according to the supplier's specifications to ensure long-term usage and consistent separations run after run, as it is an important component of the system [9].

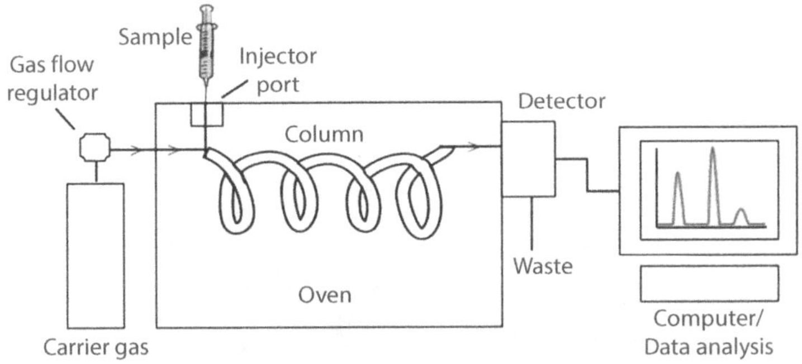

Figure 8.1 A simple diagrammatic representation of gas chromatography [53].

Oven: The column is housed in an oven (as shown in Figure 8.2), which allows the temperature of the column to be controlled. Temperature control is important for achieving optimal separation of the sample components.
Carrier gas supply: The carrier gas is typically helium or nitrogen, and is used to transport the sample through the column. The gas is supplied from a high-pressure cylinder and is regulated using a flow controller. It is important to ensure that any residual moisture or other gaseous impurities are removed with care in Gas Chromatography to prevent potential interference with the accuracy of the results.
Detector: The detector is used to measure the amount of each component that is eluted from the column. There are several types of detectors used in GC, including flame ionization detectors (FID), thermal conductivity detectors (TCD), and mass spectrometers (MS).
Data acquisition system: After passing through the detector, the output is recorded and analyzed using a data acquisition system, which can range from a simple chart recorder to a more advanced computer-based data acquisition and analysis system. Modern Gas Chromatography systems are typically computer-based, with software that controls operating factors such as carrier gas flow rate, temperature programming, injection volume, and sequence, as well as data collection and processing.
Software: The software is used to control the instrument and to analyze the data. It allows the user to set up the method parameters, such as injection volume, column temperature, and detector settings, as well as to process and analyze the data.

The choice of column, detector, and data system depends on the specific application and the properties of the sample being analyzed. Columns can

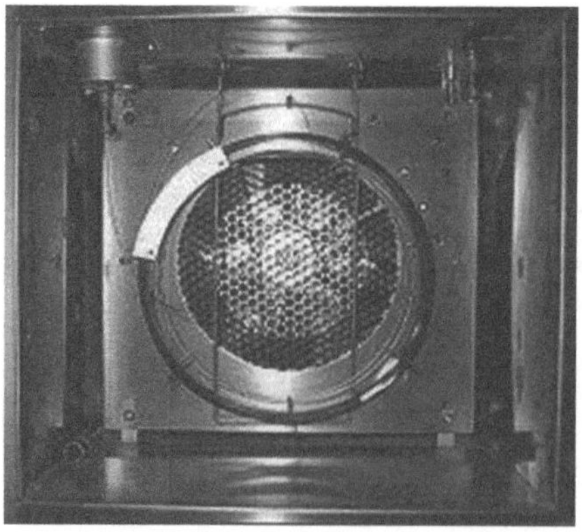

Figure 8.2 Column oven [54].

be packed or capillary, while detectors can be flame ionization, thermal conductivity, or mass spectrometry. The data system can be used to generate a chromatogram, which is a graphical representation of the separation of the components in the sample [10]. GC systems can be either gas-solid chromatography (GSC) or gas-liquid chromatography (GLC). In GSC, the stationary phase is a solid material, and the sample components adhere to its surface through intermolecular forces. In GLC, the stationary phase is a liquid that coats the surface of the column packing material. The sample components partition between the stationary phase and the mobile phase based on their solubility in each phase. GLC is the more common type of GC used in analytical laboratories [11–13].

8.5 Advancement in Gas Chromatography Technique

Gas chromatography (GC) has undergone significant advancements in recent years, improving its accuracy, efficiency, and versatility in various analytical applications [14, 15].

8.5.1 High-Resolution GC

High-resolution gas chromatography (HRGC) is a powerful analytical technique that allows for the separation and identification of complex mixtures with high precision and accuracy [16, 17]. HRGC achieves this by using columns with smaller particle sizes, which results in improved resolution, sensitivity, and peak capacity compared to traditional GC [18–20].

The HRGC system typically consists of a gas chromatograph with a high-resolution column, a sample inlet system, a detector, and a data acquisition system. The sample is introduced into the system through the sample inlet, where it is vaporized and carried by an inert gas such as helium or nitrogen into the column. The column is typically coated with a stationary phase that interacts with the sample components, causing them to separate based on their physical and chemical properties. As the sample components elute from the column, they are detected and quantified by the detector, which converts the signals into a chromatogram. HRGC can be used for the analysis of a wide range of compounds, including volatile and semi-volatile organic compounds, pesticides, drugs, and environmental contaminants. The technique is particularly useful for the analysis of trace compounds in complex matrices, such as environmental samples, foods, and pharmaceuticals. HRGC can separate compounds that are present in very small amounts, often at concentrations as low as parts per billion (ppb) or even parts per trillion (ppt) [21].

The key advantage of HRGC over traditional GC is its ability to separate compounds with similar physical and chemical properties. Traditional GC columns are typically packed with particles ranging in size from 2 to 5 μm, which limits their resolving power. HRGC columns, on the other hand, use particles that are smaller than 01 μm, which improves resolution and peak capacity. HRGC can also use columns with multiple stationary phases, such as polar and non-polar phases, which further enhances selectivity [22].

The major applications of HRGC include environmental analysis, forensic science, petrochemical analysis, and food analysis. HRGC is widely used in the analysis of environmental contaminants, such as pesticides, herbicides, and industrial chemicals, in soil, water, and air samples. In forensic science, HRGC is used to analyze trace evidence, such as arson residues, explosives, and drugs. In petrochemical analysis, HRGC is used to analyze the composition of crude oil and refined products. In food analysis, HRGC is used to identify and quantify flavor and fragrance compounds, as well as contaminants such as pesticides and mycotoxins [23]. HRGC is a powerful analytical technique that allows for the separation and identification of complex mixtures with high precision and accuracy. The technique is widely used in various industries, including environmental science, forensic science, petrochemical analysis, and food analysis, and has led to significant advancements in our understanding of complex mixtures. The continued development of HRGC technology is expected to further expand its applications and improve its sensitivity, resolution, and speed [24].

8.5.2 Fast GC

Fast GC (gas chromatography) is a technique that utilizes specialized columns and injection techniques to reduce the analysis time from several hours to just a few minutes. This technique is particularly useful for high-throughput analysis, where a large number of samples need to be analyzed quickly [25]. The traditional GC analysis involves using long, narrow columns with small particle sizes to separate and detect the different components of a sample. However, this can take several hours to complete, which can be a major bottleneck in industries such as food and beverage, pharmaceuticals, and environmental science. Fast GC utilizes shorter columns with larger particle sizes and higher flow rates to increase the analysis speed. The faster flow rate means that the sample components spend less time in the column, resulting in faster separations. Additionally, fast GC often uses specialized injection techniques, such as splitless injection or cold on-column injection, to ensure that the sample is rapidly vaporized and introduced into the column [23].

One of the main advantages of fast GC is the reduced analysis time, which allows for higher sample throughput and faster results. This makes it ideal for routine quality control testing, where large numbers of samples need to be analyzed quickly. It also reduces the risk of sample degradation or contamination during the analysis process. Another advantage of fast GC is that it can increase the sensitivity of the analysis. This is because the faster analysis times can reduce the chance of peak broadening, which can reduce the resolution of the separation. Additionally, fast GC can reduce the amount of solvent required for the analysis, which can improve the sensitivity and reduce the environmental impact of the analysis. Fast GC is a prevailing analytical tool that can significantly reduce analysis time while maintaining high resolution and sensitivity. It has applications in a wide range of industries and is particularly useful for high-throughput analysis, where speed and efficiency are crucial [26].

8.5.3 Multidimensional GC

Multidimensional gas chromatography (GCxGC) is an analytical technique that enhances the resolution and selectivity of traditional gas chromatography (GC). GCxGC involves the use of two or more chromatographic columns with different stationary phases, arranged in a series, to separate complex mixtures into individual components [27]. The first-dimension column separates the sample mixture into individual components based on their volatility and interactions with the stationary phase. The individual components are then transferred to the second-dimension column, which separates the components based on their polarities and interactions with the second stationary phase. The resulting two-dimensional separation provides a much higher resolution and peak capacity than traditional GC, allowing for the detection of trace components and the identification of complex mixtures [50]. GCxGC can be coupled with various detectors, including flame ionization detectors (FID), mass spectrometry (MS), and sulfur chemiluminescence detectors (SCD), depending on the application. The most commonly used detector is MS, which provides a high level of sensitivity and specificity for compound identification [24].

GCxGC is widely used in various fields, including petrochemicals, environmental analysis, food and beverage, and pharmaceuticals. In the petrochemical industry, GCxGC is used to analyze complex hydrocarbon

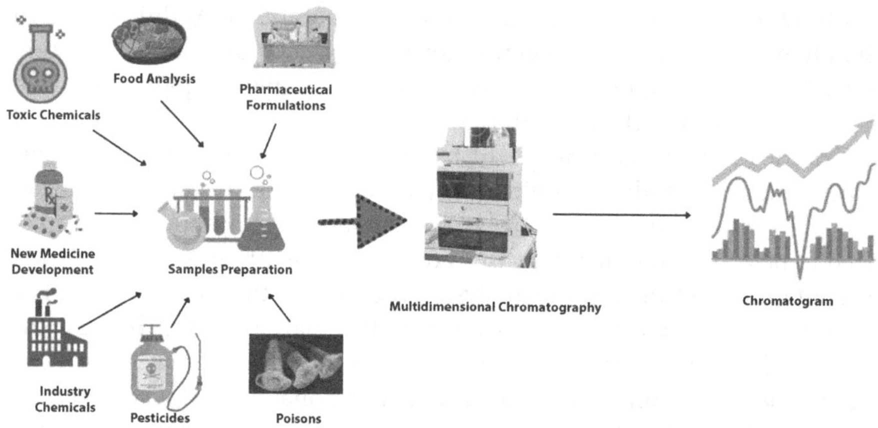

Figure 8.3 Applications of multidimensional GC [56].

mixtures and to detect trace impurities in crude oil, gasoline, and other petroleum products. In environmental analysis, GCxGC is used to identify and quantify trace levels of pollutants and contaminants in soil, water, and air samples. In the food and beverage industry, GCxGC is used to analyze complex flavor and aroma profiles in wine, coffee, and other products. In pharmaceuticals, GCxGC is used to analyze complex drug formulations and to identify impurities and degradation products [50]. GCxGC is a prominent analytical tool that provides enhanced resolution and selectivity, making it an ideal technique for analyzing complex mixtures in various fields. Its ability to detect trace components and identify complex mixtures makes it a valuable tool in research, quality control, and regulatory compliance (as represent in Figure 8.3) [27].

8.5.4 Mass Spectrometry (MS) Detection

Mass spectrometry (MS) detection is a technique that can be coupled with gas chromatography (GC) to provide enhanced compound identification and quantification. The combination of GC-MS allows for the analysis of volatile and semi-volatile compounds with high sensitivity and specificity. MS detection in GC works by separating compounds based on their chemical and physical properties using GC, and then detecting and analyzing them using MS. In this technique, the separated compounds are ionized, typically by electron impact or chemical ionization, to produce ions that are then separated by their mass-to-charge ratio using a mass analyzer.

The resulting mass spectrum is a unique "fingerprint" of the compound, which can be used to identify the compound and quantify its concentration in the sample [28].

The benefits of using MS detection in GC include:

Enhanced sensitivity: MS detection can detect compounds at very low concentrations, even in complex matrices. The high sensitivity of MS allows for the detection of trace levels of impurities, degradation products, and contaminants in samples.

Increased specificity: The mass spectrum produced by MS provides unique information about the molecular structure of the compounds, allowing for their identification with high specificity. This is particularly useful when analyzing complex mixtures of compounds, where traditional GC detectors may not be able to differentiate between them.

Quantification: MS detection in GC can be used to quantify the concentration of compounds in a sample, allowing for accurate determination of their levels. This is particularly useful for monitoring product quality and safety in industries such as food and pharmaceuticals.

Structural information: MS detection can provide information about the structure of the compounds, such as their molecular weight, fragmentation patterns, and functional groups. This information can be used to identify unknown compounds and elucidate reaction pathways. Thus, MS detection in GC is a significant analytical technique that has revolutionized the field of chemical analysis. The combination of GC-MS allows for the analysis of a wide range of compounds, making it a valuable tool in various fields, including environmental science, forensic science, pharmaceuticals, and food and beverage analysis [25].

8.6 Miniaturization and Automation in GC

Miniaturization and automation are two significant advancements in GC that have revolutionized the field of analytical chemistry. These advancements have enhanced the repeatability of GC analysis as well as its efficiency and sample consumption.

8.6.1 Miniaturization

The miniaturization of GC instruments involves using smaller columns, lower sample volumes, and reduced gas flow rates, which allows for faster analysis times and increased sensitivity. The miniaturization of GC has resulted in the development of microscale GC or micro-GC, which is a miniaturized GC system that is capable of analyzing small samples or performing high-throughput analysis. Micro-GC uses small columns with low sample volume requirements, which allows for the analysis of samples that were previously too small to be analyzed with conventional GC systems Micro-GC is particularly useful in industries such as pharmaceuticals and food and beverage, where rapid analysis of small samples is required. In addition, the miniaturization of GC instruments has also led to the development of portable GC systems, which are compact, lightweight, and easily transportable, making them ideal for field analysis [26].

8.6.2 Automation

The automation of GC instruments involves the use of robotic systems for sample preparation and injection, which reduces human error, increases efficiency, and improves the reproducibility of GC analysis. Automated sample preparation systems can extract, purify, and concentrate samples, making them ready for analysis. Automated injection systems ensure that the sample is injected accurately and reproducibly into the GC system. The automation of GC instruments has led to increased sample throughput, reduced sample consumption, and improved precision and accuracy. In addition, automated GC systems are less labor-intensive, which reduces the workload of the analyst and increases productivity. Automated GC systems are widely used in the pharmaceutical, environmental, and food and beverage industries, where large numbers of samples need to be analyzed rapidly and accurately [27].

In conclusion, miniaturization and automation are two significant advancements in GC that have transformed the field of analytical chemistry. The miniaturization of GC instruments has led to the development of micro-GC systems and portable GC systems, which have improved the efficiency and sensitivity of GC analysis. The automation of GC instruments has led to increased throughput, reduced sample consumption, and improved precision and accuracy, making GC analysis more reliable and efficient.

8.7 Application of Gas Chromatography in Criminalistics

The forensic use of GC is growing rapidly because of its ability to separate and analyze complex mixtures of compounds found in a variety of forensic

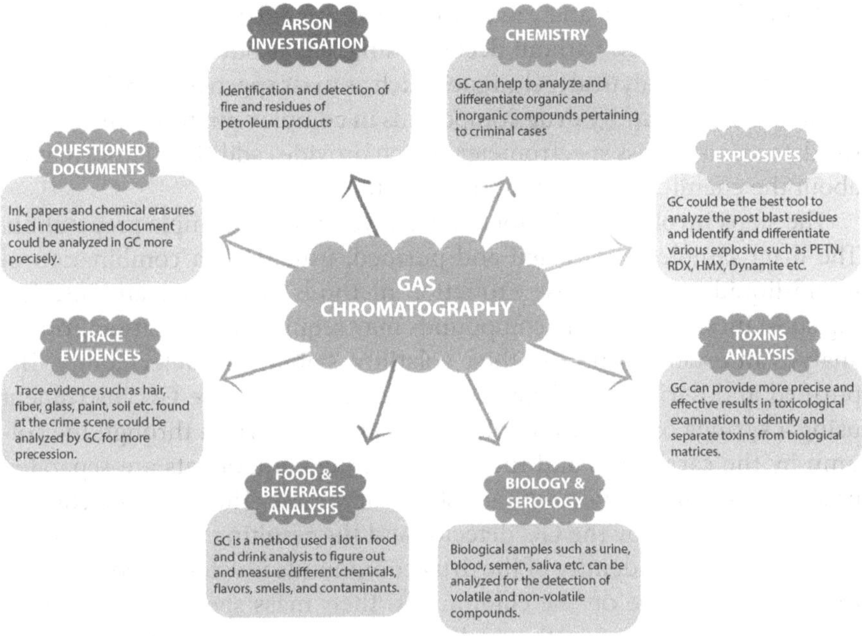

Figure 8.4 Use of GC in various fields of criminology [28].

samples (Figure 8.4). In forensic investigations, GC can be used to analyze trace evidence found at crime scenes, such as fibers, paint, and glass fragments, to identify the source or origin of the material. It can also be used to analyze blood and urine samples to detect drugs or toxins present in the body. GC is a highly sensitive technique that has been used in forensic science for decades. It is used to identify and quantify compounds in a sample, such as drugs, explosives, and volatile organic compounds (VOCs) [1, 28].

8.7.1 Drug Analysis Using GC

One of the main applications of GC in forensic science is the analysis of drugs. GC can identify and quantify drugs such as cocaine, heroin, and methamphetamine in blood, urine, hair, and other biological samples. GC can identify the purity of the drugs and determine if they have been adulterated with other substances. This information can be used to determine the source of the drugs and can help law enforcement agencies in their investigations [30]. In both forensic and pharmaceutical research, gas chromatography (GC) is frequently employed for drug analysis. GC is particularly useful for analyzing drugs that are volatile, thermally stable, and can be vaporized without decomposing. GC is often used in conjunction with other analytical techniques, such as mass spectrometry (GC-MS), to identify and quantify drug compounds in complex mixtures. In GC-MS, the detector is a mass spectrometer, which provides additional information about the chemical structure of the analyte [29].

The steps involved in GC for drug analysis include sample preparation. The drug sample is extracted and purified, usually by a combination of liquid-liquid or solid-phase extraction methods, to remove any interfering substances. Some drug compounds may require derivatization prior to analysis in order to improve their volatility, stability, or detectability. The purified and derivatized drug sample is injected into the GC instrument using a syringe or an autosampler. The sample is carried through the column by the carrier gas and the different drug components are separated based on their interaction with the stationary phase. The separated components are detected by the GC detector and the resulting signal is recorded and analyzed. The identity of the drug compounds is determined based on their retention time on the column and their mass spectra (in GC-MS). GC is commonly used in the analysis of drugs of abuse, such as cocaine, heroin, and amphetamines, as well as in the analysis of prescription drugs, such as benzodiazepines and opioids. The results of GC analysis can be used for forensic investigations, drug testing, and drug development [30].

One of the most renowned criminal cases cracked through gas chromatography for drug analysis is the "French Connection" case. It revolved around the largest heroin trafficking network in the United States during the 1960s [31]. The case involved a group of French drug traffickers who smuggled large quantities of heroin into the United States and sold it on the streets of New York City. The US Drug Enforcement Administration (DEA) worked with French authorities to intercept a shipment of heroin that was en route to New York City. The DEA was able to seize the shipment and analyze it using GC to identify the purity and composition of the heroin. GC was used to separate and analyze the different components of the heroin sample, which allowed the DEA to determine the origin and purity of the drug. The analysis revealed that the heroin was of a high purity level and contained a unique impurity that was only found in heroin from a particular region of France. This information led to the arrest and conviction of several key members of the French Connection, including the main supplier of the heroin, Jean-Baptiste "Tito" Venturi. Venturi was convicted of drug trafficking and sentenced to 15 years in prison. The use of GC in the French Connection case was a ground-breaking development in drug analysis and played a key role in the dismantling of one of the largest drug trafficking operations in US history. Today, GC is still widely used in forensic laboratories to analyze drugs and provide crucial evidence in criminal investigations [31].

8.7.2 Arson Investigation

Gas chromatography (GC) is an important analytical technique used in arson investigations to identify the presence of accelerants, which are substances used to increase the rate of combustion. Accelerants are commonly used in arson cases to start fires or to increase the intensity of fires [33]. GC can detect and identify the presence of accelerants in fire debris samples collected from the scene of a fire. Fire debris samples are collected from the scene of the fire using sterile tools and placed in airtight containers. Extraction of accelerants takes place using a suitable solvent, such as n-hexane, to extract any accelerants present in the sample. The extract is then concentrated using a technique such as solvent evaporation or solid phase microextraction (SPME) to increase the sensitivity of the analysis. Concentrated extract is injected into the GC instrument, which separates the accelerants based on their interaction with the stationary phase in the column. The separated accelerants are detected by the GC detector, and the resulting signal is recorded and analyzed (Figure 8.5). The identity of the accelerants is determined by comparing their retention time on the GC column with those of known standards or by analyzing their mass spectra (in GC-MS).

GC is a highly sensitive and reliable technique for the detection of accelerants in fire debris samples as represented in the Figure 8.5. The results of GC analysis can provide valuable evidence in arson investigations, helping to establish the presence of accelerants and the possible cause of the fire [32].

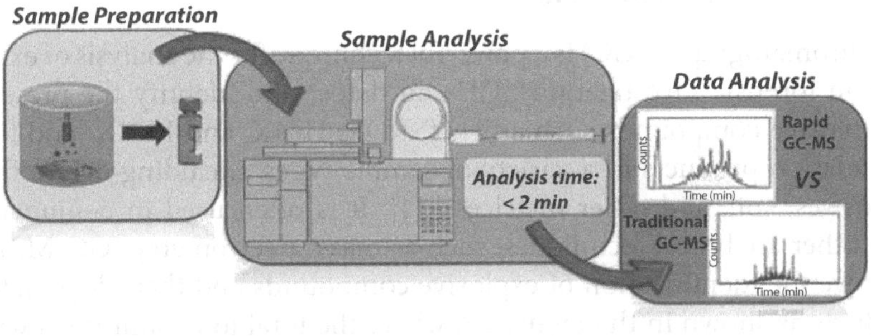

Figure 8.5 Analysis of fire debris [56].

A famous criminal case of Cameron Todd Willingham was solved using GC for arson investigation. Willingham was convicted and sentenced to death in 1992 for allegedly setting fire to his home in Corsicana, Texas, killing his three young children. At the time of the trial, the forensic evidence used to convict Willingham was based on outdated methods and assumptions about how fires start and spread. The prosecution presented testimony from a fire investigator who claimed that the presence of certain burn patterns in the house indicated that the fire had been intentionally set. However, these assumptions were later shown to be unreliable and based on outdated theories. In 2004, a team of experts in fire investigation, including several renowned scientists, reviewed the evidence in the Willingham case and concluded that the original investigation was deeply flawed. The team used advanced techniques, including gas chromatography, to re-examine the evidence and found that the original investigators had misinterpreted the evidence and made numerous errors in their analysis. In particular, the team found that the original investigators had misinterpreted the presence of certain chemical compounds as evidence of arson, when in fact these compounds were likely the result of normal household activities. Using GC, the team was able to identify the specific chemical compounds present in the fire debris and match them to common household products such as cleaning solutions, paint thinner, and gasoline [33].

The re-examination of the evidence in the Willingham case sparked widespread controversy and led to renewed scrutiny of the use of forensic science in criminal investigations. The case has been cited as a prime example of the dangers of relying on flawed or outdated forensic techniques and has led to calls for better training and oversight of forensic investigators. Ultimately, the evidence presented by the expert team helped to exonerate Willingham posthumously and shed new light on the use of GC in forensic investigations [33].

8.7.3 Explosive Analysis

Gas chromatography (GC) is a powerful technique for the analysis of explosives in forensic investigations. GC can detect and identify the presence of explosive compounds such as TNT, RDX, HMX, and PETN, and their degradation products in a variety of sample types, including debris from explosives, soil, and other matrices [34]. It is often used in conjunction with other analytical techniques, such as mass spectrometry (GC-MS), to improve the identification of explosive compounds and their degradation products as shown in the Figure 8.6 where the total ion count is shown at

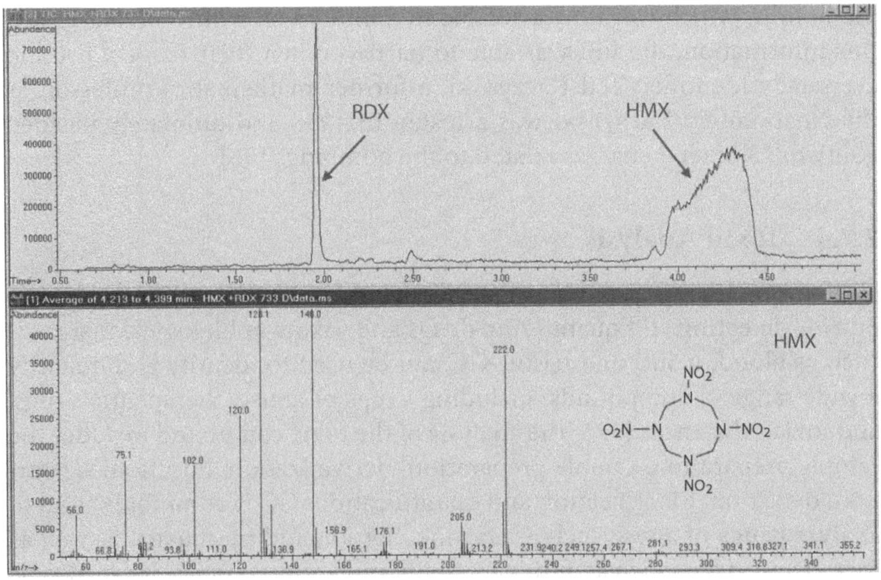

Figure 8.6 The analysis of explosives mixture with the GC-MS [58].

the upper trace while the Cold EI mass spectrum of HMX is shown at the bottom trace (Figure 8.6).

GC is a valuable tool in forensic investigations involving explosives, such as bombings or terrorism cases. The results of GC analysis can provide important evidence regarding the type of explosives used, their origin, and their method of manufacture, which can help to identify the perpetrators and build a strong case in court [35].

In 1995, the case of the Unabomber was solved using GC analysis of the explosive sample find at the bombing site. The Unabomber was a serial bomber who carried out a series of bombings between 1978 and 1995, targeting universities and airlines, killing three people and injuring 23 others. In 1995, the FBI obtained a warrant to search the Unabomber's cabin in Montana, where they found a wide variety of materials, including bomb-making materials and journals written by the Unabomber. The FBI analyzed the materials using GC, which allowed them to identify the chemicals used in the bombs and the materials used to construct them [36]. Based on the GC analysis, the FBI was able to determine that the Unabomber had used a type of polyethylene plastic to wrap his bombs, which was manufactured by only a few companies in the United States. The FBI was also able to identify the type of wood used in the construction of the bombs, which was only available in a limited area of Montana. Using this information, the FBI was able to narrow down their suspect list and eventually identified Ted Kaczynski, a former mathematics professor, as the Unabomber. Kaczynski was arrested in 1996 and ultimately pleaded guilty to 13 federal charges related to the bombings [36].

8.7.4 Toxin Analysis

Gas chromatography (GC) is an effective technique in forensic toxicology for detecting and quantifying drugs and toxins in biological materials such as blood, urine, and tissue. GC can be used to identify and quantify a wide range of compounds, including drugs of abuse, therapeutic drugs, and toxic substances [37]. The analysis of the toxic compound includes the sample preparation: sample preparation, derivatization, injection, separation, detection, identification and quantification. GC is commonly used to analyze drugs of abuse such as cocaine, heroin, and marijuana, as well as therapeutic drugs such as antidepressants and antipsychotics. It can also be used to detect toxic substances such as carbon monoxide and pesticides in biological samples. GC is a powerful tool in forensic toxicology, providing accurate and reliable results that can be used as evidence in legal proceedings. The results of GC analysis can help to establish the presence of drugs or poisons in biological samples, determine the cause of death or injury, and identify potential suspects in criminal cases [38, 39].

In 1982, GC was used is the case of the Chicago Tylenol murders for the toxicological analysis of the forensic evidence. In September 1982, seven people in the Chicago area died after taking Extra-Strength Tylenol capsules that had been laced with cyanide. This incident led to one of the largest recalls in the history of the pharmaceutical industry and resulted in major changes in the way products are packaged and sold in the United States. The toxicological analysis of the Tylenol capsules was carried out using GC. Investigators used GC to detect and identify the presence of cyanide in the capsules. Cyanide is a volatile chemical compound that can be detected using GC. The samples were dissolved in a solvent and injected into the GC instrument. The GC instrument separated the cyanide from other compounds in the sample and detected it using a specific detector. The use of GC in the Tylenol case was crucial in identifying the presence of cyanide in the capsules, which led to the recall of the product and prevented further deaths. The analysis also provided important information to investigators, which led to the identification and prosecution of the person responsible for the poisoning [40].

8.7.5 Food and Beverage Analysis

Gas chromatography (GC) is a technique frequently employed in food and beverage analysis to identify and quantify various analytes such as volatile and semi-volatile chemicals, tastes, scented products, pollutants, aroma and flavors, or contaminants such as pesticides, mycotoxins, and heavy metals which help in the examination of the composition and quality of different products, GC is a powerful tool in food and beverage analysis, providing accurate and reliable results that can be used to ensure compliance with regulatory standards and to maintain product quality and safety. The results of GC analysis can help to identify potential issues with food and beverage products, allowing for corrective action to be taken before they reach consumers [41, 42, 55].

8.7.6 Trace Evidences Analysis

Forensic science frequently employs the technique of gas chromatography (GC) to analyze traces of evidence such as fibers, hair, paint, and glass fragments and provide information about the chemical composition of these materials, which can help forensic scientists identify their source and origin [43].

Hair analysis: Hair is an important source of evidence in forensic investigations because it can provide information about an individual's drug use, toxic exposure, or environmental exposure. GC can analyze the chemical composition of hair, which can provide valuable information for forensic investigations. When hair is analyzed using GC, it is first cleaned and then pulverized into a fine powder. The powder is then extracted using a solvent, such as methanol, and the resulting solution is injected into the GC instrument (Figure 8.7). The GC separates the compounds in the solution based on their chemical properties, and the resulting chromatogram provides information about the chemical composition of the hair sample [44]. One of the main applications of GC in hair analysis is the detection of drugs. Many drugs, such as cocaine, amphetamines, and opioids, can be detected in hair samples. When drugs are ingested or metabolized in the body, they are deposited in the hair shaft. GC can analyze the chemical composition of the hair sample and detect the presence of these drugs. This information can be used to determine if an individual has used drugs and, if so, when they used them [44].

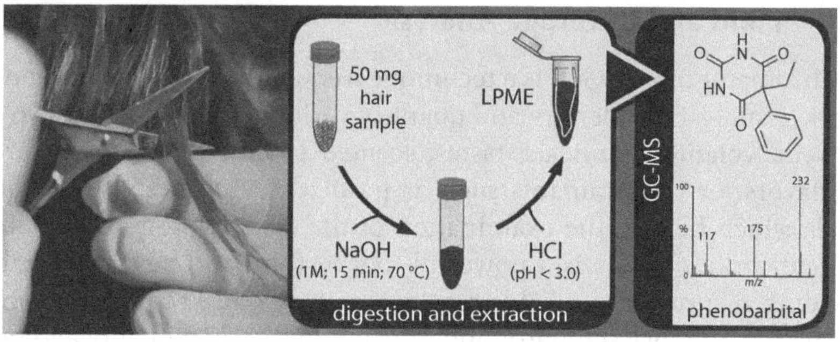

Figure 8.7 Determination of phenobarbital in hair matrix by GC-MS [57].

As shown in the Figure 8.7 GC-MS is utilized to or identification and quantification of phenobarbital in hair samples by liquid phase microextraction (LPME) and gas chromatography–mass spectrometry (GC–MS). The detection limit is 0.1 g/g and the quantification limit is 0.25 g/g. This method has been demonstrated to be effective for the detection and quantification in hair samples. This method can be quickly adapted for other applications whenever needed.

GC can also be used to analyze the stable isotopes of carbon and nitrogen in hair samples. Stable isotopes can provide information about an individual's diet and geographic origin. The ratios of stable isotopes in hair can vary depending on the individual's diet and the geographic region where they lived [45].

Paint analysis: Paint evidence can be found at crime scenes, in hit-and-run accidents, and in cases of vandalism. Analysis of paint using GC provides the chemical composition of paint, which can help forensic scientists to determine its origin, match it to a particular manufacturer, and link it to a particular vehicle or suspect [46]. Paint is a complex mixture of organic and inorganic compounds. When paint samples are analyzed using GC, the sample is first extracted using a solvent, and then it is injected into the GC system. The GC system consists of a column, a detector, and a computer that records and analyses the data and provides valuable information in paint analysis, such as the presence of certain additives, pigments, and solvents. The presence of specific compounds in the paint can also be used to link it to a particular vehicle or suspect [46, 47]. However, GC also has limitations in paint analysis. The method is destructive and requires a sample to be taken from the evidence, which can limit the amount of evidence available for further analysis [47].

Glass analysis: Glass is a common material found at crime scenes, such as in cases of vandalism, burglary, or homicide. The use of GC in glass analysis can provide valuable information about the origin and source of the glass fragments, which can aid in forensic investigations. When applied to glass fragments, GC can detect and analyze the presence of organic compounds, such as paint or adhesive residues, on the surface of the glass. These organic compounds can provide valuable information about the origin and source of the glass, such as the make and model of a car, the type of adhesive used in construction, or the type of paint used in a building [48]. GC is often used in conjunction with other techniques, such as Scanning Electron Microscopy (SEM), to provide a more complete analysis of the glass fragments. SEM is used to analyze the physical properties of the glass, such as its color, texture, and fracture patterns, which can provide information about the type of glass and how it was broken. GC is used to analyze the chemical composition of the glass, which can provide information about the source and origin of the glass. However, GC also has limitations. GC can only identify organic compounds, which means that it cannot analyze the glass itself. GC is also limited in its ability to analyze complex mixtures of compounds. In some cases, other analytical techniques, such as Fourier Transform Infrared Spectroscopy (FTIR) or Inductively Coupled Plasma Mass Spectrometry (ICP-MS), may be used in conjunction with GC to overcome these limitations [48].

Fiber analysis: Fibers are a common type of trace evidence that can be found at crime scenes and can provide valuable information to forensic investigators. GC is a highly sensitive technique that can separate and identify compounds present in the fiber sample [49]. The analysis of fibers using GC involves several steps. First, the fiber is extracted from the sample and prepared for analysis. This may involve heating the fiber to release the compounds that are present. Next, the compounds are separated using GC, which involves the use of a stationary phase and a mobile phase. The stationary phase is a column that is packed with a material that can separate the compounds based on their chemical properties. The mobile phase is a gas that is used to move the compounds through the column. As the compounds move through the column, they are separated based on their chemical properties and detected by a detector at the end of the column.

Different types of fibers have different chemical compositions, which means that GC can be used to identify the type of fiber that is present and also identify additives that may be present in the fiber, such as dyes or coatings. This information can be used to identify the source and origin of the fiber, which can help forensic investigators narrow down the pool of potential suspects [50–52].

8.8 Conclusion

Gas chromatography technique has a wide range of applications and offers several advantages that make it indispensable in criminalistics such as GC can detect and quantify even trace amounts of substances, making it suitable for forensic analysis, where small quantities of evidence can be crucial. It can separate and identify complex mixtures of compounds, ensuring accurate analysis and reducing the likelihood of false positives or negatives and its analyses are relatively quick, allowing forensic laboratories to process large volumes of cases efficiently. This technique of precise quantitative data is essential for legal proceedings and scientific rigor. Most importantly GC typically requires only a small amount of sample, which is advantageous when dealing with limited or irreplaceable evidence. In this context, the role of gas chromatography in criminalistics has had a profound impact on the criminal justice system. Its contributions include accurate and scientifically valid evidence obtained through GC analysis can strengthen cases, leading to higher conviction rates for offenders. This technique has played a crucial role in exonerating wrongfully convicted individuals by reevaluating evidence and providing a more precise analysis of samples and the ability to analyze and identify substances used in crimes, such as arson or explosives, helps prevent future incidents and protect public safety.

However, GC also has some limitations. GC can only identify compounds that can be vaporized, which means that it cannot analyze solid samples. GC is also limited in its ability to analyze complex mixtures of compounds. In some cases, other analytical techniques, such as liquid chromatography (LC), may be used in conjunction with GC to overcome these limitations.

GC is an important analytical technique that has helped law enforcement agencies in their investigations and has contributed to the advancement of forensic science.

References

1. Adebo, O. A., Oyeyinka, S. A., Adebiyi, J. A., Feng, X., Wilkin, J. D., Kewuyemi, Y. O., ... & Tugizimana, F. (2021). Application of gas chromatography–mass spectrometry (GC-MS)-based metabolomics for the study of fermented cereal and legume foods: A review. *Int. J. Food Process. Technol.*, 56(4), 1514-1534.

2. Kolomnikov, I. G., Efremov, A. M., Tikhomirova, T. I., Sorokina, N. M., & Zolotov, Y. A. (2018). Early stages in the history of gas chromatography. *J. Chromatogr. A*, 1537, 109-117
3. Marriott, P.J. (2016). *Gas chromatography: a practical approach*. CRC Press
4. Mudge, E., & Shaw, M. J. (2013). An introduction to gas chromatography. *Chemistry Education Research and Practice*, 14(4), 483-497.
5. Poole, C. (Ed.). (2021). *Gas chromatography*. Elsevier
6. Poole, C. F. (2012). *The essence of chromatography*. Elsevier.
7. Wang, Y., & Zeng, E. (2013). Recent developments in gas chromatography for forensic analysis. *Anal. Bioanal. Chem.*, 405(9), 2673-2688.
8. Wilson, R. B. (2012). *Novel Injection Techniques to Enable Fast, High Peak Capacity Gas Chromatography Separations*. University of Washington.
9. Grob, R. L., & Barry, E. F. (Eds.). (2004). *Modern practice of gas chromatography*. John Wiley & Sons.
10. Eiceman, G. A. (2006). *Instrumentation of gas chromatography*. Encyclopedia of Analytical Chemistry: Applications, Theory and Instrumentation.
11. Wenclawiak, B. W., & Poole, C. F. (1996). *The practice of gas chromatography*. Wiley-VCH.
12. Smith, P.A. (2002). A review of fast gas chromatography. *J. Chromatogr. A*, 965(1-2), 3-14.
13. Karasek, F. W., & Clement, R. E. (2012). *Basic gas chromatography-mass spectrometry: principles and techniques*. Elsevier.
14. Lohse, B. (2017). *The essential guide to gas chromatography*. Lohse Consulting.
15. Lehotay, S. J., & Hajšlová, J. (2002). Application of gas chromatography in food analysis. *TrAC - Trends Anal. Chem.*, 21(9-10), 686-697.
16. Liao, H., Zhang, Q., & Ding, Y. (2016). Recent developments in sample preparation and analytical techniques for the analysis of pharmaceuticals in environmental and human matrices. *TrAC Trends Anal. Chem.*, 76, 62-77.
17. Rotzsche, H. (1991). *Stationary phases in gas chromatography*. Elsevier.
18. Mahdavifar, Alireza & Navaei, Milad & Hesketh, Peter & Dimandja, Jean-Marie & Stetter, Joseph & Mcmurray, Gary. (2015). Implementation of a Polysilicon Micro Electro-Thermal Detector in Gas Chromatography System with Applications in Portable Environmental Monitoring. *ECS J. Solid State Sci. Technol.*, 4. S3062-S3066. 10.1149/2.0151510jss.
19. Colón, L. A., & Baird, L. J. (2004). Detectors in modern gas chromatography. *Modern practice of gas chromatography*, 275-337.
20. de Oliveira, L. P., Rocha, D. P., de Araujo, W. R., Muñoz, R. A. A., Paixão, T. R. L. C., & Salles, M. O. (2018). Forensics in hand: new trends in forensic devices (2013–2017). *Anal. Methods*, 10(43), 5135-5163.
21. Górecki, T., Panić, O., & Oldridge, N. (2006). Recent Advances in Comprehensive Two-Dimensional Gas Chromatography (GC×GC). *J. Liq. Chromatogr. Relat.Technol.*, 29(7-8), 1077-1104.

22. Ouyang, G., & Pawliszyn, J. (2014). Recent developments in solid-phase microextraction for food analysis by gas chromatography-mass spectrometry. *J. Chromatogr. A*, 1353, 1-18.
23. Zhang, Y., Pan, L., & Qiu, B. (2019). Recent advances in gas chromatography-mass spectrometry for metabolomics. *J. Sep. Sci.*, 42(1), 304-314.
24. Xu, J., & Chen, C. (2015). A review of recent developments in gas chromatography-mass spectrometry analysis of polycyclic aromatic hydrocarbons in environmental samples. *J. Environ. Sci.*, 34, 1-21.
25. Wang, Y., & Zeng, E. (2013). Recent developments in gas chromatography for forensic analysis. *Anal. Bioanal. Chem.*, 405(9), 2673-2688.
26. Tretzel, J., & Heger, M. (2016). Advances in gas chromatography for clinical analysis. *J. Sep. Sci.*, 39(1), 16-33.
27. Seeley, J. V., & Seeley, S. K. (2013). Multidimensional gas chromatography: fundamental advances and new applications. *Anal. Chem.*, 85(2), 557-578.
28. Jing, W., Wang, J., Kuipers, B., Bi, W., & Chen, D. D. Y. (2021). Recent applications of graphene and graphene-based materials as sorbents in trace analysis. *TrAC Trends Anal. Chem.*, 137, 116212.
29. Costa, R., Dugo, P., Santi, L., Dugo, G., & Mondello, L. (2010). Advances of modern gas chromatography and hyphenated techniques for analysis of plant extracts. *Curr. Org. Chem.*, 14(16), 1752-1768.
30. Wiederhold, J. G. (2017). Critical review of analytical methods used in forensic chemistry for the determination of drugs of abuse in biological fluids. *J. Chromatogr. B*, 1042, 3-12.
31. Wikipedia contributors. (2023, August 8). French Connection. In *Wikipedia, The Free Encyclopedia*. Retrieved 05:01, September 10, 2023, from https://en.wikipedia.org/w/index.php?title=French_Connection&oldid=1169252284
32. Sutherland, D.R. (2013). *Gas chromatography of petroleum products*. CRC Press.
33. Wikipedia contributors. (2023, June 27). *Cameron Todd Willingham*. In Wikipedia, The Free Encyclopedia. Retrieved 04:42, September 10, 2023, from https://en.wikipedia.org/w/index.php?title=Cameron_Todd_Willingham&oldid=1162111621
34. Zeichner, A., Eldar, B., Glattstein, B., Koffman, A., Tamiri, T., & Muller, D. (2003). Vacuum collection of gunpowder residues from clothing worn by shooting suspects, and their analysis by GC/TEA, IMS, and GC/MS. *J. Forensic Sci.*, 48(5), JFS2002390.
35. Zhong, W., Wang, D., Chen, J., Zhang, X., & Jiang, S. (2019). Advances in gas chromatography in China. *TrAC Trends Anal. Chem.*, 116, 217-228.
36. Wikipedia contributors. (2023, September 9). *Ted Kaczynski*. In Wikipedia, The Free Encyclopedia. Retrieved 05:16, September 10, 2023, from https://en.wikipedia.org/w/index.php?title=Ted_Kaczynski&oldid=1174522660
37. Aerts, G., & Everaerts, F. M. (1989). Gas chromatography in forensic toxicology. *Anal. Chem.*, 61(10), 569A-576A.

38. Molina, D. K., & Hargrove, V. (2018). *Handbook of forensic toxicology for medical examiners*. CRC press.
39. Popescu, R. (2019). Gas chromatography-mass spectrometry in forensic analysis of drugs of abuse. In *Clinical Applications of Mass Spectrometry* (pp. 183-200). Springer.
40. Wikipedia contributors. (2023, September 7). *Chicago Tylenol murders*. In Wikipedia, The Free Encyclopedia. Retrieved 05:27, September 10, 2023, from https://en.wikipedia.org/w/index.php?title=Chicago_Tylenol_murders&oldid=1174272715
41. Ye, M., & Zhao, Y. (2019). Advances in gas chromatography-based methods for food analysis. *TrAC Trends Anal. Chem.*, 115, 74-88.
42. Friedman, M. (2003). Chemistry, biochemistry, and safety of acrylamide. A review. *J. Agric. Food Chem.*, 51(16), 4504-4526.
43. Skoog, D.A., West, D.M., & Holler, F.J. (2013). *Fundamentals of Analytical Chemistry* (9th ed.). Cengage Learning.
44. Baez, H., Castro, M. M., Benavente, M. A., Kintz, P., Cirimele, V., Camargo, C., & Thomas, C. (2000). Drugs in prehistory: chemical analysis of ancient human hair. *Forensic Sci. Int.*, 108(3), 173-179.
45. Uhl, M. (1997). Determination of drugs in hair using GC/MS/MS. *Forensic Sci. Int.*, 84(1-3), 281-294.
46. Zięba-Palus, J., Zadora, G., Milczarek, J. M., & Kościelniak, P. (2008). Pyrolysis-gas chromatography/mass spectrometry analysis as a useful tool in forensic examination of automotive paint traces. *J. Chromatogr. A*, 1179(1), 41-46.
47. De Roy, G., & Köhler, L. Examination of Paint. In *17th Interpol International Forensic Science Managers Symposium*, Lyon 8 th-10 th October 2013 (Vol. 526, p. 129).
48. Caddy, B. (Ed.). (2001). *Forensic examination of glass and paint: analysis and interpretation*. CRC press.
49. van Asten, A., van Veenendaal, N., & Koster, S. (2000). Surface characterization of industrial fibers with inverse gas chromatography. *J. Chromatogr. A*, 888(1-2), 175-196.
50. Rabel, W. (2014). *Gas Chromatography in Environmental Chemistry*. Springer.
51. "Column Chromatography - Solid-Phase Extraction [SPE]" *Waters.com*, 15 May 2023, https://www.waters.com/nextgen/au/en/education/primers/beginner-s-guide-to-liquid-chromatography.html
52. Vranes, M., "New highly-sensitive method for H2 measurement" *Applied Bioenergetic Lab*, 15 May 2023, https://www.appliedbioenergetics.org/robust-gas-chromatography-that-detects-even-0-001-mg-of-h2-in-a-solution-2/
53. Polimerek., November 2005, "*Gass chromatographer - oven with capliary column inside*." https://commons.wikimedia.org/wiki/File:GC_Oven_inside.jpg

54. Warwick, Thomas., Ocober 2022, *Schematic drawing of a gas chromatograph.* By https://bitesizebio.com/28687/carrying-gas-chromatography/
55. Amin, R., Alam, F., Dey, B. K., Mandhadi, J. R., Bin Emran, T., Khandaker, M. U., & Safi, S. Z. (2022). Multidimensional Chromatography and Its Applications in Food Products, Biological Samples and Toxin Products: A Comprehensive Review. *Separations*, 9(11), 326. https://doi.org/10.3390/separations9110326
56. Capistran, B. A., & Sisco, E. (2022). Rapid GC–MS as a screening tool for forensic fire debris analysis. *Forensic chemistry*, 30, 100435.
57. Roveri, F. L., Paranhos, B. A. P. B., & Yonamine, M. (2016). Determination of phenobarbital in hair matrix by liquid phase microextraction (LPME) and gas chromatography–mass spectrometry (GC–MS). *Forensic Sci. Int.*, 265, 75-80.
58. Aviv A. "Explosives Analysis with the 5975-SMB GC-MS with Cold EI" *Aviv Analytical Advanced GC-MS Blog Journal.* 18 December 2013. http://blog.avivanalytical.com/2013/12/explosives-analysis-with-5975-smb-gc-ms.html

9

HPLC and HP-TLC

Lovlish Gupta[1], Abhiramy S. Shenoy[1] and Divya Bajpai Tripathy[2*]

[1]School of Forensic Sciences, LNJN National Institute of Criminology and Forensic Sciences, National Forensic Science University, Delhi Campus, Rohini, Delhi, India Ministry of Home Affairs, Government of India

[2]School of Basic Science, Galgotias University, Greater Noida, UP, India

Abstract

A several ranges of instrumentations and methodologies are used in order to analyze various samples or evidence found at the crime scene. Such analytical instrumentation has had great significance in forensic science. There are 'n' number of instruments which are sensitive, fast, accurate and time efficient to detect any unwanted impurities, in checking the efficacy of a drug product, or in analyzing the samples. One such technique or analytical methods are High Performance Liquid Chromatography (HPLC) and High-Performance Thin-Layer Chromatography (HP-TLC). HPLC is an enhanced form of liquid chromatography whereas HP-TLC is an enhanced form of Thin Layer Chromatography. HP-TLC is abundantly used in several qualitative and quantitative estimations. All chromatographic separations, including HPLC and HP-TLC, work under the common basic principle i.e., separation of a specific samples into its constituent parts because of the differences in their relative affinities of specific molecules for the mobile phase and the stationary phase used in the separation. The most important features of both these techniques prominently use Reverse Phase Chromatography in HPLC and Normal Phase Chromatography (unmodified silica gel G) in HPTLC which results in partition chromatography and adsorption chromatography respectively. The application of HPLC is mainly used for analyzing the concentration of certain biogenic substances like drug levels in body and it also helps forensic scientist in analyzing the contents used in explosive, gunpowder residue, fibers and toxin and HP-TLC is mainly used in biomedical analysis, active ingredient quantification, phytochemical, fingerprinting of formulation and checking adulterant in the sample. HPTLC is also used in the detection of chemicals for forensic findings.

**Corresponding author*: divyabaj@gmail.com

Priyanka Chhabra, Divya Bajpai Tripathy, Anjali Gupta, Rajeev Kumar, Kajol Bhati and Shruti Shukla (eds.) Advances in Analytical Techniques for Forensic Investigation, (241–270) © 2024 Scrivener Publishing LLC

***Keywords*:** Chromatography, HPLC, HP-TLC, instrumentation, forensic sample analysis

9.1 Introduction

Chromatographic Techniques have been used since the early 1900s after the research of Mikhail Semenovich Tsvett in 1906. He was a botanist and he derived this technique for the separation of leaf pigments. He named it as 'chromatography' because of its results of analysis being 'written in color' along the length of the adsorbent column. In the term chromatography, 'chroma' means 'color' and 'graphein' means 'to write'. Chromatography is a physical methodology of separation in which components are to be separated or distributed between the two phases, i.e., stationary phase, which remains intact into the column, and the other is the mobile phase, which passes along the stationary phase packed in the column [1]. The separation in the column occurs due to the differences in the distribution constant of individual samples. Various Chromatographic Techniques have been developed since then, such as, adsorption chromatography, partition chromatography, molecular exchange chromatography, column chromatography, thin layer chromatography, etc. Later, 1970 began with the modification of a new modified technique called High Performance Liquid Chromatography (HPLC), the technique is associated with high pressure due the small particle size of the stationary phase. Since then, the HPLC technique has been preferably used as the most powerful separation technique in analytical chemistry for analysis of a wide range of samples. HPLC and HPTLC are modifications of chromatography which uses high pressure under the column in order to force the introduction and passage of mobile phase and analytes through the stationary phase of micro sized particles compactly packed in the column. Nowadays, a major modification in HPLC is UHPLC i.e., Ultra High' Performance Liquid Chromatography [1–3].

High Performance Liquid Chromatography has been known from various other names as well, which are based on their mode of action such as 'High Speed Liquid Chromatography', ' High Resolution Liquid Chromatography', 'High Pressure Liquid Chromatography'. High performance in HPLC instrumentation is a combined result of factors such as uniform and micro pore size, packing of column using slurry under high pressure, accurate volume of sample or analyte of interest, highly sensitive detector and most importantly the pump and degasser system. Reduction in the particle size of the stationary phase induces two subsequent conditions in the column, one, it leaves lesser space for the mobile phase to pass through, secondly, it decreases the flow rates of liquid mobile phase. Hence, a high pressure of about 1000 to 5000 psi (68–340 atm) per round square inch is applied in order to overcome the obstructive effects of small size of particles [2, 3]. HPLC instrumentation is typically constituted of mobile phase reservoir, solvent delivery system, solvent injection system, column, post column apparatus, detectors, and read out devices. The process of separation in the HPLC column begins with injecting the solute in the column, separation of components of solute in the column, and the process is sustained till the detection of components by detector to form a chromatogram. HPTLC on the other hand is the most précised instrument which is capable of applying a specified amount of sample by spraying it with the help of nitrogen gas. Hence, so called an auto sampler device. Similarly, a computer system or readout device is attached to deceive the analysis about the amount of sample applied, number of bands along with the position and width of the bands formed. HPTLC is however an improvisation of TLC which utilizes TLC in an optimized manner. It is also considered as planar Chromatography or flatbed Chromatography. The major purpose of using HPTLC for forensic analysis is better comparative analysis of forensic samples as it allows multiple sample handling [4]. There are several other forms of HPLC, and each one of them have various significances in forensic sciences as well as in pharmaceuticals. The forms of HPLC are represented in Figure 9.1. This classification is based upon its use and mechanical separation of solute particles [5].

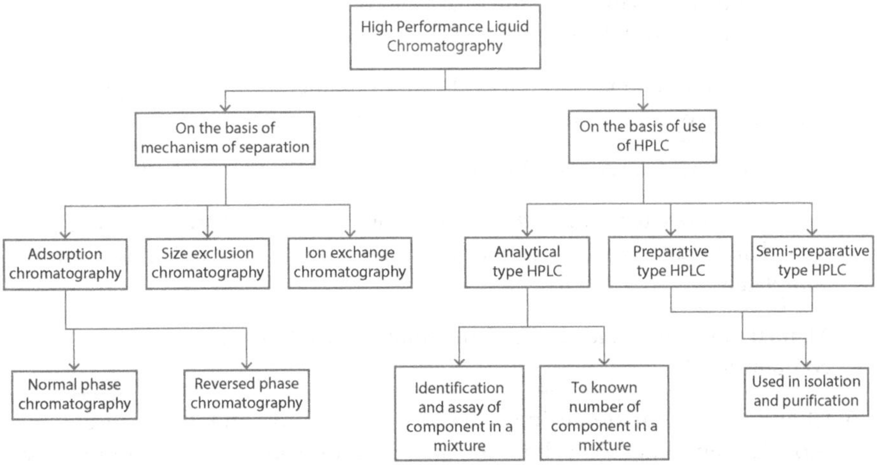

Figure 9.1 Classifications of HPLC.

The major advantages of HPLC over other Chromatographic Techniques, which increases its reliability of analysis of forensic samples, are mentioned in Table 9.1 [6].

A variation of thin-layer chromatography (TLC) known as high-performance thin-layer chromatography (HPTLC) provides for quick, low-cost analysis in both the lab and the field while also providing better separation power. The contemporary HPTLC technology is sensitive and entirely dependable, appropriate for use in both qualitative and quantitative analysis. It is paired with automated sample application and densitometric scanning. Because it can produce chromatographic fingerprints that can be seen and preserved as computer images, HPTLC is a useful technique for accurate identification. The unique benefits of HPTLC include high sample throughput, low cost per analysis, simultaneous separation of multiple samples and standards, and minimal sample preparation requirements due to the disposable nature of the stationary phase and the ability to pack the particles more densely and produce a more homogeneous stationary phase. It also includes the storage of the separation, containing all sample components, on the layer for identification and quantification later by *in situ* or elution methods, as well as static, off-line zone detection using a wide range of complementary post-chromatographic universal and selective detection methods that are frequently applied sequentially [7].

Table 9.1 Advantages of HPLC over other chromatographic techniques.

1. Highly sensitive to even minute quantities of analyte sample, hence very effective for quantitative estimations of forensic samples.
2. High resolution, hence, produces clear chromatograms of the samples analyzed, so produced highly qualitative results.
3. High speed, which reduces the effective time of quantitative analysis.
4. Non-destructive technique, therefore, samples are not destroyed and can be reused and reanalyzed for forensic analysis because the sample is recovered completely.
5. Manual power is reduced as instrumentation is automatic and computerized.
6. Quantitative estimation using HPLC is more sensitive and it therefore provides better method validation, quality control and quality assurance for sample analysis in forensics.

Table 9.2 Advantages of HPTLC over other chromatographic techniques [8].

1. Better separation of bands because of the rectangular area and it is highly precise.
2. Response time is faster and the responses are generally immediate due to the presence of a densitometer in the instrument.
3. Large quantities of sample can be analyzed in less time because of multiple sample handling, and gives better quantitation.
4. Because of multiple sample handling systems, HPTLC permits simultaneous analysis of test and reference/standard samples for better accuracy and precision.
5. Solvents in HPTLC are used without any prior technical treatment such as degassing or filtration.
6. Reduces the travel distance for solvent, i.e., 3–5 cm from 10–15 cm (TLC), shortens development time.

Various advantages of HP-TLC over other chromatographic techniques are reflected in Table 9.2.

The Instrumentation of HPLC includes single or multiple solvent systems, a degasser, a mixing vessel, high pressure pump, a pre column, a sample injector port and an HPLC column, also the detectors and read out devices are attached to it. The entire instrumentation is very sophisticated and allows separation of various components at a faster rate. The instrumentation of HPLC is also shown in Figure 9.2. The instrumentation shown in Figure 9.2 however, belongs to M/S Shimadzu Corporation of model, Shimadzu Prominence–ILC-2030C 3D Plus

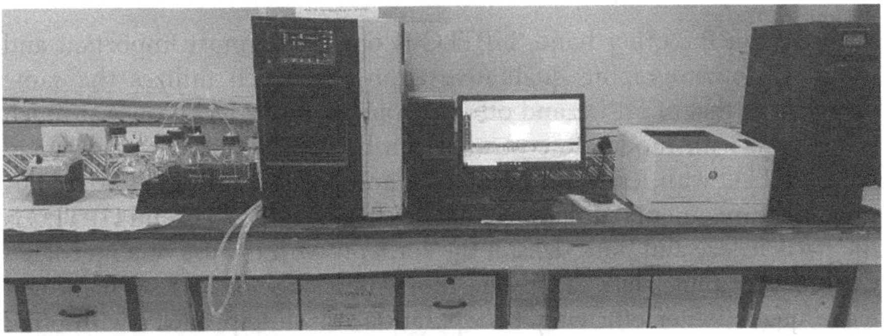

Figure 9.2 The HPLC instrument.

HPLC and HPTLC are chromatographic techniques used in forensic analysis major for quantification, recognition, segregation and discernment of various forensic samples such as drugs and other toxicants. These techniques are now a days most preferably used by Forensic Science Laboratories for the examination various categories of evidences recovered from crime scene such as examination of age of documents, analysis of heavy metals in cosmetic products, component analysis of cosmetics, for examination of alcohol and petroleum products, analysis of adulteration in food items and analysis of explosive materials [9].

9.2 Principle

9.2.1 Basic Principle of HPLC

The entire instrumentation and working of HPLC is based on the distribution separation of the analyte by its distribution between the two phases of the chromatographic column. The entire procedure depends upon two major factors, one, the chemical composition of the analytes added, two, the affinity of the analyte towards the stationary phase, because of which the molecules are retarded while passing through the mobile phase. The intermolecular interactions between the analyte's molecules and the molecules of stationary phase are responsible for their time of separation within the column. This is why different components are eluted at different times. Analytes that have been separated are then recognized by the detectors or the detection device such as UV detectors. The signals are interpreted in the read-out devices with the help of a data management system or computer software which are represented in the form of a chromatogram [10, 11].

9.2.2 Basic Principle of HP-TLC

Whereas, on the other hand, HPTLC is one of the most important and useful Chromatographic qualitative approach which utilizes the same principle as that of HPLC and other chromatography techniques at much faster pace with moderate cost or it can be considered as the advancement of TLC with lesser time duration and production of better resolution. The fundamental difference that lies between the TLC and HPTLC is the particle size and pore sizes of the sorbents with the use of a precoated Chromatographic plate [12]. One more advantage of this sophisticated technique is better efficiency of separation of solute particles with often better limit of detection, which sometimes serve as an alternative even for

HPLC and Gas chromatography (GC). The separation of analyte can either be due to absorption or can also be due to partition or sometimes by both the phenomenon, this entirely depends upon the nature of solute used along with the solvent system [13].

9.2.3 Basic Parameters and Steps Involved

In HPLC, the separation of analytes is dependent upon the chemical nature of solute, the affinity of solute towards the stationary and mobile phase and most importantly the high pressure used in the HPLC column. These separated analytes which are transported by mobile phase are recorded by the detectors as peaks, collectively called a chromatogram. Each peak constitutes certain qualitative and quantitative measures of the analytes. These quantitative peaks generally appeared as a Gaussian bell shaped curve. Basic chromatographic parameters of HPLC and HPTLC collectively are Delay time, Retention time, Peak width, Tailing factor which have equal importance in forensic sample analysis [14].

• ***Delay time (T_0):***
This measurement refers to the time which is required to transport a non retarded analyte from the injection port to within the detection device. This time is basically the sum total of the time taken by the sample to travel exclusively within the mobile phase and the time for which the substance was adhered to the stationary phase. This is an essential approach in forensic chemistry and toxicological examination which lead to the identification of various drugs samples, various alcoholic beverages and other exhibits recovered from the crime scene, this is because different exhibits have different chemical properties and affinities towards mobile phase and stationary phase and systems have set database for specific range of frequently found samples such as cocaine, barbiturates, opiates, alcohol, paint chips etc [14, 15].

• ***Retention time (t_R):***
This time ranges particularly from the moment of introduction of injection till the moment it gets deceived by detectors. This overall time is essential and very helpful in qualitative estimations of forensic exhibits because the retention time for specific sample will always have the same values under same optimum conditions which further ensures repeatability and reproducibility testing, hence, provides a quality assurance of the results obtained [14, 16].

- ***Peak width (w):***

The peaks for different samples have different size, width and amplitude, hence, this is a very peculiar parameter for the identification and differentiation of two or more samples, also, this has been useful in quantifying mixtures and production of qualitative results. The peak width is basically the entire space or period covered from the initiation of the signal slope till it reaches the baseline even after repeated drops in the detector signals [14–16].

- ***Tailing factor (T):***

Tailing factor is the measure of the degree of tailing obtained by an imperfect peak, as ideally symmetrically perfect peaks are not formed. The measure of peak Tailing is described as peak asymmetry or in other words, it can be said that, the more the tailing effect will be, the less the symmetry of the peak will be seen. i.e., the tailing effect is inversely proportional to the symmetry in the peak. This factor again has similar indices when it comes to the analysis of various forensic samples. Different samples have different tailing edge at the peak apex [16, 17].

HPTLC validation process since ancient times has gone through Quality control and Quality assurance checks which have helped in the total quality management for the particular instrument. These analyses included specificity, selectivity, sensitivity, precision, accuracy, ruggedness.

Limit of detection (LOD), limit of quantitation (LOQ) and most importantly the stability of the instrument. Some other, important fundamentals have been implemented in planar chromatography as well as HPLC which are helpful and important to be theoretically considered for analysis of samples are separation efficiency, partition coefficient, retention factor (or retardation factor, as discussed above), capacity factor, spot capacity and plate height (only in case of HPTLC), resolution and selectively [7, 18, 19]. The validation and analytical criteria is not only required to produce accurate or precise results, but are also essential because the evidences found on the crime scene are many a times, in very minute quantities, where an analysts requires special care in order to prevent the evidence from contamination, and also to ensure the repeatable use of sample for analysis, hence, the techniques need to highly calibrated and non-destructive for the samples [18–20]. The essential method validation and calibration criteria for any instrument which is so far essentially being done before the analysis of any Forensic or pharmaceutical species, are shown in Figure 9.3.

On the other hand, the general steps of HPLC and HPTLC procedures from the introduction of samples till the separation and detection of samples is represented in Figures 9.4 and 9.5, respectively [21, 22].

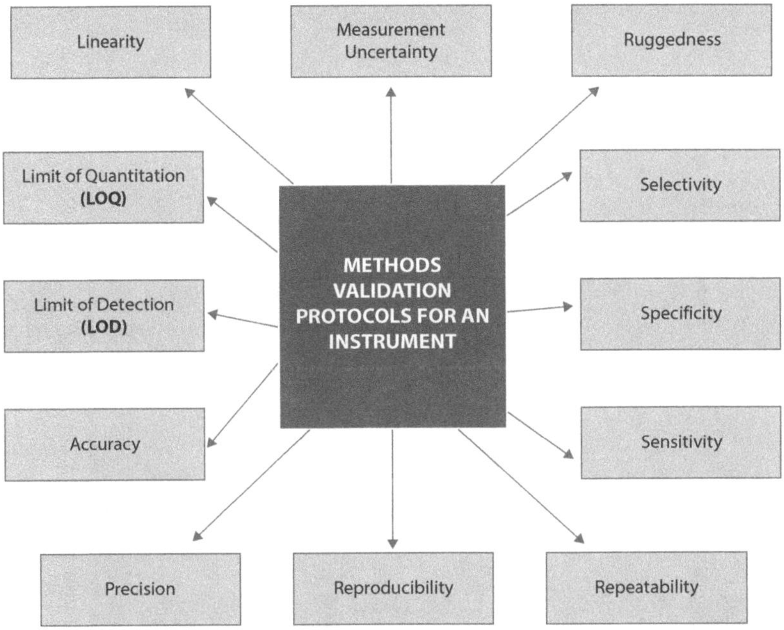

Figure 9.3 Various protocols for method validation for an analytical instrument.

9.3 Applications of HPLC and HP-TLC in Forensic Sciences

HPLC and HPTLC are hyphenated chromatographic techniques that have been used so far for the analysis of forensic samples. Recent students have proven the use of these Chromatographic techniques to be validated in forensic and legal consultations. HPLC has become highly popular for the qualitative and quantitative analysis in the field of forensic chemistry and toxicology mainly. However, document examination, determination of blood stain age, identification of various kinds of narcotics substances, drugs, inks, various poisons and pesticides, explosive materials and propellants, can also be favorably done using HPLC because of its high-resolution power, higher sensitivity, and reduced time for the detection of the chromatogram [23]. HPLC have also been found to possess various meaningful applications when coupled with other hyphenated technologies such as diode array detection (DAD), HPLC coupled with atmospheric pressure ionization mass spectrometry (HPLC-API-MS). These coupled techniques find their wide applications in emergency toxicology [24].

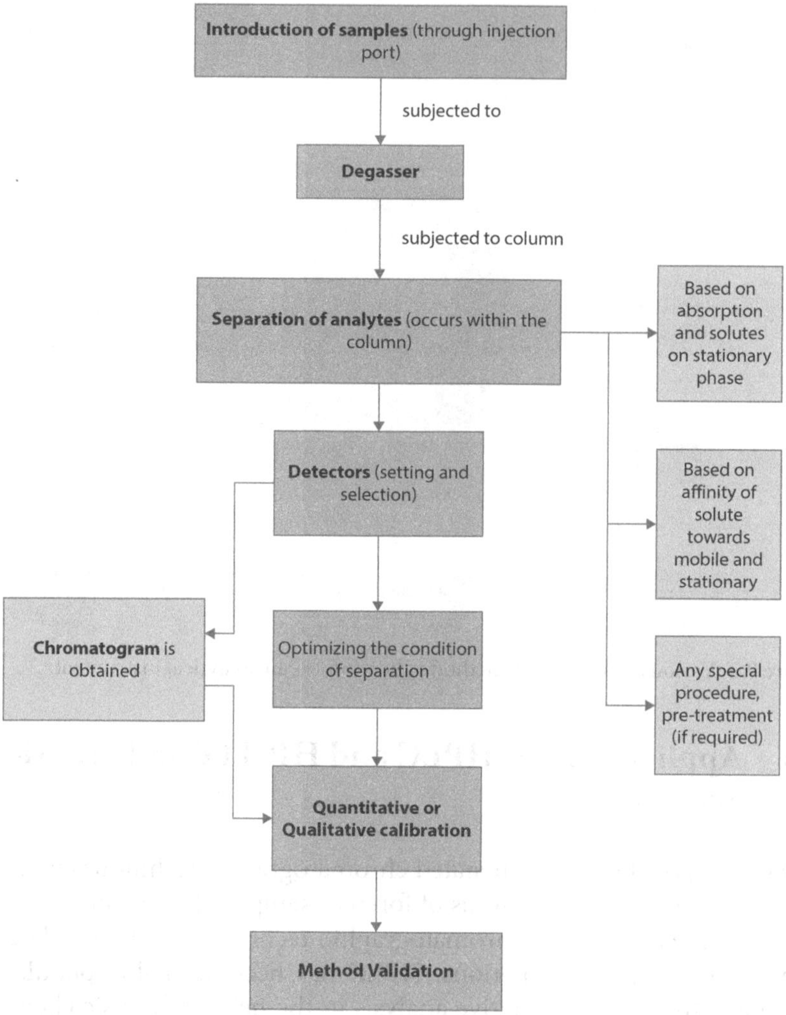

Figure 9.4 General workflow for HPLC process.

9.3.1 Forensic Examination of Samples Using HPLC

9.3.1.1 Forensic Examination of Toxicological Samples

Various toxicological samples or poison analysis are done on the basis of their chemical nature, toxicants such as ammonium phosphide, various noxious gases, various autopsy samples, or viscera, or other bodily fluids are found to have poison concentrations. A case of systemic toxicity of aluminium phosphide has been also reported in a 39-year-old man, who

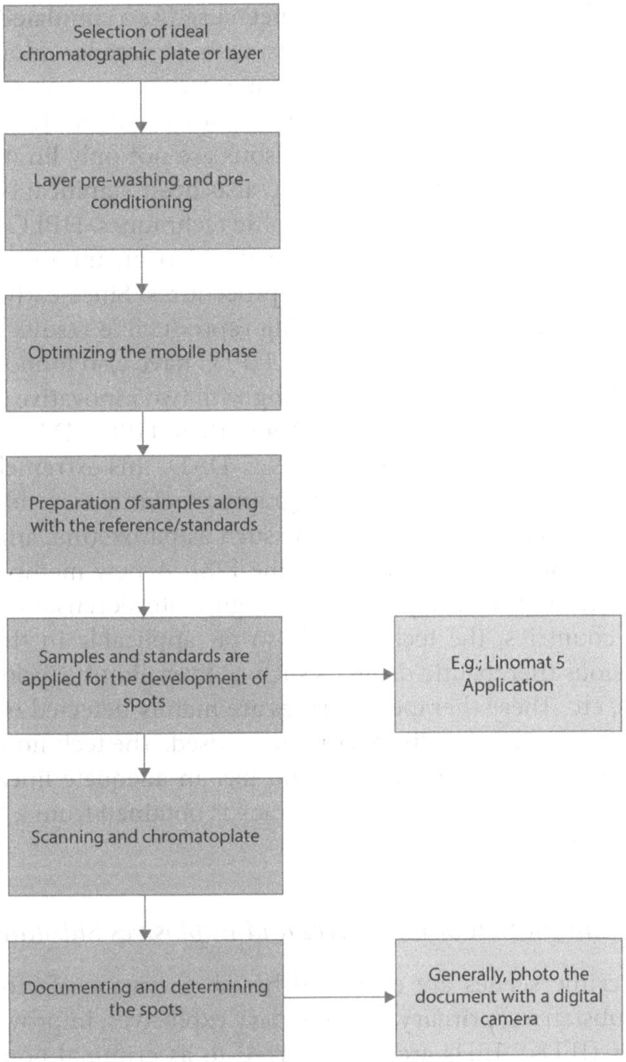

Figure 9.5 General workflow for HPTLC process.

committed suicide by its ingestion, the toxicity was determined by the use of HPLC. However, in HPLC sufficient quantities of hydrogen phosphine (PH3) gas was determined but not the presence of aluminium. This phenomenon has occurred due the conversion of aluminium phosphide into hydrogen phosphine, a very toxic gas, in reaction with humidity [25]. Various researchers have revealed that HPLC have determined various organophosphorus pesticides, which are responsible for causing acute poisoning in humans. HPLC DAD has been used as a simulated technique for the detection of pesticidal toxicants such as organo-chloro, organo-phosphorus, ricin, etc. and the technique serves as a non-destructive technique for qualitative and quantitative measurements [26]. The toxicological examination of drugs and poisons are not only limited till this, whereas the animal-based poisons have also been significantly analyzed by the use of hyphenated Chromatographic techniques. HPLC techniques have been seen to give sensitive detection of anticoagulant properties when it gets coupled with various extraction procedures. Since early time only, the methods are applicable in producing reproducible results hence, it is more suitable for forensic analysis [27]. HPLC have also found to have its applications in forensic field after coupling with two innovative techniques, one HPLC with DAD i.e., HPLC-DAD, and then, HPLC-DAD with fabric phase sorptive extraction i.e., FPSE-HPLC-DAD, this extremely hyphenated and advanced form of chromatographic technique is able to detect the presence of various antidepressants such as paroxetine, amitriptyline, etc. even from biological fluids like urine [28]. A new methodology i.e., HPLC-MS/MS is now a days a part of legitimate Forensic examination in various countries, the technique is so far applicable in the development of various therapeutic drugs as such as Everolimus, Cyclosporine A, Tacrolimus, etc. These therapeutic drugs are mainly detected in the blood samples of the deceased or live victim or accused. The technique has been validated under various parameters and has an adequate linearity range along with this high precision and accuracy is obtained from a large range of samples [29].

9.3.1.2 Examination of Explosives and Explosives Substances

Explosion crime scenes are evaluated based on various factors such as explosive substances, primary, or secondary explosives, improvised explosive devices (IEDs). IEDs are also referred to as criminal bombs, which are planned by the perpetrators or offenders, for mass homicides, and bulk damage of properties. Since it can be in any shape, size or can be equipped, embedded, filled in any type of explosion causing material or chemicals. Hence, these chemicals are needed to be fully recognized in order to detect the nature of explosives, its property and thereby the motive of explosion and nature of crime. HPLC and HPTLC are two hyphenated Chromatographic techniques that help in better detection and estimation of explosives for crime reconstruction [32]. Explosives can however be either a single or a mixture of chemicals which, on provision of sufficient energy, undergo rapid decomposition and due to high amounts of pressure of gases explode into the air, creating various blast and shock waves resulting in release of high heat and production of large volumes of gases. Various explosive compounds such as gunpowder, black powder, smokeless powder, semi smokeless powder, Trinitrotoluene, Mercury fulminate, Cyclotrimethylenetrinitramine (RDX) can be detected and analyzed using HPLC and HPTLC both [32, 33]. Cases have also been reported where, trace amounts of extracts of explosives from clothing or hands or anybody swabs of the victim or perpetrators can be detected by HPLC, however, in this case HPLC examination act as the preliminary examination for the trace explosives which can be further confirmed by their analysis in Gas chromatography [34]. Generally, cyanopropyl phase is used for the detection of nitroaromatic explosives using HPLC. Various nitro based explosive substances possess different retention time, which are determined using different composition of solvents [35].

In both forensic and environmental applications, analysis of hazardous explosive substances like 2,4,6-trinitrotoluene (TNT) and pentaerythritol tetranitrate (PETN) is crucial. Thin layer chromatography (TLC), infrared spectroscopy (IR), gas chromatography (GC), high-performance liquid chromatography (HPLC), and high-performance thin layer chromatography (HPTLC) combined with mass spectroscopy are a few important techniques that were employed for the investigation of explosives. When compared to HPLC, the HPTLC method offers various benefits, including higher throughput, reduced costs, and a need for less solvent per sample. The literature provides information on the physical, chemical, and thermodynamic properties of PETN and TNT. Using a double development procedure, PETN and TNT were separated on Silica gel 60 F254 plates. The study of the chromatogram peak regions acquired from the TLC-S was done using the least-squares calibration method [36].

9.3.1.3 Examination of Textile and Fabrics

Presence of fabrics in forensic cases have been seen in majority in various criminal acts such as murders, homicides, sexual assaults, stab wounds or injuries, fabrics can also be found deposited on weapons and all the shop objects used for stabbing. Textiles and fabrics can be analyzed for the chemical properties, for the manufacturing, for any pattern of damages, this can help linking the suspects and the victims to each other, also to the weapon of offence and the crime scene. Sometimes, the composition of dye can also help in corroborating the case. HPLC, here also has so far served as an essential tool for its examination. The examination of fiber includes not only their chemical properties. However, it can also reveal its physical structure, its production or manufacturing details, dye variability, physical and mechanical deterioration of fibers may also help in revealing time Since death, sometimes manner of death, this approach is very helpful in burial conditions [38–40]. Hyphenated techniques such as HPLC-DAD-MS have been used for the identification of dyes present in the textiles or fabrics. This technique has been proven as the best technique to provide the qualitative detection of dyes even when very minute quantities of fabrics are present, such as polyester, cotton, etc. Dye mixtures are variable and can be separately identified, this increases the evidentiary value [41]. Fabrics collected from the crime scene are subjected to HPLC mainly for the determination of dyes. These dyes can be of various chemical compositions such as organic or inorganic dyes. The analysis can be done using various techniques coupled with HPLC such as HPLC-DAD-MS, HPLC-MS/MS [42], HPLC combined pH/organic solvent gradient, etc. [43].

9.3.1.4 Examination of Questioned Documents and Variable Inks

Since the turn of the 20th century, writing inks on contested documents have been subjected to forensic analysis. The pigments, which make up most of the inks, are one of many ingredients that increase the inks' properties. UV radiation is one environmental factor that can age inks and induce some chemical changes to their makeup. So, while attempting to determine the origin of questioned ink specimens, forensic ink examiners are confronted with the extremely wide variety of pairings between ink compositions and writing tool brands or models.

Analysis of ageing of paper as well as inks are well established not only by HPTLC, however, other chromatographies like HPLC and GC have also played a very significant role in it. HPLC has been used to detect the deterioration of different dyes and inks, by analysis of degradation kinetics of the compounds. Both natural and artificial ageing of paper can be examined, it has been significantly observed that criminals with the intention of forgery acts into inducing artificial ageing of related questioned documents by relative heating or by application of light. Whereas, for the analysis of pen inks, TLC has been playing significant role since decades, whereas, separation techniques such as HPLC or GC combined with scanners (used as detectors) is very helpful for multivariate and statistics analysis of ink which serves as best alternative of a spot test on TLC [46]. Certain significant researches have also revealed that a modification in HPLC by coupling it with an ions pairing (IP) i.e., IP HPLC is capable of examining the correct chemical composition of fountain pen inks, as well as dating of fountain pens. These hyphenated technologies are now majorly in use because of the low efficiency of separation and lesser quantitation abilities of thin layer chromatography [47]. Relative dating of ball point pen inks can be determined but only when there is a significant similarity or difference in the writing surfaces. HPLC when used for the analysis of ink, it was producing certain significant results, such as age of document, age or dating of the ballpoint pen inks, along with the quantity of ink with which the text is being written, this intern proves HPLC to be a validated and appropriate method for such analysis protocols [48]. On the other hand, non-ball point pen inks were analyzed by a simple isocratic HPLC system coupled with multivariate detectors, and produces highly sensitive and precise spectra [49].

9.3.1.5 *Examination of Narcotics, Psychotropic Substances and Pharmaceutical Substances*

Analysis of narcotic drugs can not only be done when the drugs are obtained in a realistic manner, however specialized techniques can also help diagnose seized narcotic substances. One such advanced hyphenated technique is HPLC-UV, where HPLC is coupled with ultraviolet, this technique is a validated method and has been utilized in detection of seized narcotic substances in different manner such as narcotic substances in grains tablets, in metallic boxes, etc. Generally, an Arcus EP-C18, 5 μm, 4.5 × 250 mm column has been used with the rate of flow to be 1.2 ml/min at 25°C and the wavelength of UV being more susceptible to the drugs is 275 to 300 nm. Hence, the mixture of various drugs will produce various significant peaks. In recent systems of forensic investigation, HPLC and GC-MS are the most sensitive and globally accredited methods for examination of narcotic substances and Psychotropic drugs [50]. HPLC coupled with DAD have specialized effects in the diagnosis of various psychotropic drugs, such as phenothiazines, various antidepressants. The technique was found to have accurate validation parameters such as relative retention times, detection limits for specific psychotropic drugs, linearity ranges [51]. Some medicinal psychotropic substances such as diazepam, medazepam, Olanzapine, Clorazepate, Escitalopram, and oxazepam and sometimes their mixtures are also analyzed using HPLC. The analysis of degraded drugs substances is to be done majorly in two manners, i.e., photodegradation and biodegradable, which is subsequently achieved by Xe and UV lamps and HPLC, representatively [52]. Not only the detection of degraded substances, whereas psychotropic substances that have been bio transformed and have converted into new transformed products are also analyzed as these transformation may serve as more severe and damage causing. The best example where HPLC have set remarkable targets is the analysis and distinguishing of Trimipramine (TMP), chlorprothixene (CPTX) and Desipramine (DMI) which have chemically similar structures but gives separate peaks in the chromatogram [53].

9.3.1.6 Examination of Cosmetic Products

Cosmetic products have been used since early times by both men and women, as well as children to some extent, and the use of cosmetics is not just limited to normal activities, however, they have been used in various industries. People use cosmetics, apply on their skin for various reasons, sometimes, for the pre-treatment of skin, for the protection of skin, for enhancing the external features of an individual. However, these cosmetics are not safe because of the presence of various contaminants and unwanted materials that sometimes increases toxicity of the cosmetics, which can even possess local toxicities or may result in systemic toxicity which further causes neurotoxicity, hepatotoxicity, cardiotoxicity, etc. Because of the presence of toxicants like preservatives, organic and inorganic colorants, phthalates, parabens, and most importantly determination of heavy metals in the cosmetics [64, 65].

Preservatives can be of various classes such as phthalates, parabens, etc. However, parabens are preservatives with broad spectrum which possess antimicrobial activities and are used in cosmetics on large scale, also found their applications in food industries, and pharmaceuticals. These parabens are found to have effects on estrogenic activities of an individual, also disrupting various cyclic functions. The paraben used in cosmetics can easily be determined using HPLC coupled with fluorescence detection because of its higher sensitivity and selectivity (in a range of wavelengths from 254 nm and 310nm). However, HPLC incorporated with Mass Spectrometry tends to produce better and confirmatory results [64, 66]. Various other Preservatives such as methylisothiazolinone (MI), benzyl alcohol, potassium sorbate, sodium benzoate, can be profoundly detected and separated in HPLC column, the best column for this separation is Develosil RP Aqueous AR-5 RP-30 (250× 4.6 mm) column, and 0.1% of aqueous solution and acetonitrile are used as gradient elution [67]. Gradient elution using a mobile phase of citrate buffer in HPLC instrumentation followed by DAD is found to be a corrective technique for the identification of organic colorants extracted from the cosmetic matrices. Different colorants used have significantly different retention time and possess variant UV vis range, which are responsible for different peaks of the chromatogram [68].

Researchers have estimated that general exposure of phthalates to human derma is 0.0006 µg/kg body weight for a phthalate known as di(2-ethylhexyl) phthalate (DEPH), whereas, concentration for diethyl phthalate (DEP) is found to be 0.6 µg/kg bw/d. But it's exposure through cosmetics is subsequently increased to 0.026 µg/kg bw/d for DEHP, 81.471 µg/kg bw/d for DEP, which served to be a hazardous range causes various acute toxicities such as teratogenicity, endocrine toxicity, etc. The analysis of these compounds are essential for the safe usage of cosmetics and to ensure whether the cosmetics are of usable range or not [69]. A wide range of heavy metals such as arsenic, Mercury, and lead, have been more subsequently used in cosmetics such as lipsticks, creams, eyeliners, etc. The analysis of these hazardous heavy metals is essential to ensure the safety before use. As these heavy metals are subsequently causing chronic toxicity such as hepatotoxicity, cardiotoxicity, neurotoxicity, etc. For the analysis of these heavy metals various instrumental analysis required which include capillary electrophoresis, induced coupled plasma mass spectroscopy (ICP MS), atomic absorption spectrometry (AAS) and HPLC are fundamentally used [70]. Cosmetics like lipstick, eyeliner, eyeshadow, nail polish, and vermilion are likely to be found during criminal investigations, especially in cases of crime against women, as they are frequently used in daily life and are easily transferred to clothing, drinking cups, handkerchiefs, tissue paper, cigarette butts, and other surfaces through contact during crime [71–73]. Cosmetic evidence, which can be used as important forensic evidence, can be discovered on such substrates, and would suggest physical touch between people and with items. Cosmetic products are easily transferable and remain persistent on the transferred object, they are useful and crucial as trace evidence in forensic situations. Since it cannot be seen with the naked eye, the criminal does not remove or damage it. In forensic science, finding and identifying the source of trace evidence is crucial because it could establish a connection between the suspect, the victim, and the crime scene and therefore serve as significant corroboration evidence [75].

9.3.2 Forensic Examination of Samples Using HP-TLC

9.3.2.1 Forensic Examination of Toxicological Samples

Chemicals known as pesticides are typically used to either kill or protect against pests. Insecticides, herbicides, fungicides, and rodenticides are some of the regularly utilized pesticides. It goes without saying that pesticides could be hazardous to humans and other non-target animals. As a result, it is important to use them responsibly and dispose of them correctly.

In order to manage pests like fungi, insects, and bacteria, early insecticides used fumigants like hydrogen cyanide and very deadly arsenic compounds like calcium arsenate and lead arsenate. Bordeaux mixes, which are concoctions of sulphur, copper sulphate, lime, and water, were additionally employed as pesticides. Pesticides are divided into four groups by the World Health Organization (WHO) based on their toxicities, including organochlorines, organophosphorus, carbamates, pyrethrins, and pyrethroids [30]. Due to its efficiency, affordability, and adaptability, HPTLC (High-performance Thin Layer Chromatography) is used as an analytical technique to analyze poisoning caused by these pesticides while screening biological samples. A new spraying reagent for the straightforward HPTLC approach of identifying toxic visceral samples via profenofos. The tested several spraying agents to determine which profenofos toxins were present in biological (visceral) samples. By performing a hydrolysis process, profenofos reacts with cupric acetate spraying reagent to produce an intensely brown-colored chemical in the presence of sodium hydroxide. Organochlorine, carbamate, and pyrethroid pesticides do not react with the chromogenic reagent. Visceral substances such as proteins, lipids, peptides, amino acids, etc. Do not obstruct the spraying reagent's ability to analyze the sample's constituent parts [31].

9.3.2.2 HP-TLC Fingerprinting to Detect Medicinal Merits

After the introduction of several new products, the market for natural products underwent a significant change. These products were characterized by both novelty and confusion, and they were given a variety of creative names, such as nutraceuticals, food supplements, botanicals, dietary supplements, medical devices, multifunctional foods, herbal drug preparations, and others. These are contemporary methods of using natural materials, inheriting their natural origins from the past like herbal medicines and herbalist products, and providing remedies for the treatment of escalating minor illnesses or maintaining good health. The requirement for proper analytical controls is to be ensured solely by quality evaluations by checking the precise determination of the composition, in order to prevent the natural goods from being eliminated from society. For the separation and identification of plant elements, chromatography was used as the analytical method. HPTLC continues to be the immediate, simplest, and most trustworthy analytical friend in the organic chemistry lab today due to the numerous applications TLC and its advanced form, such as HPLC, have for determining the presence and identity of known marker compounds, monitoring the development of a synthesis, and testing column fractions separation trends. The technique HPTLC is poised to rank among the finest for verifying the composition of intricate botanical goods by controlling quality, purity, stability, and identification. Due to the use of smaller silica gel, which increases surface area, the effectiveness has significantly increased. Additionally, thanks to new, specialized equipment, it is now possible to perform high-quality HPTLC analytical determinations and thereby finally achieve the required reliability, repeatability, and flexibility. The speed and ability to analyze many samples simultaneously under the same chromatographic conditions were two benefits of HPTLC. Because HPTLC just requires chamber saturation and runs for a short period of time, the mobile phase is consumed less and the results appear faster. Thus, that interferences can be removed, costs can be kept to a minimum, and all the sample components can be viewed collectively as part of the chromatogram, the mobile phase is entirely removed from the plate during detection. On the same plate and under the same conditions, reference materials can be chromatographed side by side. The major characteristic is in the flexibility and complexity: HPTLC can provide a chromatographic fingerprint in the form of a distinct series of peaks that fully represent the sample that was tested. Using a computerized digitalis data bank, the goal is to produce fingerprints that can be compared in terms of the quantity, order, location (Rf), and color of the divided zones, as well as in relation to a data bank. Hence, utilizing their fingerprint and the detection of adulterants, botanicals may be compared quickly and easily. The use of HPTLC fingerprinting provided a significant benefit in examining adulteration, substituting botanical species, and comparing extracts of the same species that were prepared in various ways [37].

9.3.2.3 Examination of Textile and Fabrics

A large component of all forensic trace evidence analyses are fiber comparisons. Given that color, thickness, and form are the most obvious features to identify when looking for target fibers through a stereomicroscope, color is possibly the most significant optical property displayed by evidence fibers. This method is more adaptable to the sample size restrictions imposed by normal forensic casework samples because of the introduction of high-performance thin-layer chromatography (HPTLC) plates, which have higher resolution and fewer sample requirements than standard plates. In forensic casework, investigative HPTLC can offer precise information about a sample that cannot be obtained by using only other analytical techniques (e.g., MSP, FTIR, Raman, etc.). Based on these outcomes in the separation and analysis of dyes extracted from textile fibers, the HPTLC technique is anticipated to have the largest potential for impact on the quality of the resulting data. This process includes steps like plate selection, pre-elution, tank saturation, developing distance, and eluent stability. The analytical method that can produce repeatable HPTLC separations has benefits, including the ability to assess the quality of the dyes on different plates, collected at various points in time, to establish tolerances for forensically comparing questioned and known HPTLC data, and, in the end, to create and assess the quality of databases of HPTLC data from a collection of reference dyes. As a result, it is possible to identify dyes in forensic analysis samples more effectively and practically [44].

9.3.2.4 Examination of Questioned Documents and Variable Inks

The ink analysis is a crucial forensic method that can provide essential details about a document under investigation. The destructive and non-destructive analytical approaches can be used to distinguish between two pieces of writing that may have been produced using the same writing instrument. The goal is to create an easy, affordable, and trustworthy solution for document authentication and ink fingerprinting. The separation technique used, such as HPTLC, provides critical data for differentiating ballpoint inks and pen inks retrieved from cartridges and sheets. The combination of fingerprints discovered using visible light detection and UV light at 366 nm enables a thorough description of samples while being sufficiently selective to highlight unique qualities of in. Further evidence that the pigments from the studied inks are highly different even though they are produced by the same manufacturer is provided by the fact that the HPTLC fingerprints of blue ballpoint inks are very different from the fingerprints of blue pen inks. Although the retention parameter alone is insufficient to differentiate samples, the color of the spots can help to accomplish this task. One such instance is the second ballpoint ink, where some of the compounds have different colors despite having the same retention parameter, indicating that they are distinct from the other inks' compounds. This might be the case because some pigments are retained on paper due to the solidification and polymerization of resins, the evaporation of volatiles from inks, and the solidification and polymerization of resins. Hence, it was virtually impossible to extract all the pigments. The scenario with ballpoint inks was the exact reverse. In the case of inks recovered from exposed paper, HPTLC separation revealed the emergence of novel compounds together with a decrease in the intensity of colored bands like those from ink cartridge samples. The types and manufacturers of the ink affect the HPTLC fingerprints. Also, the HPTLC fingerprints and the constituents' retention characteristics could be utilized to confirm the age of papers [45].

9.3.2.5 *Examination of Narcotics, Psychotropic Substances and Pharmaceutical Substances*

An essential analytical separation technique is HPTLC. The primary benefit of HPTLC is the simultaneous separation of several samples on a single plate, which only requires a minimal quantity of developing solvent to separate milligram-sized samples. HPTLC tool and other devices can be used to increase sensitivity of analyte detection using automatic sample application device, UV/fluorescent detectors, densitometer scanner (which turns the spot on a layer into a chromatogram with series of peaks), and software [54–56]. The study of several chemicals, medications, and colors can be done using the flexible approach known as high performance thin layer chromatography (HPTLC). For routine quality control analysis, the technique is simple and practical [57, 58]. Narcotic drugs are those that relieve pain and induce sleep but are not socially acceptable. Drugs and psychoactive chemicals can be natural, semi-natural, or manufactured. When ingested, they affect the central nervous system, alter mental status, and cause physical and mental dependence on the substance [59]. When forensic laboratories receive samples that have been tampered with, the psychotropic drugs are found and identified by misting Dragondroff's reagent on an HPTLC plate, which produces orange spots with various Rf. The various Rf values of the medicines allow for their detection and identification. It established Noscapine as an adulterant in heroin and described how stable heroin is in methanol. They also discussed profiling street drugs by high performance liquid chromatography, simultaneous detection of adulterants and coextract ants in illicit heroin, and caffeine and paracetamol as the primary adulterants in heroin and brown sugar, respectively. According to the, alcohol is regularly discovered in post-mortem forensic toxicology, both by itself and in combination with other substances [60].

The technique is also used in both qualitative and quantitative analytical applications, including those for nutraceuticals, herbal and dietary supplements, and many types of medications. It is utilized in quality control and purity checks, clinical applications such as drug screening and metabolic studies, forensic poisoning investigations, and the detection and identification of pharmaceutical raw materials, active pharmaceutical ingredients, and their metabolites in biological medium [61]. HPTLC is also used to determine the purity of lab-prepared mixes and tablets, as well as to analyze dose forms and dosage purity. Similarly, lamivudine, stavudine, and nevirapine HPTLC technique samples. A sensitive, straightforward, focused, exact, and accurate HPTLC technique of analysis for famotidine, diclofenac potassium, and paracetamol both as a bulk drug and in tablet format was created and validated. For the quantitative analysis of omeprazole in capsule dose form, a novel HPTLC approach has been created and validated [62]. The construction of a quality assurance program has been reported to use HPTLC, which is highly suitable for evaluating and monitoring the cultivation, harvesting, and extraction processes as well as testing for stability in herbal medicinal products [63].

9.3.2.6 Examination of Cosmetic Products

In cases where the connection could not be made, cosmetic evidence could be used to exclude the suspect exhibits [74]. The approach Separation, identification, and quantification are all possible using HPTLC. By utilizing HPTLC to separate the active ingredients, each one can produce a distinct fingerprint that can be compared to a reference fingerprint to determine whether the active ingredient is present or absent. Hence, analytical techniques utilizing HPTLC are created for standard quality assurance in order to identify the active components and excipients in cosmetics. The color of cosmetic evidence in forensic cosmetic examination enables speedy separation between questioned and recovered samples, however when identical colors are displayed, a subjective interpretation is required. Consequently, instrumental analysis is carried out on cosmetic evidence, with objective outcomes [75, 76].

9.4 Conclusion

HPLCs and HPTLCS are advanced hyphenated techniques of chromatography, and have been used for decades for the analysis of various pharmaceuticals, industrial, chemical and forensic samples. These techniques are widely used today for their better efficiency, and validated method in approach for the maintenance of quantitative and qualitative results with high accuracy and precision. The techniques are so far used for the analysis of chemical composition of various forensic exhibits found at the Crime scene. For both HPLC and HPTLC, the validation process since ancient times has gone through various Quality control and Quality management checks which have helped in the total quality management for these instruments in order to analyze samples. These analyses included specificity, selectivity, sensitivity, precision, accuracy, ruggedness, limit of detection (LOD), limit of quantitation (LOQ) and most importantly the stability of the instrument. Both the techniques work on the principle of adsorption chromatography which is practiced to analyze both quantitative and qualitative analytes and to detect the impurity in the sample. It has the quality to perform complex analysis as it consists of a large number of theoretical plates in the minimum area of plates, analysis time also gets reduced due to shorter migration distance and higher efficiency due smaller particle size. At present these instruments are widely used in discipline forensic sciences for the identification, determination and comparison of drugs, alcohol, ink, disputable documents, explosives, toxicological and biological examination are majorly encountered and analyzed with great degree of accuracy. They are also used for the examination of pharmaceutical industries and in clinical trail applications to check the quality control, metabolism studies and drug screening evaluation. The approach is widely used for processing the sample for better precision and accuracy consisting of lower analyzing time, cost efficient, easier sample preparation, low mobile phase consumption per sample and high possibility of clear visual detection of sample which help the forensic investigators to analyze thoroughly and provide opinion to present in court of law.

Consent for Publication

Consent of all authors

Conflict of Interest

No conflicts

Acknowledgement

All the authors have contributed to the chapter with interest.

References

1. LaCourse, M. E., LaCourse, W.R. (2017). General instrumentation in HPLC. *Liq. Chromatogr.* Elsevier. 417-429. http://dx.doi.org/10.1016/B978-0-12-805393-5.00017-8

2. Zotou, A. (2012). An overview of recent advances in HPLC instrumentation. *Cent. Eur. J. Chem.*, 10(3), 554-569. http://doi.org/10.2478/s11532-011-0161-0
3. Papadoyannis, J.N., Samanidou, V.F. (2004). Validation of HPLC instrumentation. *J. Liq. Chromatogr. Relat. Technol.,* 27 (5). 753-783. https://doi.org/10.1081/JLC-120029697
4. Dong, M.W. (2019). *HPLC and UHPLC for Practicing Scientists.* John Wiley & Sons.
5. Forlay-Frick. P., Fekete., J., Heberger, K. (2005). Classification and replacement test of HPLC systems using principal component analysis. *Anal. Chim. Acta,* 536(1- 2). 71-81. https://doi.org/10.1016/j.aca.2004.12.030
6. Reuhs, B.L.(2017). High-performance liquid chromatography. *Food Analysis,* 213-226.
7. Srivastava, M. M. (2011). An overview of HPTLC: A modern analytical technique with excellent potential for automation, optimization, hyphenation, and multidimensional applications. *High-performance thin-layer chromatography (HPTLC).* 3-24.
8. Loescher, C.M., Morton, D W., Razic, S , Kustrin, S.A. (2014). High performance thin layer chromatography (HPTLC) and high performance liquid chromatography (HPLC) for the qualitative and quantitative analysis of Calendula officinalis—Advantages and limitations. *J. Pharm. Biomed. Anal.,* 98. 52-59. http://dx.doi.org/10.1016/j.jpba.2014.04.023
9. Chawla, G., Chaudhary, K.K. (2019). A review of HPLC technique covering its pharmaceutical, environmental, forensic, clinical and other applications. *Int. J. Pharm. Chem. Anal.,* 6(2), 27-39. http://doi.org/10.18231/j.ijpca.2019.006
10. Hashim, H.O. (2018). Chromatography and HPLC principles. *Tech. Rep.,* http://dx.doi.org/10.13140/RG.2.2.33635.25126
11. Fornstedt, T., Forssen, P., Westerlund, D., (2015). Basic HPLC theory and definitions: retention, thermodynamics, selectivity, zone spreading, kinetics, and resolution. *Anal. Sep. Sci.,* 5(2). 1-22. https://doi.org/10.1080/10826070802126429
12. Pereira, L., (2008). Porous graphitic carbon as a stationary phase in HPLC: theory and applications. *J. Liq. Chromatogr. Relat. Technol.,* 31(11-12). 1687-1731.
13. Ramu, B, Chittela, K.B., (2018). High Performance Thin Layer Chromatography and Its Role Pharmaceutical Industry: Review. *Open Sci. J. Biosci. Bioeng.,* 5(3). 29-34.
14. Meyer, V.R., (2010). *Practical High Performance Liquid Chromatogryphy.* 5. Aufl. Chichester: WILEY.
15. Böcker, J., (1997). *Chromatographie.* Würzburg. Vogel Buchverlag.
16. .Kromidas, S.; Kuss, H.J., (2008). *Chromatogramme richtig integrieren und bewerten: Ein Praxishandbuch für Die HPLC und GC.* Weinheim. WILEY-VCH Verlag GmbH & Co. KGaA.
17. Dolan, J. W., (2002). *Peak Tailing and Resolution.* LC GC Europe.

18. Wille, S.M.R., Baere, T.D., Peters, F.T., (2017). Update of standard practices for new method validation in forensic toxicology. *Curr. Pharm. Des.*, 23(36). 5442-5454. https://doi.org/10.2174/1381612823666170714154444
19. Peters, F.T., Drummer, O.H., Musshoff, F., (2007). Validation of new methods. *Forensic Sci. Int.*, 165. 216-224. https://doi.org/10.1016/j.forsciint.2006.05.021
20. Variyar, P.S., (2011). Chatterjee, S., Sharma, A., Fundamentals and Theory of HPTLC-Based Separation. High-Performance Thin-Layer Chromatography (HPTLC). *Springer-Verlag Berlin Heidelberg*. 27-40. https://doi.org/10.1007/978-3-642-14025-9_2
21. Singh, R., (2013). HPLC method development and validation-an overview. *J. Pharm. Educ. Res.*, 4(1). 26-33.
22. Srivastava, M.M., (2011). An Overview of HPTLC: A Modern Analytical Technique with Excellent Potential for Automation, Optimization, Hyphenation, and Multidimensional Applications. High-Performance Thin-Layer Chromatography (HPTLC). *Springer-Verlag Berlin Heidelberg*. 3-26. https://doi.org/10.1007/978-3-642-14025-9_1
23. Inoue, H., Takaeb, F., Iwasa, M., Maeno, Y., Seko, Y., (1992). A New Marker for Estimation of Bloodstain age by High Performance Liquid Chromatography, *Forensic Sci. Int.*, 57. 17-27. https://doi.org/10.1016/0379-0738(92)90041-T
24. Bogusz, M.J., (1999). Hyphenated liquid chromatographic techniques in forensic toxicology. *J. Chromatogr. B*, 733. 65-91. https://doi.org/10.1016/s0378-4347(98)00520-9
25. Anger, F., Paysant, F., Brousse, I.L.N., Develay, P., Galliard, Y., Baert, A., Gueut, M.A.L., Pepi , G., Anger, J P., (2000). *J. Anal. Toxicol.*, 24(2). 90-92. https://doi.org/10.1093/jat/24.2.90
26. Cho, Y, Matsuoka, N., Kamiya, A., (1997). Determination of Organophosphorus Pesticides in Biological samples of Acute Poisoning by HPLC with Diode-Array Detector. *Chem. Pharm. Bull.*, 45(4). 737-740.
27. Meiser, H., (2005). Detection of Anticoagulant Residues by a New HPLC Method in Specimens of Poisoned Animals and a Poison Control Case Study. *J. Anal. Toxicol.*, 29. 556-563. https://doi.org/10.1093/jat/29.6.556
28. Lioupi, A., Kabir, A., Furton, K.G., Samanidou, V., 2019. Fabric phase sorptive extraction for the isolation of five common antidepressants from human urine prior to HPLC-DAD analysis. *J. Chromatogr. B*, 1118. 171-179. https://doi.org/10.1016/j.jchromb.2019.04.045
29. Krnac, D., Reiffova, K., Rolinski, B., (2019). A new HPLC-MS/MS method for simultaneous determination of Cyclosporine A, Tacrolimus, Sirolimus and Everolimus for routine therapeutic drug monitoring. *J. Chromatogr. B*, 1128. 121772. https://doi.org/10.1016/j.jchromb.2019.121772
30. Ullah, Q., Fatema, N., & Mohammad, A. (2020). Detection reagents used for on-plate identification of organic pesticides in biological samples with preliminary separation by TLC/HPTLC. *JPC–Journal of Planar Chromatography–Modern TLC*, 33, 533-546.

31. Pawar, U. D., Pawar, C. D., Kulkarni, U. K., & Pardeshi, R. K. (2020). Development method of high-performance thin-layer chromatographic detection of synthetic organophosphate insecticide profenofos in visceral samples. *JPC–Journal of Planar Chromatography–Modern TLC*, 33, 203-206.
32. Moorthy, T.N., Vicente, R , Haron, A.B., Nagayah, S., (2013). Identification of Explosives in Improvised Explosive Device (IED) Explosions for use in Crime Scene Investigation. *Journal for Bloomers of Research*, 5 (2). 637- 642.
33. Brown, G.W., Giambra, A.M., (2014). HPLC-MS examination of impurities in pentaerythritol tetranitrate. *J. Energ. Mater.*, 32(2). 117-128. https://doi.org/10.1080/07370652.2013.794887
34. Lloyd, J.B.F., (1991). Forensic explosives and firearms traces: Trapping of hplc peaks for gas chromatography. *J. Energ. Mater.*, 9(1-2). https://doi.org/10.1080/07370659108019857
35. Kaiser, M., HPLC Investigation of Explosives and Nitroaromatic Compounds with a Cyanopropyl Phase. (1999). *Propellants Explos. Pyrotech.*, 23(6). 309-312. https://doi.org/10.1002/(SICI)1521-4087(199812)23:6<309::AID-PREP309>3.0.CO;2-L
36. Chaloosi, M., Nejad-Darzi, S. K. H., & Ghoulipour, V. (2009). Separation and Determination of PETN and TNT by HPTLC. *Propellants, Explosives, Pyrotechnics: An International Journal Dealing with Scientific and Technological Aspects of Energetic Materials*, 34(1).
37. Nicoletti, M. (2011). HPTLC fingerprint: a modern approach for the analytical determination of botanicals. *Revista Brasileira de Farmacognosia*, 21, 818-823.
38. Kemp, S.E., Carr, D.J., Kieser, J., Nivem, B.E., Taylor, M.C., (2009). Forensic evidence in apparel fabrics due to stab events. *Forensic Sci. Int.*, 191 (1-3). 86-96. https://doi.org/10.1016/j.forsciint.2009.06.013
39. Robertson, J, Roux, C., Wiggins, K.G., (2017). *Forensic Examination of Fibres*. CRC press.
40. Mitchell, J L., Carr, D.J., Niven, B.E., Harrison, K., Girvan, E., (2012). Physical and mechanical degradation of shirting fabrics in burial conditions. *Forensic Sci. Int.*, 222 (1-3). 94-101. https://doi.org/10.1016/j.forsciint.2012.05.005
41. Schotman, T.G., Xu, X., Rodewijk, N., Weerd, J.V.D., (2017). Application of dye analysis in forensic fibre and textile examination: Case examples. *Forensic Sci. Int.*, 278. 338-350. https://doi.org/10.1016/j.forsciint.2017.07.026
42. Hu, C., Zhu, J., Mei, H., Shi, H., Guo, H., Zhang, G., Wang, P., Lu, L., Zheng, X., (2018). A sensitive HPLC-MS/MS method for the analysis of fiber dyes. *Forensic Chem.*, 11. 1-6. https://doi.org/10.1016/j.forc.2018.08.001
43. Wiczling, P., Markuszewski, J., Kaliszan, M., Galer, K., Kaliszan, R., (2005). Combined pH/organic solvent gradient HPLC in analysis of forensic material. *J. Pharm. Biomed. Anal.*, 37 (5). 871-875. https://doi.org/10.1016/j.jpba.2004.06.031

44. Groves, E., Palenik, S., & Palenik, C. S. (2018). Reproducibility of high-performance thin-layer chromatography (HPTLC) in textile dye analysis. *Forensic Chem.*, 8, 104-110.
45. Hosu, A., Pop, B., & Cimpoiu, C. (2015). The forensic analysis of pigments from some inks by HPTLC. *J. Liq. Chromatogr. Relat. Technol.*, 38(11), 1109-1112.
46. Calcerrada, M., Ruiz, C.G., (2015). Review on the Analysis of Questioned Documents. *Anal. Chim. Acta*, 853. 143-166. https://doi.org/10.1016/j.aca.2014.10.057
47. Wang, X.F., Yu, J., Xie, M.X., Yao, Y.T., Han, J., (2008). Identification and dating of the fountain pen ink entries on documents by ion-pairing high-performance liquid chromatography. *Forensic Sci. Int.*, 180. 43-49. https://doi.org/10.1016/j.forsciint.2008.06.008
48. Hofer, R., (2004). Dating of ballpoint pen ink. *J. Forensic Sci.*, 49(6). 1353-1357.
49. Tebbett, I.R., Chen, C., Fitzgerald, M., Olson, L., (1992). *The Use of HPLC with Multiwavelength Detection for the Differentiation of Non Ball Pen Inks.* Larry Olson ASTM International.
50. Salman, H.N.K.A., Jasim, E.Q., (2018). Analytical methods for diagnosis a mixture of narcotic substances in seized materials. *Int. J. Green Pharm.*, 12(3). 216-226. https://doi.org/10.22377/ijgp.v12i03.1955
51. Al-Salman, H.N., (2017). Analysis methods and qualitative diagnosis chromatographic for mixture of narcotic substances in seized materials. *Eur. J. Sci. Res.*, 147. 403-411.
52. Madej, K., Parczewski, A., Kala, M., (2003). HPLC/DAD screening method for selected psychotropic drugs in blood. *Toxicol. Mech. Methods,* 13(2). 121-127. https://doi.org/10.1080/15376510309842
53. Khaleel, N.D.H., *Fate of Psychotropic Drugs in the Aquatic Environment,* Leuphana University Luneburg.
54. United Nations. Division of Narcotic Drugs. (1988). *Recommended Methods for Testing Opium/crude Morphine: Manual for Use by National Narcotics Laboratories.* UN.
55. Butler William, P. (1987). *Method of Analysis for Alkaloids.* Opiates, Marihuana, Barbiturates & Miscellaneous Drugs, Bureau of Narcotics & Dangerous Drugs, Department of Justice, US, 59.
56. Stevens, H. M., & Moffat, A. C. (1986). *Clarke's Isolation and Identification of Drugs (in Pharmaceuticals, Body Fluids, and Post-Mortem Material).*
57. Gunn John, W. (1986). In *Analytical Manual of Bureau of Narcotics & Dangerous Drugs.* Department of Justice, US (By Stenely P Sobol & Richard A Moore): Page, (121).
58. Reddy, M. M., Suresh, V., Jayashanker, G., Rao, B. S., & Sarin, R. K. (2003). Application of capillary zone electrophoresis in the separation and determination of the principal gum opium alkaloids. *Electrophoresis,* 24(9), 1437-1441.

59. United Nations. Division of Narcotic Drugs. (1986). Recommended Methods for Testing Heroin: Manual for Use by National Narcotics Laboratories (Vol. 6). UN.
60. More, B. P., Doundkar, B. B., Toche, R. B., & Shinde, D. B. (2013). Separation and identification of alprazolam from diacetylmorphine along with other opium alkaloids by HPTLC. *Int. J. Pharm. Bio. Sci.*, 3, 204-208
61. Ramu, B., & Chittela, K. B. (2018). High Performance Thin Layer Chromatography and Its Role Pharmaceutical Industry. *Open Sci. J. Biosci. Bioeng.*, 5(3), 29-34.
62. Attimarad, M., Ahmed, K. M., Aldhubaib, B. E., & Harsha, S. (2011). High-performance thin layer chromatography: A powerful analytical technique in pharmaceutical drug discovery. *Pharm. Methods*, 2(2), 71-75.
63. Sherma, J. (2010). Review of HPTLC in drug analysis: 1996-2009. *Journal of AOAC International*, 93(3), 754-764.
64. Almeida, A., Sarmwnto, B., Rodrigues, F., (2017). Insights on *in vitro* models for safety and toxicity assessment of cosmetic ingredients. *Int. J. Pharm.*, 519 (1-2). 178-185. https://doi.org/10.1016/j.ijpharm.2017.01.024
65. McRill, C., Boyer, L.V., Flood, T.J., Ortega, L., (2000). Mercury toxicity due to use of a cosmetic cream. *J. Occup. Environ. Med.*, 42(1). 4-7.
66. Grześkowiak, A.Z., Werner, J., Skowron, J., Goslinska, B.C., (2016). Determination of parabens in cosmetic products using high performance liquid chromatography with fluorescence detection. *Anal. Methods*, 8(19). 3903-3909.
67. Baranowska, I, Wojciechowska, I, (2013). The Determination of Preservatives in Cosmetics and Environmental Waters by HPLC. *Pol. J. Environ. Stud.*, 22(6). 1609-1625.
68. Rastogi, S.C., Barwick, V.J., Carter, S.V., (1997). Identification of organic colourants in cosmetics by HPLC-diode array detection. *Chromatographia.*, 45(1). 215-228.
69. Koo, H.J., Lee, B.M., (2004). Estimated exposure to phthalates in cosmetics and risk assessment. *J. Toxicol. Environ. Health, Part A*, 67 (23-24). 1901-1914.
70. Lee, S.M., Jeong, H.J., Chang, I.S., (2008). Simultaneous determination of heavy metals in cosmetic product. *J. Cosmet. Sci.*, 59 (5). 441-448.
71. Valet, B., Mayor, M., Fitoussi, F., Capellier, R., Dormoy, M., & Ginestar, J. (2007). Colouring Agents in Decorative and other Cosmetics. Analytical Methods. *Analysis of cosmetic products*, 141-152. 10
72. Saferstein, R. (2004). *Criminalistics: An introduction to forensic science.*
73. Andrasko, J. (1981). Forensic analysis of lipsticks. *Forensic Sci. Int.*, 17(3), 235-251.
74. Shimamoto, G. G., Terra, J., & Bueno, M. I. (2013). Use of portable X-ray fluorescence to discriminate brands of nail polishes: a potential forensic tool. *J. Braz. Chem. Soc.*, 24, 731-735.

75. López-López, M., Vaz, J., & García-Ruiz, C. (2015). Confocal Raman spectrocopy for the analysis of nail polish evidence. *Talanta*, 138, 155-162.
76. Chophi, R., Sharma, S., Sharma, S., & Singh, R. (2019). Trends in the forensic analysis of cosmetic evidence. *Forensic Chem.*, 14, 100165.

10

Forensic Aspects of Hyphenated Techniques

Nisha[1], Priyanka Singh[1] and Priyanka Chhabra[2*]

[1]*Amity Amity Institute of Forensic Sciences, Amity University, Noida, Uttar Pradesh, India*
[2]*Centre of Medical Biotechnology, Amity Institute of Biotechnology, Amity University, Noida, Uttar Pradesh, India*

Abstract
Hyphenated techniques are a blend of chromatographic and spectral methods for the analysis of various forensic samples with more accuracy and precision. Chromatography generates pure or nearly pure fractions of chemical constituents within a mixture, while spectroscopy provides specific identification information using established standards or library spectra. Over the past two decades, hyphenated analytical methodologies have undergone remarkable advancements, greatly broadening their utility in scrutinizing various forensic samples, such as drugs, toxins, fire residue, explosives, trace materials, paint, ink assessments, illicit substances, volatile and organic substances, as well as the metabolites of various drugs or poisons. These advancements have proven valuable in crime scene investigations, aiding both the medico-legal and criminal justice systems. In this chapter, we will discuss most used hyphenated techniques used in forensic science and their practical applications for the analyses of various forensic samples.

Keywords: Analysis, detection, techniques, hyphenated, forensic, application

**Corresponding author*: pchhabra188@gmail.com

Priyanka Chhabra, Divya Bajpai Tripathy, Anjali Gupta, Rajeev Kumar, Kajol Bhati and Shruti Shukla (eds.) Advances in Analytical Techniques for Forensic Investigation, (271–306) © 2024 Scrivener Publishing LLC

10.1 Introduction to Hyphenated Techniques in Forensic Science

Over the past century, numerous novel chemical compounds have been investigated and examined across various scientific domains to drive technological progress. In recent years, analytical chemists have increasingly employed methods such as electrochemistry, chromatography, spectroscopy, and others to thoroughly investigate the composition and characteristics of diverse materials and chemical compounds. Traditionally, these techniques were done separately to identify and quantify the components of intricate mixtures, such as pollutants in the environment or drugs in the bloodstream [1]. Nowadays, Hyphenated approaches have drawn more and more attention as the primary method for resolving challenging analytical issues. The effectiveness of integrating separation technologies with spectroscopic methods has been showcased, enabling the comprehensive examination of unknown compounds within forensic samples, both quantitatively and qualitatively. This new approach is evolving at a rapid speed [2]. Liquid chromatography-mass spectrometry (LC-MS), gas chromatography-mass spectrometry (GC-MS), and capillary electrophoresis-mass spectrometry (CE-MS) are commonly used analytical chemistry techniques that combine the separation abilities of chromatography or electrophoresis with the sensitive and specific skills of mass spectrometry. These methods facilitate the precise identification and quantification of a diverse array of chemicals, becoming increasingly vital in various fields for their enhanced accuracy, precision, specificity, and sensitivity provided by the combined instruments. It finds relevance in various domains such as pharmaceutical research, environmental analysis, and forensic science and represents the cutting-edge of analytical instrumentation, advancing our comprehension of intricate chemical systems [3].

Hyphenated techniques can be applied to much forensic evidence as they present abilities to separate, identify, and quantify complex mixtures of compounds. Forensic scientists utilize (GC-MS) extensively and frequently to analyze narcotics, poisons, explosives, and other volatile substances. When combined with MS, GC, a separation technique that offers both qualitative and quantitative information on the molecules contained in a sample, produces the most reliable results, making it a perfect tool for toxicology, arson investigations, and drug testing [4]. Another commonly used method in forensic chemistry for analyzing non-volatile substances such metabolites, narcotics, poisons, and pesticides is (LC-MS). Its great sensitivity and specificity enable it to identify tiny quantities of chemicals in complicated mixes and matrices. The detection of tiny molecules, peptides, and proteins is often accomplished using (CE-MS). The instrument is being exploited by forensic professionals to evaluate bodily fluids for the identification of drugs, metabolites, and proteins. The GC-IR technology (gas chromatography-infrared spectroscopy-infrared spectroscopy) combines the analytical skills of IR with the separation capacity of GC and used to evaluate organic compounds in a range of materials, including fibers, paint, and soil. A tandem technique for finding and detecting pharmaceuticals and their metabolites in biological samples is (LC-MS/MS). Hyphenated procedures are essential for analyzing trace and forensic evidence, detecting illegal compounds, and characterizing unknown molecules [5].

10.2 Hyphenated Techniques Used in Forensic Science

10.2.1 Gas Chromatography-Mass Spectrometry (GC-MS)

GC-MS is an exceptional technique used for the separation of components in a mixture which is combined with detection and identification capabilities, serving two roles at once. Several forensic samples such as drug, drug metabolites, fire debris, explosives investigation, and identification of unknown samples found at crime scenes rely on GC-MS. Gas chromatography separates mixtures of volatile compounds into individual components according to their physical and chemical properties. The segregated components pass through a detector which records the presence and amount percentage of each component in a mixture on the basis of their mass-to-charge ratio and provide mass spectra that yield increased structural insights through the interpretation of fragmentations [5]. GC-MS is a powerful analytical tool that combines gas chromatography and mass spectrometric analysis to identify and measure the concentration of components in a mixture [6].

10.2.1.1 Principle and Instrumentation

There are two fundamental phases in the GC-MS method: firstly, gas chromatography is used to separate the molecules and secondly, mass spectrometry detects and delivers the spectra for examination. Gas chromatography can discriminate between distinct components of a sample based on their physical and chemical characteristics, such as boiling point and polarity. The stationary phase is a thin coating put inside of the column. The sample is injected into the column which undergoes vaporization and is transported through the column by an inert gas like helium. As the different components of the sample interact with the stationary phase, it results in the separation and elution of the sample at different times. After the separation of chemical components by gas chromatography, they are injected into the mass spectrometer. The separated components are ionized by the bombardment of high-energy electrons which leads to the fragmentation of those compounds into smaller ions or charged particles. The ions or charged particles are separated according to their mass-to-charge ratio and are detected by a detector, such as an electron multiplier [7]. This technique provides a mass spectrum enabling the identification and measurement of the sample components. Each component provides a separate mass spectrum, which is compared to a library of known spectra for the identification of compound.

Gas chromatography (GC) utilizes a fused silica capillary column coated with a stationary phase to effectively separate components [8]. Initially, an unknown sample is introduced into the GC column's inlet via a syringe located at one end of the column, where it is vaporized and separated. A carrier gas, including gases like argon, helium, nitrogen, or hydrogen, transports the sample through the column, resulting in the separation of mixture elements over time. Subsequently, a Mass spectrometer (MS) is employed to ionize the separated sample components, utilizing various ionization sources like chemical ionization (CI), Electron ionization (EI),

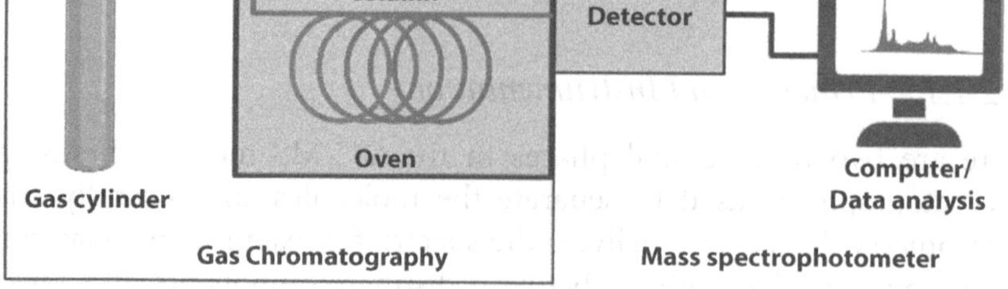

Figure 10.1 Gas chromatography–mass spectrometry: Instrumentation [1].

and electrospray ionization. Identification of ionized components is based on their mass-to-charge ratios, with commonly used analyzers in GC-MS being quadrupole, ion trap, and Time-of-flight (TOF) analyzers. These analyzers generate signals transmitted to detectors for component identification and quantification [8]. Detector signals are converted into mass spectra, displayed on the screen (Figure 10.1). The resulting mass spectra from this combined technique provide enhanced structural insights through the interpretation of fragmentations, enabling comparison with library spectra by evaluating fragment ions with varying relative abundances.

10.2.1.2 Applications of GC-MS in Forensic Science

Forensic materials including narcotics, explosives, poisons, trace evidence, and more are often identified and their chemical components are analyzed using the gas chromatography-mass spectrometry (GC-MS) technology.

Drug analysis: The detection and identification of drugs and their metabolites in bodily fluids, such as blood and urine, is accomplished using GC-MS. Designer benzodiazepines (DBZDs) result from blending Benzodiazepines (BZDs) and Z-drugs, commonly employed to alleviate anxiety, aid sleep, manage seizures, and relax muscles. DBZDs, a category of psychoactive substances derived from non-medically approved benzodiazepines and primarily used for recreational purposes, present a considerable challenge to toxicologists. Detecting and quantifying these substances, particularly in blood, necessitates the development of fast and reliable techniques. In one study, Laura Banaszkiewicz and colleagues established and validated GC-MS/TS (Gas chromatography-tandem mass spectrometry) for measuring 28 benzodiazepine derivatives and 3 Z-drugs [7]. In another research endeavor, Maiko and co-researchers successfully separated and identified a 63 drugs and pesticides, including barbiturates, benzodiazepines, tri/tetracyclic antidepressants, drugs of abuse, phenethylamines, and pesticides, from whole blood using GC-MS. This process involves sample preparation through modified QuEChERS extraction and dispersive solid-phase extraction (dSPE) clean-up, followed by gas chromatography-tandem mass spectrometry (GC-MS/MS). This method finds effective application in clinical and forensic toxicology analysis [8].

Methylenedioxypyrovalerone (MDPV) is a cathinone stimulant that has similarities with the drug ecstasy, often known as MDMA, which has been misused during the past several years in many parts of the world. In a case from Germany, people felt unwell after using this new medicine and its content in the blood of the patients varied a lot. Different people's biological samples, including blood and urine, were collected and analyzed using GC-MS. MDPV medication could be detected utilizing this approach which comprised its chemical makeup and its metabolites. GC-MS was also proven to be beneficial in identifying opiates, cannabis, benzodiazepines, cocaine accessible in blood and the urine collected from the individuals [9].

Fire debris: GC-MS is used to analyze any accelerants or other chemicals, residues such as soot and debris, which can be essential to ascertain the cause of fire. In a recent study, Briana A. Capistran and team successfully detected pure ignitable liquids, such as gasoline and diesel fuel in fire debris samples, within a concentration range of 0.012 mg/mL to 0.018 mg/mL. They utilized GC-MS analysis as part of their efforts to expedite the analytical process and enhance sample processing capacity. This approach has garnered significant attention in the field of forensics in recent years. The primary components present in both the liquids were identified through a combination of total ion chromatograms, relevant extracted ion profiles, and deconvolution techniques [8]. In another studies Guerrara and colleagues conducted an investigation to evaluate whether the substances found in clothing and body products could potentially disrupt the analysis of ignitable liquids They examined samples of both used and unused clothing as well as various body products using PHC and GC-MS and found that somebody products resemble to heavy petroleum distillates and contain compounds often found in ignitable liquids [10].

In an arson investigation, charred debris from a desk drawer, including some evidence that seemed to be burnt plastic, was analyzed using GC-FID and MS. Results received from GC-FID was unclear about the presence of accelerant in the sample which led to the coupling of MS with the GC system and the results revealed the existence of heavy petroleum distillate in the sample. The sample is made up of a diene, an alkene, and an n-alkane, with the alkene having the most noticeable peak, according to the analysis of the mass spectra. The Sample matched burnt polyethylene bag standards that confirmed that the components in the chromatogram were typical of polyethylene. Finally, the results e GC-MS study showed peaks in the chromatogram were caused by debris pyrolysis rather than by the presence of an accelerant [11].

Trace evidences: In recent years GC-MS is used for the identification and quantification of dye components in hair samples. This application can potentially aid in distinguishing human hair samples discovered at crime scenes. The process involves extracting diamines and aminophenols from the hair samples and subjecting them to GC-MS analysis. Specifically, five components commonly found in oxidation hair dyes—namely, p-phenylenediamine, toluene-2,5-diamine, o-aminophenol, m-aminophenol, and p-aminophenol—were successfully detected and identified by *Tanada et al.* [11].

Paint analysis: Gas Chromatography-Mass Spectrometry (GC-MS) is a highly analytical technique employed for the fractionation of constituents found within paint, including pigments, binders, solvents, and additives. This separation process occurs via gas chromatography. Subsequently, the technique employs mass spectrometry to identify and elucidate the molecular structures of these components. The acquired data is instrumental in discerning the formulation and provenance of the paint, rendering GC-MS particularly indispensable in scientific disciplines such as forensic science. In a study Sabaradin and their research team conducted an analysis of 80 simulated automotive paint samples by employing Pyrolysis-Gas Chromatography-Mass Spectrometry (Py-GC-MS) [12]. Their primary focus was on assessing the ability to distinguish between paint transfers of two distinct layers: the base coat and the primer. The study involved a detailed examination of the chemical composition of the different components within the paint samples. Subsequently, this analysis resulted in the categorization of the samples into three distinct classes through the utilization of Principal Component Analysis (PCA) and cluster analysis techniques [11].

Food and beverage analysis: The GC-MS method has versatile applications in the identification and categorization of various contaminants, encompassing pesticides, toxins, and additional substances, within food and beverage specimens. In a specific investigation conducted by Gulyaim N. Sagandykova and colleagues, the research team employed GC-MS in conjunction with Solid-Phase Microextraction (SPME) to detect and quantify the presence of propylene glycol, sorbic acid, and benzoic acid in 25 wine samples, which were employed as adulterants. Therefore, the suggested approach is advocated for wine quality assessment and the identification of adulterated samples [13].

Gunshot residue analysis: Gunshot residue (GSR) comprises minuscule metallic particles discharged from a fired firearm, and these particles can be detected on the hands and clothing of a shooter. Rapid identification and characterization of both organic and inorganic GSR are crucial in investigations related to firearm incidents. In a study conducted by Ellen Goudsmits and colleagues, they present a technique for extracting and identifying a comprehensive range of organic and inorganic compounds from a single GSR sample. This method employs solid-phase microextraction gas chromatography-mass spectrometry (SPME-GC-MS). It successfully categorized organic GSR compounds like ethyl centralite, diphenylamine, and 2-nitrodiphenylamine, as well as distinctive inorganic GSR components. Since the identified organic GSR compounds are significant for confirming GSR materials, this method effectively its capability to generate a comprehensive chemical profile from a solitary GSR sample therefore potentially enhancing the evidential value of GSR findings [14].

In another study, Arie Zeichner and colleagues gathered GSR from the attire of individuals who had discharged firearms. They employed vacuum collection techniques and subjected the collected residues to analysis using gas chromatography/thermal energy analyzer (GC/TEA), ion mobility spectrometry (IMS), and gas chromatography/mass spectrometry (GC/MS) and identify the constituents of gunshot residue within the provided sample [15].

Skeletal analysis: The analysis of DNA in skeletonized human remains can be quite challenging, particularly when the remains have been exposed to substances that hinder DNA processing during decomposition. These substances can impede efficient DNA extraction or interfere with subsequent PCR-based procedures. In a research study conducted by Suni M. Edetson and their team, they developed a gas chromatography/mass spectrometry (GC/MS) protocol to assess the substances present in skeletonized human remains recovered from the field, as well as the DNA extracted from these materials. They assessed twenty-one bone samples and seventeen DNA extracts using three different solvents and various GC/MS parameters to determine the optimal conditions for recovering trace DNA materials present in the samples [16].

GC-MS offers significant advantages compared to other analytical methods. Its high sensitivity allows for the detection and differentiation of substances even in complex mixtures, due to its selectivity in producing distinct spectra for compounds. Furthermore, it is non-destructive, making it suitable for examining small or valuable samples without causing harm. In the realm of analytical chemistry, GC-MS is emerging as an invaluable tool for forensic experts due to its ability to detect, identify, and analyze trace amounts of chemicals in complex compound mixtures [2].

10.2.2 Head Space–Gas Chromatography (HS-GC)

Head-space gas chromatography (HS-GC) is a modern, fast and easily automated technique that has achieved much interest for the identification and determination of range of concentration volatile compound such as toxicological agents, medications, and accelerators, as well as volatile organic compounds (VOCs) in solid and liquid samples. HS-GC also aid in determining thermodynamic properties like partition coefficients, activity coefficients at infinite dilutions [17]. The demand of headspace analysis lies in its easiness and the fact that it offers a very clean way for introducing volatile analytes into a gas chromatograph, as the injector system and column hardly need any maintenance [18]. In HS-GC a sealed container holds a small sample portion, and the headspace above it is examined for compounds which contain volatile compounds that have evaporated from the sample. The volatile compounds are then heated to migrate into the gas phase and injected into the Gas Chromatograph (GC) section for component separation and analysis. The analysis in HS-GC involves toxicological samples for pharmaceuticals and volatile toxins in biological samples including blood, urine, and tissues as well as the examination of fire debris samples gathered from arson investigations [19]. The findings from the analysis may be utilized for diagnosing the cause of death of an individual, combatting drug trafficking and misuse, and pinpointing the cause and origin of fire. Gas Chromatography combined with Head Space sampling has proven to be a crucial tool in forensic science for swiftly, precisely, and sensitively detecting volatile compounds in various forensic materials. It plays a vital role in crime investigations, toxicological analysis, and upholding the principles of law and public safety [20].

10.2.2.1 Principle and Instrumentation

In HS-GC (Gas Chromatography with Headspace sampling), volatile chemicals present in a sealed sample vial's headspace are selectively separated and identified. A small portion of the sample is placed into a sealed container, allowing its volatile components to equilibrate with the headspace. Upon heating, these volatile substances in the vial evaporate, entering the headspace as a gas phase. This headspace gas, containing volatile compounds, is then extracted from the vial and introduced into the Gas Chromatograph (GC) for separation and analysis on the basis of varying physical and chemical properties of the compounds (Figure 10.2). These volatile compounds move through the chromatographic column at distinct rates, resulting in the formation of individual peaks on the chromatogram. These peaks are identified by their retention time and the mass spectra obtained from the Mass Spectrometer (MS) detector connected to the GC. To identify and quantify the volatile compounds in the forensic

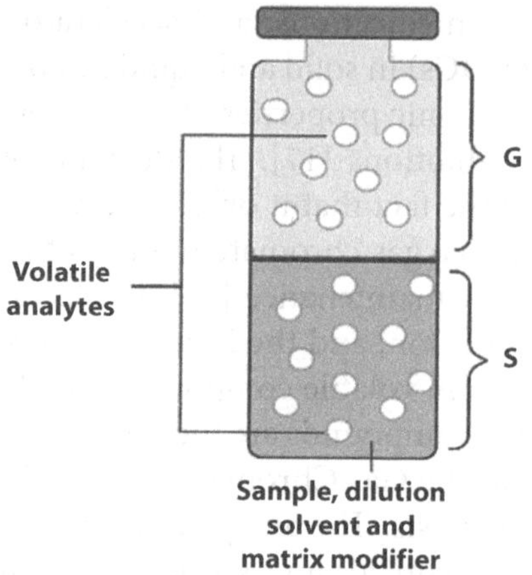

Figure 10.2 Phases of the headspace in the vial are shown schematically [2].

sample, the acquired data is compared with reference standards or spectral databases [21].

The sample vial employed in HS-GC is specially crafted with a polytetrafluoroethylene (PTFE)-lined septum to ensure compatibility with the analytical system and withstand the elevated temperatures necessary for analysis. HS-GC incorporates an autosampler, an automated apparatus that loads sample vials into the HS-GC system, offering the capability to

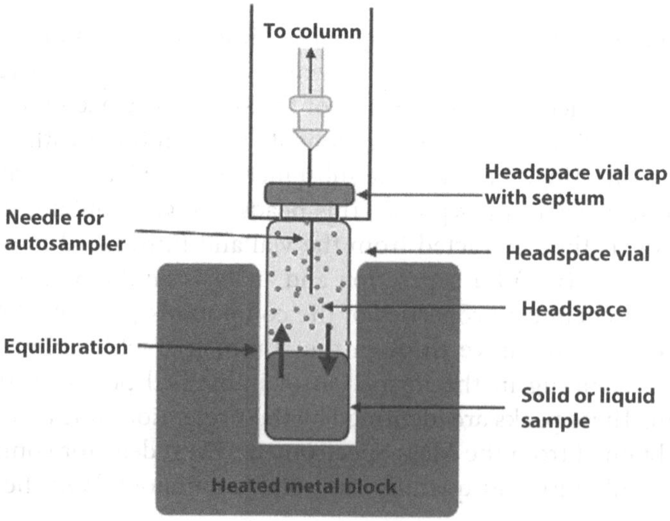

Figure 10.3 Gas chromatography–headspace: instrumentation [3].

handle multiple samples simultaneously, thus enhancing laboratory efficiency. A critical component of HS-GC is the Headspace Sampler, which generates the headspace above the sealed vial by warming it, causing volatile chemicals to transition into the gas phase [17]. Within the GC Column, the headspace gas holds and separates volatile substances, undergoing a separation process as they traverse the column (Figure 10.3). Typically, a Mass Spectrometer (MS) serves as the detector in HS-GC, aiding in the identification and quantification of the separated compounds by generating mass spectra for each compound. The data system captures and processes signals from the detector, converting them into chromatograms and mass spectra, which are then interpreted for analytical purposes [18].

10.2.2.2 Applications of HS-GC in Forensic Science

Gas chromatography (GC) and headspace sampling (HS) are two analytical procedures used jointly in forensic science for the investigation of distinct forms of evidence.

Drug and Poison Analysis in Biological Fluids: HS-GC is largely employed for the detection of drug, pesticide, and poison analysis in biological samples such as blood, urine, and saliva, since it facilitates the identification of volatile chemicals that would otherwise be lost during sample preparation.[19] A case from India focuses on the forensic analysis of Sevoflurane, an anesthetic drug using the GC-HS technique. Sevoflurane is a volatile and non-flammable anesthetic drug with potential health risks such as cardio-respiratory depression and hypotension. In this case, a bottle of suspected narcotics was submitted to the Punjab Forensic Science Agency. The suspected substance was analyzed using HS-GC-MS. The results displayed a single peak on the chromatogram which matched with the reference spectrum of Sevoflurane, confirming its presence in the sample. This case study demonstrates the efficacy and efficiency of the HS-GC-MS method in detecting Sevoflurane and other potentially harmful drugs [22].

To find instances of cyanide poisoning and fire exposure in post-mortem biological matrices, a study was conducted. For the research of dangerous compounds using GC-HS, biological samples comprising blood, aqueous solutions, and gastrointestinal contents were collected. The experiments were run to see how stable cyanide was in the blood, and the findings revealed that at 4 or 20 °C, the concentration did not fluctuate much over a two-week period. This proof demonstrates the technique's applicability in forensic investigations involving cyanide poisoning and fire exposure [23].

Fire and Explosive Residue Analysis: HS-GC is a valuable analytical technique widely used in the fields of arson and explosive analysis. In their research, María José Aliaño-González and colleagues successfully employed an advanced and rapid analytical method known as HS-GC, combined with the utilization of chemometric tools in the analysis of 80 fire debris samples. This innovative approach holds promise for the detection of ignitable liquid residues within samples of fire debris. The team conducted experiments using four distinct substrates like pine wood, cork, paper, and cotton sheet and four different ignitable liquids with varying compositions like gasoline, diesel, ethanol, and paraffin. In this study they a achieved a high level of accuracy, with a 95% correct discrimination rate in identifying specific ignitable liquid residues present in the samples [24].
Biological Sample Analysis: Headspace gas chromatography (HS-GC) combined with mass spectrometry offers a means to detect a variety of volatile organic compounds within different biological samples like whole blood vitreous humor and urine and found practical application in forensic cases. In a study, C. Monteiro and colleagues focused on qualitatively and quantitatively analyzing a set of 11 volatile organic substances such as ethyl acetate, 2-propanol, acetaldehyde, ethyl acetate with diverse physicochemical properties in biological sample. The developed method demonstrated high selectivity and sensitivity, even with small sample volumes (100 μL). Notably, no extraction procedure was required, as the sample was directly injected using the HS injection technique [25].

10.2.3 Gas Chromatography-Infrared Spectroscopy (GC-IR)

A dynamic analytical approach called gas chromatography-infrared spectroscopy combines the power of GC to separate compounds with the ability of IR to identify molecules. Several disciplines, including chemistry, forensic science, pharmacology, and environmental science, have adopted this method. Gas chromatography separates and analyses the volatile substances based on their molecular weight and boiling point. The sample is vaporized and separated into individual components which traverse through the infrared spectrometer. The components of the sample are then analyzed and identification is done based on individual infrared spectra generated [23].

Infrared spectroscopy is a method employing the interaction of infrared radiation with matter to detect and quantify different chemical species in a sample. When infrared radiation is applied to the sample, the molecular bonds of the sample absorb radiation at distinct frequencies, resulting in a unique infrared spectrum that can be used to identify the sample components [26].

GC-IR allows the identification and separation of complex mixtures of compounds in a single analysis making it a very useful technique in different fields, including the analysis of complex mixtures of organic compounds in forensic samples. Additionally, GC-IR offers a wide range of advantages due to its ability to detect unknown compounds in complex mixtures. The spectra obtained are compared with a library of known spectra and the unknown compounds of the sample can be confidently identified. Another advantage of GC-IR is its sensitivity. The limit of detection (LOD) of GC-IR can be as low as parts per billion, due to which it is an ideal instrument for analyzing the trace amount of components in a sample evidence [27].

10.2.3.1 Principle and Instrumentation

The fundamental principle of GC-IR is rooted in the distinct absorption of infrared light at specific wavelengths by various chemical substances. The GC-IR process involves several stages, including sample injection, separation, and detection. Initially, the sample is introduced into a gas chromatography column equipped with an internal stationary phase. A carrier gas, typically helium or nitrogen, vaporizes the sample and conveys it through the GC column. The individual compounds within the mixture start to separate based on their physical and chemical properties, such as boiling point, polarity, and molecular size, as they interact with the stationary phase. Subsequently, these separated compounds enter an infrared (IR) detector, where they each generate a unique spectrum depending on the amount of IR light they absorb [28].

GC-IR is comprised of essential elements, including a Gas Chromatography column and an injector responsible for introducing the sample along with a carrier gas, typically helium or nitrogen. Various techniques, such as liquid injection, headspace analysis, or solid-phase microextraction, can be employed for sample introduction. The composition of the stationary phase within the GC column can be tailored to specific applications. Precision in the separation of sample components is achieved through adjustments in gas flow rate and pressure. As the sample traverses the column, it is subjected to IR radiation, detected and quantified by a detector consisting of a sample cell, an infrared source, and a detecting element that transforms absorbed radiation into an electrical signal. Data generated by the detector undergoes processing and analysis via specialized software on a computer, facilitating compound identification and quantification based

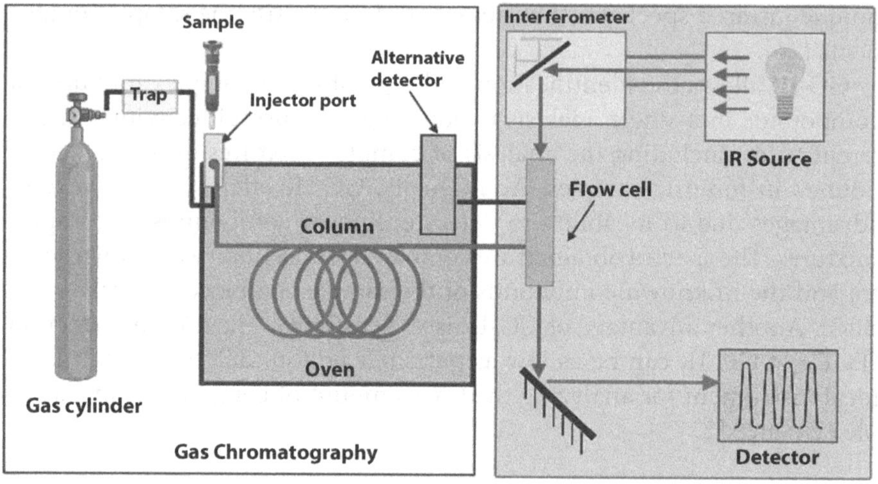

Figure 10.4 Gas chromatography–infrared spectrophotometry: instrumentation [4].

on the spectra produced. Additionally, some GC-IR systems may incorporate supplementary components like a thermal modulator to enhance sample component separation or a mass spectrometer for comprehensive sample composition analysis (Figure 10.4) [27].

10.2.3.2 Applications of GC-IR in Forensic Science

A variety of items, such as drugs, explosives, arson leftovers, and trace evidence, can be investigated using GC-IR.

Drug Analysis: Gas chromatography Fourier transform infrared spectroscopy (GC/FT-IR) has been explored as an innovative technique for forensic drug identification. This method proves to be highly specific, even when dealing with closely related isomers. GC/FT-IR enables precise identification through infrared fingerprinting, routinely detecting substances in the parts per billion (ppb) range. Researchers are currently developing GC/FT-IR methods capable of detecting extremely low picogram quantities of materials. The primary advantage of employing GC/FT-IR lies in its data specificity, offering fingerprint-like identification, significantly enhancing the confidence level of the analysis. This technique can differentiate isomers and facilitate the detection of designer drugs as part of routine analysis. In a study led by Tania Maria Grazia Salerno and her colleagues, they successfully elucidated the structure of 1-pentyl-3-(1-naphthoyl) indole, commonly known as JWH-018, a synthetic cannabinoid found in illegal "incense blends." The accurate identification of such compounds, despite their chemical similarities, underscores the effectiveness of this approach for reliably analyzing complex mixtures of illicit drugs, presenting a viable alternative to widely used mass spectrometry-based methods [29].

Arson and Explosive Analysis: Explosive residues in debris and post-blast materials can be identified and quantified using GC-IR. It can also be used to analyze explosive residues present in the air at a scene of crime or on surfaces of objects. The accelerants can be analyzed with their chemical composition using GC-IR [28].

Analysis of Chemicals in Biological Samples: In toxicology, GC-IR is used to identify and measure the presence of poisonous substances in biological samples [30]. In research concentrating on detecting and identifying clandestinely synthesized fluoro-methoxy-substituted amphetamines 1–5 using gas chromatography–mass spectrometry (GC-MS). IR-spectroscopy employing solid- or vapor-phase IR-spectra effectively recognized and discriminated all tested fluoro-methoxy amphetamines 1–8 without difficulty. These findings suggest that GC-IR is undoubtedly a fantastic tool for examining complicated compounds at once and producing the desired results. Another study involved the investigation of the usefulness of GC-IR in discovering the distinction of positional isomers of fentanyl-related compounds. In this work, GC-IR was examined to replace GC-MS due to its constraints of limited discrimination between different kinds of Forensic Reference Standards. GC-IR proved its capacity to discriminate precisely [29]. New libraries of reference standards for 212 FRS were produced and made available to the forensic science community. When the GC-IR library, comprising all 212 FRS, was utilized for identification, a 100% success rate was attained. Three laboratories examined blind FRS samples using the GC-IR library and got flawless match correlations. The study also estimated the LODs (Limit of Detection) and LOQs (Limit of Quantification) for the GC-IR techniques. The findings significantly support employing GC-IR in evaluating unknown chemicals, notably FRS and other complicated drug structures with multiple isomer configurations. It delivers the best confidence in detecting novel psychoactive substances (NPS) molecules when both GC-MS and GC-IR are used simultaneously [31].

Forensic Anthropology: Drugs and other compounds that may have contributed to the person's death can be found using GC-IR in the study of skeletal remains. Additionally, it can be used to examine bone samples for isotopic signatures, which reveal details about a person's diet and place of origin [30].

10.2.4 Liquid Chromatography-Mass Spectrometry (LC-MS)

LC–MS is an integrated scientific approach that combines liquid chromatography (LC) with mass spectrometry (MS), uniting LC's capacity for physical separation with MS's remarkable specificity and sensitivity [32]. This amalgamation is extensively applied across diverse industries, encompassing forensic analysis, pharmaceuticals, the food and beverage sector, cosmetics, fingerprint examination, and the scrutiny of toxicological, biological, and serological samples. In LC-MS, an interface plays a crucial role due to the inherent incompatibility between liquid chromatography and mass spectrometry devices. LC employs a pressurized liquid as the mobile phase, while mass analyzers typically function under vacuum conditions (around 10–6 Torr). This disparity necessitates the use of a switching valve to facilitate a harmonious integration of these two techniques [2]. The LC-MS method consists of three pivotal stages: separation, ionization, and detection. During the separation phase, the sample is introduced into the LC system, where it undergoes separation based on its distinct physical and chemical properties. Subsequently, the separated components are ionized using an ion source, such as electrospray ionization (ESI) or air pressure chemical ionization (APCI). The mass analyzer then detects these ionized components by analyzing their mass-to-charge ratio (m/z), constructing a spectrum of masses [31]. LC-MS stands as a remarkably sensitive and precise technology, enabling the identification and detection of minute quantities of compounds within complex mixtures. Its significance is pronounced in forensic sample analysis, where the identification and quantification of low-abundance compounds hold paramount importance. Furthermore, LC-MS boasts exceptional selectivity and robustness, capable of distinguishing between substances with closely related chemical structures, even under varying pH conditions, including acidic, basic, and neutral environments [32].

10.2.4.1 Principle and Instrumentation

In LC-MS, components are segregated through liquid chromatography (LC) and subsequently identified via mass spectrometry (MS) by examining their mass-to-charge (m/z) ratios. In this process, the sample is introduced into the LC column and fractionated into distinct constituents based on their physical and chemical attributes, encompassing characteristics like molecular size, polarity, charge, and hydrophobicity (Figure 10.5).

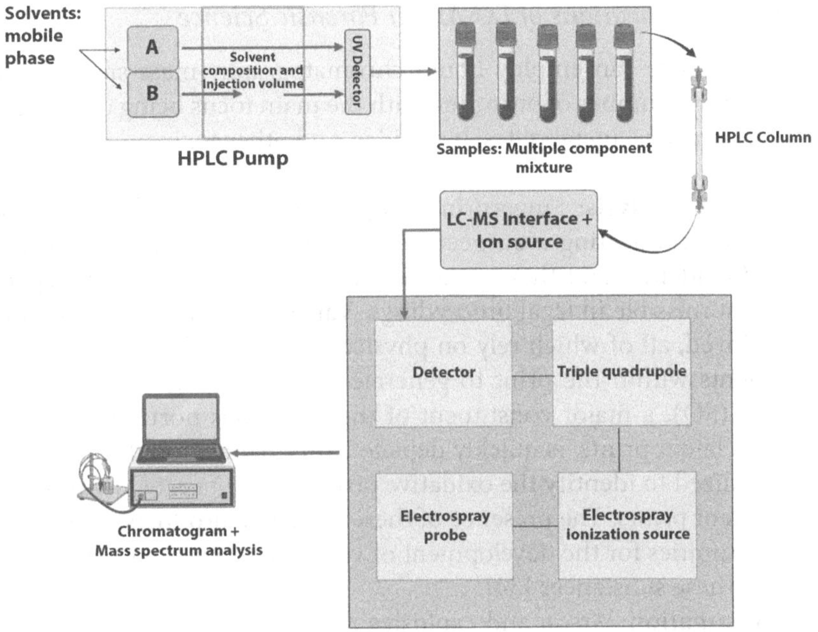

Figure 10.5 Liquid chromatography–mass spectrometry: instrumentation [5].

To ensure seamless integration of these two methodologies, various interfaces such as moving belt Interface, direct liquid introduction interface, thermospray interface, and FAB-based interfaces are employed [33]. These interfaces serve to nebulize and vaporize the liquid, ionize the sample, eliminate excess solvent vapor, and transport the ions into the mass analyzer [34]. Once the sample reaches the MS phase, its components undergo ionization through an ion source, which may involve techniques like electrospray ionization (ESI), air pressure chemical ionization (APCI), or other ionization methods [36, 37]. The mass analyzer, which can be a quadrupole, time-of-flight (TOF), ion trap, or Fourier transform ion cyclotron resonance (FTICR) mass spectrometer, is then employed to scrutinize the ionized constituents. The resulting mass-to-charge (m/z) ratio spectrum displayed on the computer screen is employed to assess and identify the components. Utilizing the mass spectrum's insights into molecular weight, structure, and fragmentation pattern, these segregated constituents can be recognized and quantified [39]. This qualitative analysis facilitates the reconstruction of unknown compounds based on MS data [35].

10.2.4.2 Applications of LC-MS in Forensic Science

Forensic science can employ liquid chromatography-mass spectrometry (LC-MS) for a number of purposes, with the main focus being on the identification of drugs, metabolites, pesticides, and other toxins.

Fingerprint Analysis: Fingerprints play a central role in forensic investigations by connecting a suspect to a crime scene, a weapon, or other pieces of evidence, and they are widely acknowledged as highly dependable and admissible in legal proceedings. Various visualization techniques are employed, all of which rely on physical or chemical interactions with components within the print to generate an image of the ridge pattern. Squalene (SQ), a major constituent of the sebaceous portion of recently deposited latent prints, is quickly depleted after deposition. LC/APCI-MS can be utilized to identify the oxidative product of SQ i.e. SQ hydroperoxides in latent prints. The presence of these oxidative products of SQ opens up opportunities for the development of visualization reagents specifically targeting these substances [34].
Fire investigation: Arson and explosive residues can also be determined using LC-MS. Different types of accelerants and explosive materials are present in samples, such as soil, clothes, etc. from the scene of the crime. LC-MS provides an analytical method for the identification of intact triglycerides within fire debris, which can serve as the ignition sources for fires. In a scientific study conducted by Craig M. Bryant and colleagues, they utilized LC-MS to successfully identify 22 distinct triglyceride-based oils and fats within fire debris, which contributes significantly in fire investigation cases [35].
Trace evidence analysis: Various types of trace pieces of evidence, including fibers, glass, cosmetics, paint, ink and soil, and the small amounts of organic compounds present in it can be determined using this technique. LC-MS serves as a tool for the identification of carcinogenic aromatic amines found in trace evidence. In a research study conducted by Urs Hauri and colleagues, more than 30 aromatic amines, such as 1,3-diphenylguanidine, O-toluidine, 1,3-di-o-tolylguanidine, and aniline are screened, specifically in the inks and dyes used in pens and tattoos using LC-MS [36].
Food and beverage analysis: Forensic scientists may be involved in investigating cases of food and drug adulteration which includes examining food, beverages, pharmaceuticals, and dietary supplements for the presence of unauthorized or harmful substances. Adulteration in these products can lead to health risks or even fatalities. LC-MS also comes with a great potential to identify the presence of contaminants, adulterants, and

other harmful substances in food and beverage samples [37]. In an investigation led by Manjun Tay, LC-QTOF–MS (Liquid chromatography-Qtrap and mass spectrometry) was successfully utilized in conjunction with chemometrics to identify the presence of the adulterant detergent Dodecylbenzenesulfonate (C12-LAS) in infant milk formula, ultimately aids in the detection of these instances of economic deception and incidents of poisoning [38].

10.2.5 Fourier Transform Infrared Spectroscopy-Mass Spectrometry (FTIR-MS)

FTIR spectroscopy and mass spectrometry (MS) are two frequently employed analytical methodologies in the domains of chemistry, biology, and materials science. These techniques are synergistically combined to form a unified approach, taking advantage of the distinctive attributes of both FTIR and MS instruments. This amalgam proves valuable for the examination of intricate samples. The FTIR component employs infrared radiation to stimulate the vibrational modes of the analyte, followed by the separation and detection of ions generated from the sample. FTIR-MS proves highly effective in swiftly identifying unknown samples through its integrated capabilities. Moreover, it serves as a valuable tool for elucidating a sample's chemical composition and structure [39]. Notably, FTIR-MS facilitates the determination of molecular weight and fragmentation patterns of ions derived from the sample. The spectrum of applications encompasses the identification of unfamiliar compounds, polymer analysis, and the scrutiny of biological specimens. Although extensively employed in diverse scientific disciplines, FTIR-MS is a relatively novel coupled technique within the realm of forensic science [40].

10.2.5.1 Principle and Instrumentation

In FTIR-MS, the sample is exposed to infrared radiation, as a result of the energy absorbed, excites the molecular vibrations within the sample and produces distinctive absorption spectra that are unique to the chemical makeup of the sample. Using MS, ionization of analytes occurs, followed by their segregation according to their m/e ratio. The sample's molecular weight and structure can be determined using the mass spectrum that was collected. The Fourier transform component of FTIR converts the recorded time-domain signal into a frequency-domain spectrum, allowing for speedy and precise data collection and analysis. FTIR-MS gives full information on the sample's molecular composition and structure by combining the data received from IR and MS systems [41].

IR radiation is produced by an infrared source in the mid-infrared region of the electromagnetic spectrum, which occurs between 4000 and 400 cm^{-1} in wavelength. The sample, which will be analyzed, is put within a sample chamber in a cuvette or tube. For further analysis, thin film or a solution of the sample is taken. The interferometer is an important part of the FTIR technique which is used to split the infrared radiation into two beams that pass through the sample and a reference material (or control material) before being recombined to produce an interference pattern. The intensity of the interference pattern is detected by the detector [42]. This intensity is converted into a time-domain signal. The interferometer, detector, and other components are connected to a computer and the time-domain signal produces a frequency-domain spectrum using the Fourier transform. Using the mass to charge ratio of the ions formed in MS, separation of ions occurs. A computer is used to record and analyze the ions' mass spectrum. In forensic science, data analysis software is typically used to compare sample spectra to a library of standards to determine the sample's chemical makeup, structural details, and eventually its constituent parts (Figure 10.6) [43].

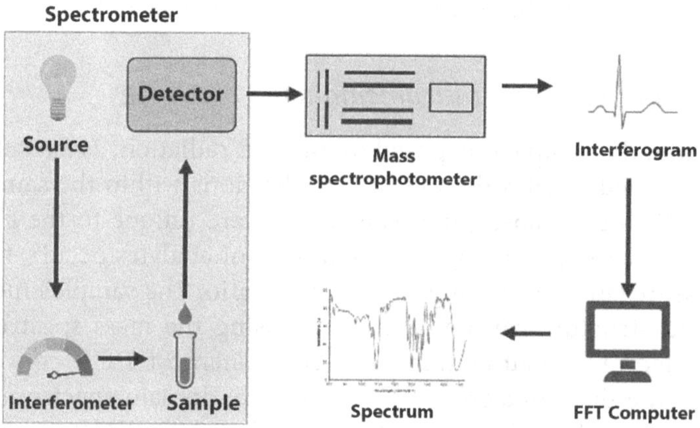

Figure 10.6 Instrumentation of FTIR-MS [6].

10.2.5.2 *Applications of FTIR-MS in Forensic Science*

Fourier-Transform Infrared Mass Spectrometry (FTIR-MS) is an advanced analytical technique with applications of drug analysis in various biological samples.

Drug analysis: The main function of FTIR-MS in forensic samples is to locate and measure drugs. The method is very helpful for analyzing complicated drug mixes, such as drug samples that have been confiscated. By combining the benefits of the linked instrument, GC-FTIR/MS is employed for research to improve chemical identification. Although the molecular and fragment ion mass values are provided by MS, occasionally false-positive substances can be proposed. When accurate mass spectral data isn't available, FTIR can offer further confirmation by comparing experimental and synthetic spectra, enhancing the identification of chemical functions and isomer information. When there is a shortage of information in the database, the GC capabilities physically separate the compounds, the MS offers distinctive m/z values to aid in identification, and the FTIR verifies the functional group patterns and molecular geometry by looking at hypothesized structures. For chemical identification and more assurance in analytical data, GC-FTIR/MS has shown to be a useful and adaptable approach and found to be a potent method for identifying constituents within intricate organic mixtures and delivers concurrent data from both GC-FTIR and GC-MS analyses following a single sample injection [44, 45].

10.2.6 Liquid Chromatography-Tandem Mass Spectrometry (LC-MS/MS)

LC-MS/MS is sophisticated hyphenated analytical technology which is being used widely nowadays in many different areas, including forensics, the pharmaceutical industry, and environmental monitoring. This technology combines the strong separation power of liquid chromatography (LC) with the efficient accuracy and precision tandem MS (MS/MS), making it simple for identification and analysis of the components from complicated mixtures. The LC component of LC-MS/MS separates sample components according to their physical and chemical characteristics, such as size, charge, and hydrophobicity. Dissolution of sample in solvent takes place initially, followed by injection into an LC column filled with the stationary phase, which is typically comprised of silica or a polymer material [46]. As a result of different components' interactions with stationary phase in the column of LC and their timing for elution, the separation of components takes place. Following the separation of the molecules, the mass spectrometer is used to ionize and fragment the components into smaller bits. The ions collide with gas molecules in a collision cell to cause collision-induced dissociation (CID), which leads to fragmentation. The mass spectrometer then divides those pieces depending on their m/z ratio and finds them [47].

Compared to MS methods, the tandem mass spectrometry component offers several benefits. First, by performing two steps of mass analysis, it increases the study's specificity. Based on its m/q ratio, separation of ions take place in the first MS, followed by their further fragmentation in other MS, creating a distinctive pattern of smaller ions. This unusual pattern, which is unique to the chemical, makes it possible to identify it with certainty. With higher specificity and sensitivity, LC-MS/MS is being used for identification and quantification of compounds at considerably lower concentrations than standard MS methods. If we talk about forensic science, LC-MS/MS has played an important role in demonstrating a broad variety of applications, including the examination of biological material, traces of evidence, ballistic, and ink analysis. Later in the chapter, other applications are covered [46].

10.2.6.1 Principle and Instrumentation

LC and MS/MS are two highly developed analytical techniques that are combined to form LC-MS/MS. When using this technique, the sample is placed into the LC column, where the process starts. Based on the components of the sample's individual components' physio-chemical characteristics, the process is then completed. The separated components are added to the mass spectrometer, which analyses each component's molecular structure in the sample. The sample molecules are ionized by the mass spectrometer into charged ions, which are then separated using an electric field according to their m/z ratios [48]. Utilizing the spectrum that the detector produces, the ions are found and quantified. To improve the specificity, accuracy, and recovery of the method used, tandem mass spectrometry employs two or more mass spectrometry stages in succession. Based on its m/z ratio, selection of precursor ion is done while performing first step, followed by their collision by slamming into neutral gas molecules. The fragments are recognized and arranged according to their m/z ratio in the following stage. Each precursor ion's fragmentation pattern is unique to the component's molecular structure and may be utilized to identify the substance accurately and precisely. The strength of the signal produced by the detector directly depends on the concentration of the analyte ions in the samples [49].

In LC-MS/MS, an injector is utilized for introduction of the sample to the LC column. Direct manual injection or an automated sample handling system can be used to introduce samples.LC system divides the sample's components according to their physicochemical characteristics. A pump, an injector, a chromatographic column, and a detector are components of the LC system. Mass spectrometer ionizes the sample's separated components, separate the sample based on m/e ratio and identify the unknown sample. The separated components of the sample are ionized using an ionization source [50]. Ionization sources that are frequently used include ESI and APCI. Analyte ions are separated using it based on m/e ratio. Ions produced by the ionization source are broken up by the collision cell. To fragment the ions, collision-induced dissociation (CID) is frequently used (Figure 10.7). The detector like electron multiplier is used to measures the concentration of ions that ionization source produces [51].

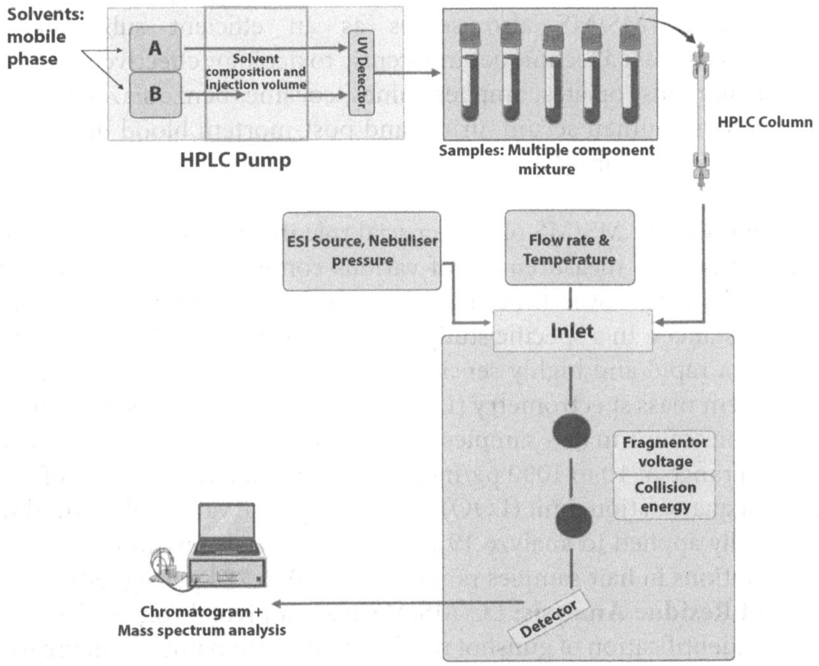

Figure 10.7 Liquid chromatography-tandem mass spectrometry (LC-MS/MS): instrumentation [7].

10.2.6.2 Applications of LC-MS/MS in Forensic Science

Liquid Chromatography-Mass Spectrometry/Mass Spectrometry (LC-MS/MS) is a highly versatile analytical technique used in various applications within the field of forensic science. Various forensic applications of LC-MS/MS are as follows:

Drug analysis: LC-MS/MS allows for the examination of drugs and their metabolites in biological specimens like blood, urine, and hair. The analysis of antipsychotic drugs in biological samples holds importance in both clinical and forensic medicine. In drug analysis, there has been a growing interest in keratinized tissues such as hair and nails due to their extended detection windows compared to blood. In a study led by Huanhuan Yang and their team, developed an LC-MS/MS based method for simultaneously measuring 10 antipsychotics in blood, hair, and nails and found high percentage of drug in the different biological matrix with low limit of detection ranging from 5-10 pg/mL. They applied this method to samples from 54 patients under long-term therapy, revealing significant correlations between drug concentrations in blood and hair [52].

Further, LC-MS/MS also serves as an efficient substitute for immunoassay-based techniques in forensic toxicology, effectively identifying cannabinoids, opiates, amphetamines, cocaine, benzodiazepines, and methadone in human serum, urine, and post-mortem blood during preliminary examinations [53].

Hair analysis: LC-MS/MS plays a crucial role in hair analysis by enabling the detection and measurement of various compounds that can become embedded in hair over time, including drugs, metabolites, toxins, and other substances. In a specific study, researchers developed and rigorously validated a rapid and highly sensitive method using liquid chromatography-tandem mass spectrometry (LC-MS/MS) to accurately determine and quantify mescaline in hair samples. This method exhibited excellent linearity over a range of 10 to 1000 pg/mg, with a detection limit (LOD) of 3 pg/mg and a quantitation limit (LOQ) of 10 pg/mg. The validated method was successfully applied to analyze 19 real forensic cases, revealing mescaline concentrations in hair samples ranging from 10 to 784 pg/mg [54].

Gunshot Residue Analysis: LC-MS/MS plays a pivotal role in the detection and identification of gunshot residue (GSR) originating from firearms, assisting investigators in ascertaining an individual's presence at a crime scene. In a research endeavor led by William Feeney and his team, LC-MS/MS was employed for chromatographic separation and simultaneous detection of both inorganic and organic residues. Their study revealed the presence of macrocycle (18-crown-6-ether) complexes lead (Pb) & barium (Ba) in the discharged sample from the firearm [55].

Human remains analysis: Accurately determining the time since death (postmortem interval or PMI) is crucial in forensic medico-legal investigations for various reasons, such as identifying missing individuals or eliminating potential suspects. Lana Brockbals *et al.* conducted a study focused on comprehending the decomposition process in human remains up to three months after death. The study introduced innovative time-dependent biomarkers, specifically peptide ratios, to estimate the time of decomposition. To achieve this, an untargeted LC–MS/MS-based bottom-up proteomics method was applied to analyze skeletal muscle samples obtained at multiple intervals from nine deceased individuals decomposing in an open eucalypt woodland environment in Australia. The study successfully identified multiple peptide ratios of human origin, which offer valuable insights and assistance in comprehending and estimating the various stages of human decomposition [56].

In another study, researchers locate and classify organic and inorganic gunshot residue (GSR) contamination. Four Pittsburgh police stations were used to gather a total of 73 samples. The study includes the detection of typical inorganic GSR particles and non-crystalline particles including lead, antimony, and barium using LC-MS/MS. Analytes were extracted with phenol and taken for LC-MS/MS analysis as part of study's search for organic GSR. The findings showed that nitroglycerin, 2,4-dinitrotoluene, 2,6-dinitrotoluene, and 2-nitrodiphenylamine were among the chemical substances present. The sensitivity of the LC-MS/MS approach for detecting GSR substances was demonstrated by the determination that the LOD for its component was in the range of 0.40 to 3.78 nmol L-1 [57].

Bone analysis: Forensic toxicology faces challenges when it comes to quantifying cocaine and its metabolites in postmortem samples, especially when decomposition has progressed significantly. To address this issue, researchers, including Malorie Mella and her team, have devised a robust method for extracting and purifying cocaine and its metabolites from bone samples. They utilized LC-MS/MS, a powerful analytical technique, to achieve this goal effectively and developed approach allowed them to reach the desired limits of detection. The results of their study showed that the limit of quantitation for cocaine and benzoylecgonine was measured at 0.05 ng/g, while for ecgonine methyl ester, it was 0.1 ng/g [58].

Blood stain analysis: Bloodstains are a common occurrence at crime scenes and serve as crucial pieces of evidence, providing valuable information about the incident, including details about the victim, suspect, and the timing of important events. In a research study led by Hyo-Jin Kim, utilized bloodstains to determine the age of the donor. To achieve this, they employed high-performance liquid chromatography-tandem mass spectrometry (LC-MS/MS) to analyze the markers present in the bloodstains. Through the examination of the MS/MS spectrum of these molecules, the researchers identified nine age markers: Δ2-cis eicosenoic acid, ergothioneine, adenosine 5'-monophosphate, benzaldehyde, phenacylamine, myristic acid ethyl ester, p-coumaric acid, niacinamide, and N-arachidonoyl-L-alanine. These markers can be employed to estimate the age of the donor associated with a bloodstain [59].

10.2.7 Capillary Electrophoresis-Mass Spectrometry (CE-MS)

Capillary electrophoresis-mass spectrometry (CE-MS) integrates a separation technique based on the movement of ions propelled by electrophoretic and electro-osmotic forces generated by an electric field with a mass spectrometer. CE, a method well-suited for handling complex sample compositions, particularly those containing polar and ionic substances, not only delivers precise separation but also confirms the presence of target molecules through mass spectrometry [60]. This makes it a valuable complementary tool in forensic sample analysis, enhancing the detection of trace metabolites compared to LC-MS and GC-MS. CS-MS has proven its value in providing distinctive and specialized information, particularly concerning cations, anions, and nucleotides in diverse biological specimens under varying experimental conditions and exhibits a wide range of applications for identifying and quantifying proteins and other compounds within intricate biological materials [61].

10.2.7.1 Principle and Instrumentation

CS-MS is based on the use of relatively low viscosity buffer systems where analyte molecules move in response to the combined effects of electrophoretic and electroosmotic mobility. CE-MS is a fully automated technique known for its exceptional sensitivity and selectivity. A capillary electrophoresis comprises a silica capillary covered with polyimide to prevent the silica from breaking a separating buffer, and a high-voltage power source make up the capillary electrophoresis apparatus. To improve molecular separation, the separation buffer is created using an electrolytic solution that can be altered depending on the type of sample being analyzed. A power source generating a high voltage, approximately 30 kV, is employed

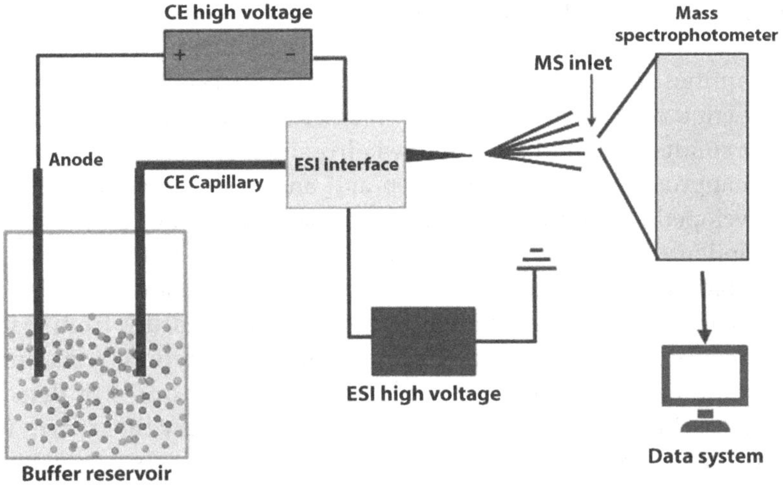

Figure 10.8 Capillary electrophoresis mass spectrometry (CE MS): Instrumentation [8].

to create an electric field within a small, fused silica capillary, serving as the primary component of the separation column (Figure 10.8) [66]. It separates species by applying voltage across buffer-filled capillaries and is generally used for separating ions that move at different speeds when voltage is applied, depending on their size and charge. Separation is achieved through channels etched on the surface of the capillary which are connected to an external high voltage power supply and delivers sample to electrospray ionization mass spectroscopy (ESIMS) or air pressure chemical ionization (APCI) [67]. The separated solutes are seen as peaks as they pass through the detector and the area of each peak is proportional to their concentration, which allows quantitative determinations. This analysis encompasses evaluations of purity, assays, and detecting minute quantities. The spectra generated also encompass details about the molecular weight, chemical composition, and structural characteristics of the substances under examination. Recently developed interfaces like the coaxial sheath liquid CE-MS interface have emerged, enabling the alternating utilization of both LC-MS and CE-MS on the same mass spectrometer [62, 68].

10.2.7.2 Applications of CE-MS in Forensic Science

Due to its high-resolution separation and detection capabilities, CE-MS has been employed in identification of forensic evidence.

Drug analysis: CE-MS, as a pivotal analytical technique, possesses the capacity to effectively handle samples that are frequently available in limited quantities at crime scene. These samples often need to be preserved for subsequent cross-analysis, especially in cases that are subject to dispute. In a study conducted by Magdalena Świądro and her colleagues developed a novel approach for the preparation and analysis of biological samples. The developed technique combines the Dried Blood Spot (DBS) method with capillary electrophoresis coupled mass spectrometry (CE-MS) to analyze blood samples obtained either *in vivo* or post-mortem. This innovative method facilitated the identification of various drugs from distinct categories, including tricyclic antidepressants, imipramine, citalopram, tetrazepam, and zolpidem. The study established the limits of detection from 1.76 – 14.7 ng/mL. It also determined the recovery rate ranges from 85.0–105.4%. Moreover, the method developed in this study exhibited selectivity, with analytes in blood applied to DBS cards remaining stable after 7 and 14 days. This innovative method was successfully applied to the analysis of both post-mortem samples and blood samples from patients undergoing treatment with the analyzed drugs and holds particular significance for samples used as evidence in legal proceedings [63].

Gunshot residue analysis: Capillary electrophoresis coupled with mass spectrometry effectively identifies handgun discharged GSR components, such as nitrite and nitrate residues. It serves as a screening tool for GSR analysis and offers a quantitative alternative to the conventional paraffin test (dermal nitrate test). Compared to contemporary techniques like flameless AAS, ICP-MS, or SEM used for gunshot residue analysis (including barium, lead, and antimony), this method is more cost-effective, efficient, and user-friendly. It has demonstrated high sensitivity and repeatability in analyzing hair and skin samples from gunshot victims [64].

Explosive and fire debris analysis: CE-MS is utilized in forensic chemistry to identify and quantify varying trace evidence including explosives, poisons, and gunpowder residue. Smokeless gunpowder, commonly used in rifle and handgun ammunition, is easily accessible and can be employed in the formation of improvised explosive devices. Identifying the specific type and origin of this powder is vital for determining those responsible for bombings. To address this challenge, De Perre and colleagues devised a technique that involves combining Capillary Electrochromatography (CEC) Time-of-Flight Mass Spectrometry (TOF-MS). This approach employs a hexyl-acrylate-based porous monolith, compatible with MS detection which detect 14 organic components found as a constituent of commercial smokeless powder [65]. CE-MS improves both sensitivity and selectivity, serving as an advanced tool for additional confirmation and facilitating precise identification of components within smokeless powder samples discovered at bombing sites and allowing for quicker and more accurate detection of evidence in criminal investigations [66]. CE-MS also enables the identification of accelerants or other chemical evidence found in arson cases.

Blood analysis: In the field of forensic science, it is critically essential to both detect and measure the levels of drugs in blood samples. This process is highly significant as it yields valuable insights into inquiries concerning drug-related offenses, accidents, and toxicology assessments as the concentration of drugs in this biological matrix is directly linked to observed biological effects. The primary objective in blood analysis is to confirm the existence of drugs or their chemical byproducts. The hyphenation of CE with MS offers concurrent identification of illegal substances and their primary metabolites in blood. Gottardo *et al.* introduced a novel approach for quantifying most common drugs of abuse and their main metabolites in post-mortem blood which include cocaine, methadone, morphine, codeine, benzoylecgonine, 6-monoacetylmorphine, amphetamine, and its metabolites using CZE-ESI-TOFMS. They achieved a sensitivity ranging from 2 to 10 ng ml−1 by employing FASS [67].

Hair analysis: Hair analysis has emerged as an established method for retrospectively examining histories of drug abuse. The combination of capillary zone electrophoresis and ion trap mass spectrometry shows great promise for accurately and sensitively quantifying major drugs of abuse and their metabolites, including 6-monoacetylmorphine, morphine, amphetamine, and methamphetamine. This approach offers advantages such as minimal sample requirements, user-friendly operation, efficiency, speed, and robustness, which are typical of capillary electrophoresis, along with the high sensitivity and selectivity provided by mass spectrometry. Researchers have successfully quantified various illicit drugs in hair samples (100 mg) with detection limits lower than the stringent cutoffs commonly used in hair analysis, typically set at 0.1 ng/mg [68].

10.3 Conclusion

Due to their capacity to deliver delicate, detailed, accurate, and exact information on any given sample, various hyphenated procedures have become an essential instrument for use in forensic science. Detection, identification, & analysis of tiny levels of chemicals in complicated matrices are made possible by the combination of two or more analytical methods, such as mass spectrometry and chromatography. Using these approaches, it is possible to identify a particular molecule or chemical, making analysis simple and advanced research which is help in diverse filed of science. Development of forensic science is aided by increasing sensitivity and selectivity of hyphenated procedures, which produce more accurate and timely findings. Hyphenated methods have also aided in the creation of fresh approaches and quick forensic investigations [69]. For instance, the combination of GC-MS, LC-MS, LC-MS/MS, and CE-MS has made it possible to identify the source and veracity of pharmaceuticals, food goods, poisonous compounds, fire, and explosive debris, as well as a variety of other materials that may be used as forensic evidence. In fraud and counterfeiting cases, hyphenated procedures are becoming more common because they can help forensic investigators by identifying minute changes in isotopic composition.

In the realm of forensic toxicology, sample analysis has significantly advanced due to hyphenated approaches. A large variety of medicines and their metabolites may be found in biological matrices and other chemicals, and they can be identified and quantified using LC-MS/MS. These tools have proven helpful in many circumstances, such as identification of small quantities of drugs in bodily fluids while driving under the influence of drugs (DUID), as they can offer crucial evidence for prosecution [70].

In conclusion, the introduction of hyphenated procedures in forensic science has made it much easier for forensic investigators to investigate more cases each day by giving them analytical tools that are both sensitive and specific. New developments are being made, and most of them may be used to analyze forensic materials more precisely and accurately.

References

1. R. Ramya, J. Adur Alaknanda, D. Raajasubramanian, S. Srinivasan, K. Narendra, and M. Manjushree, "Weed—An Alternate Energy Source," 2023, pp. 165–193. doi: 10.1007/978-981-99-3002-9_10.
2. R. B. Kumar, R. K. Varma, S. Sen, and S. Oruganti, "Head-space miniaturization techniques," *Emerging Freshwater Pollutants: Analysis, Fate and Regulations*, pp. 95–116, Jan. 2022, doi: 10.1016/B978-0-12-822850-0.00018-1.
3. M. J. Sithersingh and N. H. Snow, "Headspace gas chromatography," *Gas Chromatography*, pp. 251–265, Jan. 2021, doi: 10.1016/B978-0-12-820675-1.00012-5.
4. X. Guo and E. Lankmayr, "Hyphenated Techniques in Gas Chromatography," in *Advanced Gas Chromatography - Progress in Agricultural, Biomedical and Industrial Applications*, InTech, 2012. doi: 10.5772/31802.

5. S. Parasuraman, A. R, B. S, M. S, J. RAJA KUMAR, and V. Venugopal, "An overview of liquid chromatography-mass spectroscopy instrumentation," *Pharm. Methods*, vol. 5, pp. 47–55, Sep. 2015, doi: 10.5530/phm.2014.2.2.
6. V. Sharma and R. Kumar, "Fourier transform infrared spectroscopy and high performance thin layer chromatography for characterization and multivariate discrimination of blue ballpoint pen ink for forensic applications," *Vib. Spectrosc.*, vol. 92, pp. 96–104, Sep. 2017, doi: 10.1016/J.VIBSPEC.2017.05.006.
7. J. Ijaq, N. Bethi, and M. V. Jagannadham, "Mass spectrometry-based identification and characterization of human hypothetical proteins highlighting the inconsistency across the protein databases," *J. Proteins. Proteom.*, vol. 11, no. 1, pp. 17–25, Mar. 2020, doi: 10.1007/s42485-020-00030-1.
8. S. A. Shamsi and F. Akter, "Capillary Electrophoresis Mass Spectrometry: Developments and Applications for Enantioselective Analysis from 2011–2020," *Molecules*, vol. 27, no. 13, p. 4126, Jun. 2022, doi: 10.3390/molecules27134126.
9. Kiyatkin, E.A.; Ren, S.E. MDMA, Methylone, and MDPV: Drug-Induced Brain Hyperthermia and Its Modulation by Activity State and Environment. *Neuropharmacol. New Psychoact. Subst. Sci. Behind Headl.*, **2017**, 183–207.
10. Jackson, G.P.; Barkett, M.A. Forensic Mass Spectrometry: Scientific and Legal Precedents. *J. Am. Soc. Mass Spectrom.*, **2023**.
11. Taylor, C.M.; Rosenhan, A.K.; Raines, J.M.; Rodriguez, J.M. An Arson Investigation by Using Comprehensive Two-Dimensional Gas Chromatography-Quadrupole Mass Spectrometry. *J. Forensic Res.*, **2012**, *3*.
12. Almirall, J.; Trejos, T. Interpol Review of Paint, Tape, and Glass Evidence 2019–2022. *Forensic Sci. Int. Synerg.*, **2023**, *6*, 100306.
13. Ballabio, D.; Skov, T.; Leardi, R.; Bro, R. Classification of GC-MS Measurements of Wines by Combining Data Dimension Reduction and Variable Selection Techniques. *J. Chemom. A J. Chemom. Soc.*, **2008**, *22*, 457–463.
14. Goudsmits, E.; Blakey, L.S.; Chana, K.; Sharples, G.P.; Birkett, J.W. The Analysis of Organic and Inorganic Gunshot Residue from a Single Sample. *Forensic Sci. Int.*, **2019**, *299*, 168–173, doi:https://doi.org/10.1016/j.forsciint.2019.03.049.
15. Zeichner, A.; Eldar, B.; Glattstein, B.; Koffman, A.; Tamiri, T.; Muller, D. Vacuum Collection of Gunpowder Residues from Clothing Worn by Shooting Suspects, and Their Analysis by GC/TEA, IMS, and GC/MS. *J. Forensic Sci.*, **2003**, *48*, 961–972.
16. Edson, S.M.; Roberts, M. Determination of Materials Present in Skeletonized Human Remains and the Associated DNA: Development of a GC/MS Protocol. *Forensic Sci. Int. Synerg.*, **2019**, *1*, 170–184, doi:https://doi.org/10.1016/j.fsisyn.2019.08.002.
17. Luis, P.; Wouters, C.; Van der Bruggen, B.; Sandler, S.I. Measurement of Activity Coefficients of Mixtures by Head-Space Gas Chromatography: General Procedure. *J. Chromatogr. A*, **2013**, *1302*, 111–117, doi:https://doi.org/10.1016/j.chroma.2013.06.007.

18. Sparkman, O.D.; Penton, Z.E.; Kitson, F.G. Chapter 2 - Gas Chromatography. In; Sparkman, O.D., Penton, Z.E., Kitson, F.G.B.T.-G.C. and M.S. (Second E., Eds.; Academic Press: Amsterdam, 2011; pp. 15–83 ISBN 978-0-12-373628-4.
19. Xiao, H.; He, L.; Tong, R.; Yu, J.; Chen, L.; Zou, J.; Li, J.; Bian, Y.; Zhang, Y. Rapid and Sensitive Headspace Gas Chromatography–Mass Spectrometry Method for the Analysis of Ethanol in the Whole Blood. *J. Clin. Lab. Anal.*, **2014**, *28*, 386–390.
20. Brettell, T.A.; Lum, B.J. Analysis of Drugs of Abuse by Gas Chromatography–Mass Spectrometry (GC-MS). *Anal. Drugs Abus.*, **2018**, 29–42.
21. Green, J.D. Headspace Analysis| Static. **2005**.
22. Riasat, M.; Chaudhary, M.T.; Jamshaid, T. Sevoflurane Analysis in Forensic Cases Using Headspace-Gas Chromatography-Mass Spectrometry: A Case Study. *Toxicol. Anal. Clin.*, **2022**, *34*, S159–S160.
23. Desharnais, B.; Huppé, G.; Lamarche, M.; Mireault, P.; Skinner, C.D. Cyanide Quantification in Post-Mortem Biological Matrices by Headspace GC–MS. *Forensic Sci. Int.*, **2012**, *222*, 346–351.
24. Scholar (2).
25. Monteiro, C.; Franco, J.M.; Proença, P.; Castañera, A.; Claro, A.; Vieira, D.N.; Corte-Real, F. Qualitative and Quantitative Analysis of a Group of Volatile Organic Compounds in Biological Samples by HS-GC/FID: Application in Practical Cases. *Forensic Sci. Int.*, **2014**, *243*, 137–143.
26. Grainger, D.W.; Castner, D.G. 3.1 Surface Analysis and Biointerfaces: Vacuum and Ambient *in Situ* Techniques. **2017**.
27. Ferguson, K.; Tupik, S.L.; Haddad, H.; Perr, J.; Gilbert, M.; Newman, R.; Almirall, J. Utility of Gas Chromatography Infrared Spectroscopy (GC-IR) for the Differentiation of Positional Isomers of Fentanyl Related Substances. *Forensic Chem.*, **2022**, *29*, 100425.
28. Czichos, H.; Saito, T.; Smith, L.E. *Springer Handbook of Metrology and Testing*; Springer Science & Business Media, 2011; ISBN 3642166415.
29. Salerno, T.M.G.; Donato, P.; Frison, G.; Zamengo, L.; Mondello, L. Gas Chromatography—Fourier Transform Infrared Spectroscopy for Unambiguous Determination of Illicit Drugs: A Proof of Concept. *Front. Chem.*, **2020**, *8*, 624.
30. Reavis, M.; Goodpaster, J. Quantitative Analysis of Smokeless Powder Particles in Post-blast Debris via Gas Chromatography/Vacuum Ultraviolet Spectroscopy (GC/VUV). *J. Forensic Sci.*, **2022**, *67*, 1431–1440.
31. Joshi, M.; Sisco, E. Forensic Seized Drug Analysis: Current Challenges and Emerging Analytical Solutions. *Wiley Interdiscip. Rev. Forensic Sci.*, **2023**, e1486.
32. Trivedi, R.; Prajapati, P. Hyphenated Techniques for Forensic Investigations. In *Technology in Forensic Science*; 2020; pp. 151–174 ISBN 9783527827688.
33. Ho, C.S.; Lam, C.W.K.; Chan, M.H.M.; Cheung, R.C.K.; Law, L.K.; Lit, L.C.W.; Ng, K.F.; Suen, M.W.M.; Tai, H.L. Electrospray Ionisation Mass

Spectrometry: Principles and Clinical Applications. *Clin. Biochem. Rev.*, **2003**, *24*, 3–12.
34. Mountfort, K.A.; Bronstein, H.; Archer, N.; Jickells, S.M. Identification of Oxidation Products of Squalene in Solution and in Latent Fingerprints by ESI-MS and LC/APCI-MS. *Anal. Chem.*, **2007**, *79*, 2650–2657.
35. Bryant, C.M.; Warnica, J.M.; Chen, R.; Shepard, C. Identification of Triglycerides in Liquid and Fire Debris Samples by Triple Quadrupole Liquid Chromatography-mass Spectrometry. *J. Forensic Sci.*, **2021**, *66*, 534–546.
36. Hauri, U.; Lutolf, B.; Schlegel, U.; Hohl, C. Determination of Carcinogenic Aromatic Amines in Dyes, Cosmetics, Finger Paints and Inks for Pens and Tattoos with LC/MS. *Mitteilungen aus Leb. und Hyg.*, **2005**, *96*, 321.
37. Smith, C.D.; Katilie, C.J.; Giordano, B.C.; Collins, G.E. Assessment of Opioid Surrogates for Ion Mobility Spectrometry Testing (Part II). *Forensic Chem.*, **2022**, *28*, 100405.
38. Tay, M.; Fang, G.; Chia, P.L.; Li, S.F.Y. Rapid Screening for Detection and Differentiation of Detergent Powder Adulteration in Infant Milk Formula by LC–MS. *Forensic Sci. Int.*, **2013**, *232*, 32–39.
39. Slough, C.G. Simultaneous Mass Spectrometry and Fourier Transform Infrared Spectrometry of Off-Gases from a Thermogravimetric Analyzer. **2007**.
40. Khan, M.; Husain, Q.; Asmat, S. Synthesis, Characterization, and Applications of Nanographene-Armored Enzymes. In *Methods in Enzymology*; Elsevier, 2018; Vol. 609, pp. 83–142 ISBN 0076-6879.
41. Kumar, A.; Khandelwal, M.; Gupta, S.K.; Kumar, V.; Rani, R. Fourier Transform Infrared Spectroscopy: Data Interpretation and Applications in Structure Elucidation and Analysis of Small Molecules and Nanostructures. In *Data Processing Handbook for Complex Biological Data Sources*; Elsevier, 2019; pp. 77–96.
42. Hills, A.E. Spectroscopy in Biotechnology Research and Development. **2017**.
43. Margenot, A.J.; Calderón, F.J.; Goyne, K.W.; Dmukome, F.N.; Parikh, S.J. IR Spectroscopy, Soil Analysis Applications. In *Encyclopedia of Spectroscopy and Spectrometry*; Elsevier, 2016; pp. 448–454.
44. Abate, S.; Ahn, Y.G.; Kind, T.; Cataldi, T.R.I.; Fiehn, O. Determination of Elemental Compositions by Gas Chromatography/Time-of-flight Mass Spectrometry Using Chemical and Electron Ionization. *Rapid Commun. Mass Spectrom. An Int. J. Devoted to Rapid Dissem. Up-to-the-Minute Res. Mass Spectrom.*, **2010**, *24*, 1172–1180.
45. Demirgian, J.C. Gas Chromatography—Fourier Transform Infrared Spectroscopy—Mass Spectrometry. A Powerful Tool for Component Identification in Complex Organic Mixtures. *TrAC-Trends Anal. Chem.*, **1987**, *6*, 58–64, doi:https://doi.org/10.1016/0165-9936(87)87024-3.
46. Gieroba, B.; Matys, J.; Jóźwiak, K. Chapter 6 - Hyphenated Liquid Chromatography Techniques in Analysis of Neurotransmitters and Their Metabolites. In *Handbooks in Separation Science*; Fanali, S., Chankvetadze, B.,

Haddad, P.R., Poole, C.F., Riekkola, M.-L.B.T.-L.C. (Third E., Eds.; Elsevier, 2023; Vol. 2, pp. 223–255 ISBN 978-0-323-99969-4.
47. Korashy, H.M.; Rahman, A.F.M.M.; Kassem, M.G. Chapter Four - Dasatinib. In; *Brittain Excipients and Related Methodology*, H.G.B.T.-P. of D.S., Ed.; Academic Press, 2014; Vol. 39, pp. 205–237 ISBN 1871-5125.
48. Wolfender, J.-L.; Bohni, N.; Ndjoko-Ioset, K.; Edison, A.S. Chapter 16 - Advanced Spectroscopic Detectors for Identification and Quantification: Nuclear Magnetic Resonance. In; Fanali, S., Haddad, P.R., Poole, C.F., Schoenmakers, P., Lloyd, D.B.T.-L.C., Eds.; Elsevier: Amsterdam, 2013; pp. 349–384 ISBN 978-0-12-415807-8.
49. Silver, R.B. The Organic Chemistry of Drug Design and Drug Action 2004.
50. Čelić, M.; Farré, M.; de Alda, M.L.; Perez, S.; Barceló, D.; Petrovic, M. Environmental Analysis: Emerging Pollutants. In *Liq. Chromatogr.*; Elsevier, 2023; pp. 549–578.
51. Seger, C.; Salzmann, L. After Another Decade: LC–MS/MS Became Routine in Clinical Diagnostics. *Clin. Biochem.*, **2020**, *82*, 2–11.
52. Yang, H.; Liu, C.; Zhu, C.; Zheng, Y.; Li, J.; Zhu, Q.; Wang, H.; Fang, X.; Liu, Q.; Liang, M.; *et al.* Determination of Ten Antipsychotics in Blood, Hair and Nails: Validation of a LC–MS/MS Method and Forensic Application of Keratinized Matrix Analysis. *J. Pharm. Biomed. Anal.*, **2023**, *234*, 115557, doi:https://doi.org/10.1016/j.jpba.2023.115557.
53. Dziadosz, M.; Teske, J.; Henning, K.; Klintschar, M.; Nordmeier, F. LC–MS/MS Screening Strategy for Cannabinoids, Opiates, Amphetamines, Cocaine, Benzodiazepines and Methadone in Human Serum, Urine and Post-Mortem Blood as an Effective Alternative to Immunoassay Based Methods Applied in Forensic Toxicology for Preliminary Examination. *Forensic Chem.*, **2018**, *7*, 33–37, doi:https://doi.org/10.1016/j.forc.2017.12.007.
54. Yang, S.; Shi, Y.; Chen, Z.; Chen, M.; Liu, X.; Liu, W.; Su, M.; Di, B. Detection of Mescaline in Human Hair Samples by UPLC-MS/MS: Application to 19 Authentic Forensic Cases. *J. Chromatogr. B*, **2022**, *1195*, 123202, doi:https://doi.org/10.1016/j.jchromb.2022.123202.
55. Feeney, W.; Menking-Hoggatt, K.; Vander Pyl, C.; Ott, C.E.; Bell, S.; Arroyo, L.; Trejos, T. Detection of Organic and Inorganic Gunshot Residues from Hands Using Complexing Agents and LC-MS/MS. *Anal. Methods*, **2021**, *13*, 3024–3039.
56. Brockbals L, Garrett-Rickman S, Fu S, Ueland M, McNevin D, Padula MP. Estimating the time of human decomposition based on skeletal muscle biopsy samples utilizing an untargeted LC–MS/MS-based proteomics approach. *Anal. Bioanal. Chem.*, 2023 Jul 10:1-2.
57. Ali, L.; Brown, K.; Castellano, H.; Wetzel, S.J. A Study of the Presence of Gunshot Residue in Pittsburgh Police Stations Using SEM/EDS and LC-MS/MS. *J. Forensic Sci.*, **2016**, *61*, 928–938.
58. Brockbals, L.; Garrett-Rickman, S.; Fu, S.; Ueland, M.; McNevin, D.; Padula, M.P. Estimating the Time of Human Decomposition Based on Skeletal Muscle

Biopsy Samples Utilizing an Untargeted LC–MS/MS-Based Proteomics Approach. *Anal. Bioanal. Chem.*, **2023**, *415*, 5487–5498, doi:10.1007/s00216-023-04822-4.
59. Kim, H.-J.; Lee, Y.-R.; Lee, S.; Kwon, S.; Chun, Y.T.; Hyun, S.H.; Sung, H.J.; Lee, J.; Kang, H.-G. Discovery of Donor Age Markers from Bloodstain by LC-MS/MS Using a Metabolic Approach. *Int. J. Legal Med.*, **2022**, *136*, 297–308, doi:10.1007/s00414-021-02640-w.
60. Lai, Y.; Wang, Y. Advances in High-resolution Mass Spectrometry Techniques for Analysis of High Mass-to-charge Ions. *Mass Spectrom. Rev.*, **2022**, e21790.
61. Godzien, J.; López-Gonzálvez, Á.; García, A.; Barbas, C. Metabolic Phenotyping Using Capillary Electrophoresis Mass Spectrometry. In *The Handbook of Metabolic Phenotyping*; Elsevier, 2019; pp. 171–204.
62. Logar, J.K.; Malej, A.; Franko, M. Hyphenated High Performance Liquid Chromatography-Thermal Lens Spectrometry Technique as a Tool for Investigations of Xanthophyll Cycle Pigments in Different Taxonomic Groups of Marine Phytoplankton. *Rev. Sci. Instrum.*, **2003**, *74*, 776–778.
63. Świądro, M.; Stelmaszczyk, P.; Wietecha-Posłuszny, R.; Dudek, D. Development of a New Method for Drug Detection Based on a Combination of the Dried Blood Spot Method and Capillary Electrophoresis. *J. Chromatogr. B*, **2020**, *1157*, 122339.
64. Tagliaro, F.; Bortolotti, F.; Manetto, G.; Pascali, V.L.; Marigo, M. Dermal Nitrate: An Old Marker of Firearm Discharge Revisited with Capillary Electrophoresis. *Electrophoresis*, **2002**, *23*, 278–282.
65. de Perre, C.; Corbin, I.; Blas, M.; McCord, B.R. Separation and Identification of Smokeless Gunpowder Additives by Capillary Electrochromatography. *J. Chromatogr. A*, **2012**, *1267*, 259–265.
66. Zanda, M.T.; Fattore, L. Novel Psychoactive Substances: A New Behavioral and Mental Health Threat. In *Addictive Substances and Neurological Disease*; Elsevier, 2017; pp. 341–353.
67. Gottardo, R.; Polettini, A.; Sorio, D.; Pascali, J.P.; Bortolotti, F.; Liotta, E.; Tagliaro, F. Capillary Zone Electrophoresis (CZE) Coupled to Time-of-flight Mass Spectrometry (TOF-MS) Applied to the Analysis of Illicit and Controlled Drugs in Blood. *Electrophoresis*, **2008**, *29*, 4078–4087.
68. Gottardo, R.; Bortolotti, F.; De Paoli, G.; Pascali, J.P.; Mikšík, I.; Tagliaro, F. Hair Analysis for Illicit Drugs by Using Capillary Zone Electrophoresis-Electrospray Ionization-Ion Trap Mass Spectrometry. *J. Chromatogr. A*, **2007**, *1159*, 185–189.
69. Ruchira, C.H. Recent Applications of Hyphenated Liquid Chromatography Techniques. *Int. J. Pharm. Sci. Rev. Res.*, **2012**, *14*, 57–63.
70. Vogeser, M.; Seger, C. A Decade of HPLC–MS/MS in the Routine Clinical Laboratory—Goals for Further Developments. *Clin. Biochem.*, **2008**, *41*, 649–662.

11

Microscopic Techniques and Their Application in Forensic Science

Vaishnavi M.A., Malavika Venu, Ravshish Kaur Kohli and Pooja Puri*

Amity Institute of Forensic Sciences, Amity University, Noida, Uttar Pradesh, India

Abstract

Microscopy has emerged as an indispensable tool for forensic scientists, enabling them to examine trace evidence, analyze biological samples, and gather crucial information to solve crimes. This chapter provides a comprehensive overview of key microscopic techniques and their wide-ranging applications within the field of forensic science. The fundamental principles of microscopy highlight the different types of microscopes commonly used in forensic laboratories. It explores the significance of optical microscopy, electron microscopy, and scanning probe microscopy, emphasizing their unique capabilities and limitations. Microscopic techniques are pivotal in the analysis of biological evidence, and the chapter discusses their role in forensic biology. It explores the examination of bloodstains, semen, hair roots, and other biological samples, elucidating how microscopy assists in identifying individuals and establishing links in criminal investigations. Microscopic Techniques and their Applications in Forensic Science is a comprehensive exploration of the pivotal role played by microscopy in modern forensic science, showcasing its broad range of applications and its continued importance in advancing the field.

***Keywords*:** Biological evidence, compound microscope, court, forensic science, microscope, optical lens

**Corresponding author*: pmalik1@amity.edu

Priyanka Chhabra, Divya Bajpai Tripathy, Anjali Gupta, Rajeev Kumar, Kajol Bhati and Shruti Shukla (eds.) Advances in Analytical Techniques for Forensic Investigation, (307–338) © 2024 Scrivener Publishing LLC

11.1 Introduction to Microscopy

Microscopy is a tool that functions with creatures that are too small to be seen properly with the unaided eye. When viewing small objects through a microscope, the observer can see them more clearly, with more contrast, resolution (the ability to tell apart two nearby objects), and magnification (the capacity to recognize various parts of the specimen based on intensity or color). The microscope makes these items evident to the naked eye by enlarging an image of them. The shape of bacteria, fungi, parasites, and host cells can be examined under a microscope in various dyed and unstained preparations [1]. By magnifying an object twice with the objective and oculus lenses, a microscope may magnify the vision of an object. A bright-field microscope is the name given to this kind of microscope because the light passes through the image. In fact, there is a specific option to lessen the quantity of light that enters the specimen because the resulting image can occasionally be so bright. The only arithmetic that matters in this situation is how much larger your final image is than the original object. The letter X stands for what is known as the final magnification. It refers to the amount of enlargement. An image of the specimen that has been magnified 100 times, for instance, will be 100 times larger than the original specimen. The final magnification of a compound microscope can be calculated using a straightforward formula. It is:

$$M_{t} = M_{ob} * M_{oc}$$

M_t = Total Magnification
M_{ob} = Magnification of the objective lens
M_{oc} = Magnification of oculus lens

The objective and oculus lenses' combined powers, whose magnifications are indicated in terms of power, will determine the overall magnification [2]. If someone inquiries about the relationship between these lenses' focal lenses and their overall magnification, however, things become a little more perplexing. Based on the spacing between the lenses inside the body tube as well as their focal lengths, a computation is made. This is how it works:

$$M_t = D/f_{ob} * L/f_{oc}$$

M_t = Total magnification
f_{ob} = focal length of the objective lens
f_{oc} = focal length of the oculus lens

D = Least distance of the distant vision
L = effective length of the microscope tube

11.2 Types of Microscopes

Microscopes are essential tools for magnifying and examining objects or specimens at the microscopic level. There are several types of microscopes, each designed for specific applications and offering different levels of magnification and imaging capabilities. Here are some common types of microscopes:

11.2.1 Optical Microscope

Optical microscopy is a technique for closely examining a sample using a lens enlarged by visible light. An optical microscope, also known as a light-sensitive microscope, uses one or more lenses to enlarge the visible images of tiny materials [3]. The lenses magnify the image and make it possible for a more complete analysis to take place while keeping the specimen and the eye of the viewer apart.

An optical microscope may create a micrograph using typical light-sensitive cameras. Photographic film was primarily used to capture images. Modern optical microscopes may now capture digital pictures using CMOS (complementary metal-oxide semiconductor) and charge-couple device (CCD) cameras [4]. These digital microscopes show real-time images on a computer screen so that samples can be examined. Employing the device is more practical now that lenses are not needed. The magnification of a compound optical microscope is determined by its ocular and objective lenses. It is equal to the sum of the powers of these lenses. To operate an optical microscope effectively, it must be set up correctly. The lens that serves as the objective needs to be closer to the research sample in order for light to pass through the microscope's tube. The material has become seen as an enlarged, inverted image through the microscope's eyepiece. Several scientific domains, including microbiology, microelectronics, nanophysics, biotechnology, and pharmaceutical research, usually use optical microscopy [5]. Due to the technique's limitations, optical microscopy may not be the best choice for the task at hand. For instance, airy discs, which are fuzzy discs enclosed by diffraction rings that appears in place of point objects at very high magnifications, may be visible [6].

Principle: An optical microscope uses an objective lens to create a magnified view of an object specimen and an eyepiece to magnify the image to such an extent that the user can see it with their unaided eye. Light from the light source is directed through the condenser lens and focused onto the specimen. Proper illumination is essential for achieving high-quality images. The objective lens magnifies the specimen, producing an intermediate image. The eyepiece further magnifies this image, allowing the viewer to see fine details. Resolution is the ability to distinguish two closely spaced objects as separate entities. The resolving power of an optical microscope is determined by the wavelength of light used and the numerical aperture (NA) of the objective lens. Lower wavelengths and higher NA result in better resolution. Contrast is achieved by variations in the intensity of light or the interaction of light with the specimen [7].

Types of Optical Microscope
There are different types of optical microscopes.

11.2.2 Stereomicroscope

A stereomicroscope, also called a stereo microscope or dissecting microscope, is a tool used to make 3D objects look bigger. It helps people in

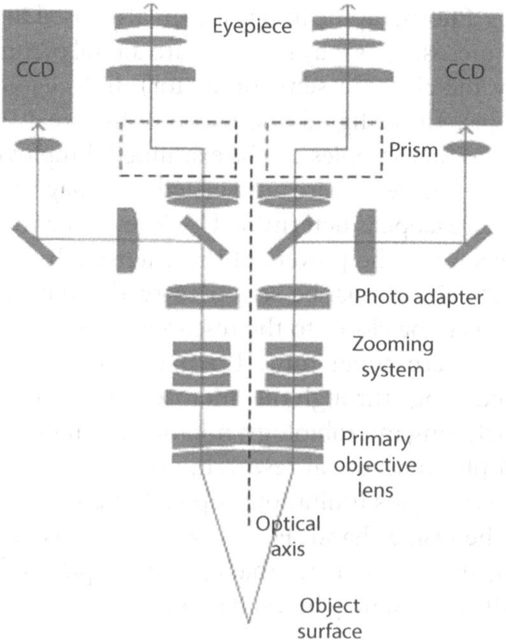

Figure 11.1 Created "*Working mechanism of Stereomicroscope*", by Biorender.com (2023).

different jobs, like scientists, engineers, and biologists, see things more clearly. This microscope is essential in many fields, such as biology, electronics, manufacturing, and materials science, because it makes objects appear three-dimensional, helping us understand them better [8]. Stereomicroscopes are typically made of a combination of various materials to ensure durability, precision, and optical clarity. The specific materials used can vary by manufacturer and model. The illustration of stereomicroscope is depicted in Figure 11.1.

Features of Stereomicroscope

Stereomicroscopes have two eyepieces (binoculars), allowing the viewer to use both eyes simultaneously. This provides a more natural and comfortable viewing experience compared to a monocular microscope, which uses only one eyepiece. Stereomicroscopes typically have lower magnification capabilities compared to compound microscopes. They usually offer magnification levels ranging from 5x to 80x, although some specialized models can go higher. The lower magnification allows for a wider field of view and a greater depth of field. Stereomicroscopes are equipped with built-in or external illumination sources to illuminate the specimen. This illumination can be transmitted (from below) or incident (from above), depending on the type of specimen and the required lighting conditions. Stereomicroscopes have a longer working distance, which is the distance between the objective lens and the specimen. This feature allows you to manipulate and work on the specimen with tools, making it suitable for tasks such as dissection or assembly. Stereomicroscopes provide a greater field depth than compound microscopes. This means that more of the specimen is in focus at once, making examining objects with uneven or 3D surfaces easier [9]. The advantages and disadvantages of stereomicroscope discussed in Table 11.1.

Application: Forensic experts use stereomicroscopes for detailed examinations of evidence, such as hair, fibers, gunshot residue, and tool marks.

11.2.3 Bright Field Microscope

A bright field microscope is a fundamental optical instrument frequently employed in laboratories, classrooms, and diverse research disciplines. Its primary purpose is to facilitate the examination of internal structures within biological specimens, cells, and other translucent or stained

Table 11.1 Advantages and disadvantages of stereomicroscope.

Advantages	**Disadvantages**
➢ Three-Dimensional Viewing ➢ Low to Moderate Magnification ➢ Long Working Distance ➢ Wide Field of View ➢ Comfortable Binocular Viewing ➢ Versatility ➢ Adjustable Magnification and Lighting	➢ Limited High Magnification ➢ Low Resolution ➢ Limited for Certain Biological Applications ➢ Bulkier Design ➢ Cost ➢ Less Precision for Certain Tasks

materials. This type of microscope is named "bright field" because when it is illuminated with transmitted light, the specimen stands out as dark against a brightly illuminated background. The working mechanism of bright-field microscope is illustrated in Figure 11.2.

Features of Bright Field Microscope

Bright field microscopes use a light source, typically a halogen bulb or LED, to provide transmitted (bottom) illumination. The light passes through the

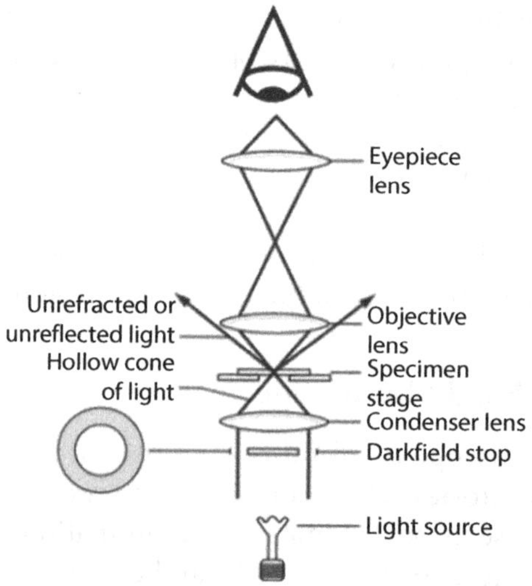

Figure 11.2 Created *"Working mechanism of Bright-field microscope"* by Biorender.com (2023).

specimen from below, making it visible. The condenser is located beneath the stage and helps focus and control the amount of light that passes through the specimen. It may have an adjustable aperture or diaphragm to regulate the light intensity. The stage is the flat platform where the specimen is placed for observation. It often has clips or a mechanical stage for securely holding slides or specimens in place. Bright field microscopes have multiple objective lenses with different magnification levels. These lenses are responsible for magnifying the specimen and forming the initial image. It can be rotated to switch between different objective lenses, allowing for various levels of magnification. The eyepiece is the lens at the top of the microscope that you look through. Typically, bright field microscopes have binocular eyepieces (two eyepieces for both eyes) for comfortable viewing. The knobs are used for precise focusing. The body tube connects the eyepiece to the objective lenses and helps maintain the correct distance between them. The illuminator is the light source housing, and it can be adjusted to control the angle and intensity of the light directed at the specimen. Some bright field microscopes have an iris diaphragm, which can be adjusted to control the amount of light entering the condenser and, therefore, the specimen [10]. The advantages and disadvantages of stereomicroscope discussed in Table 11.2.

Application: Bright field microscopy plays a crucial role in forensic science, aiding forensic investigators and experts in various aspects of their work. Hair and fiber analysis, bloodstain analysis, tool mark examination, document examination, firearm and ballistics analysis, trace evidence analysis, drug analysis, serology and bodily fluid analysis, entomology, and crime scene investigation.

Table 11.2 Advantages and disadvantages of bright field microscope.

Advantages	Disadvantages
➢ Widespread Use ➢ Simple to Use ➢ Cost – Effective ➢ General Observation ➢ Compatibility ➢ Real-Time Observation	➢ Low Contrast ➢ Limited Resolution ➢ Specimen Preparation ➢ Inability to Observe Unstained Specimens ➢ Depth of Field ➢ Limited for Certain Applications ➢ Limited Magnification

11.2.4 Confocal Microscope

A confocal microscope is a specialized optical microscope used in scientific research and various fields to obtain high-resolution, three-dimensional images of specimens. It achieves this by selectively eliminating out-of-focus light, resulting in improved image clarity and depth information [11]. The term "confocal" refers to the use of a pinhole aperture to ensure that only light originating from a specific focal plane is detected.

Principle: The primary principle of confocal microscopy is the elimination of out-of-focus light, achieved through the combination of laser scanning and the pinhole aperture. The laser beam scans across the specimen, illuminating each point in a sequential manner. If the specimen contains fluorescent markers or reflects light, the laser light interacts with these markers, causing them to emit fluorescence or reflect light. The emitted or reflected light from each illuminated point passes through the pinhole aperture, which selectively allows only the light originating from the focal

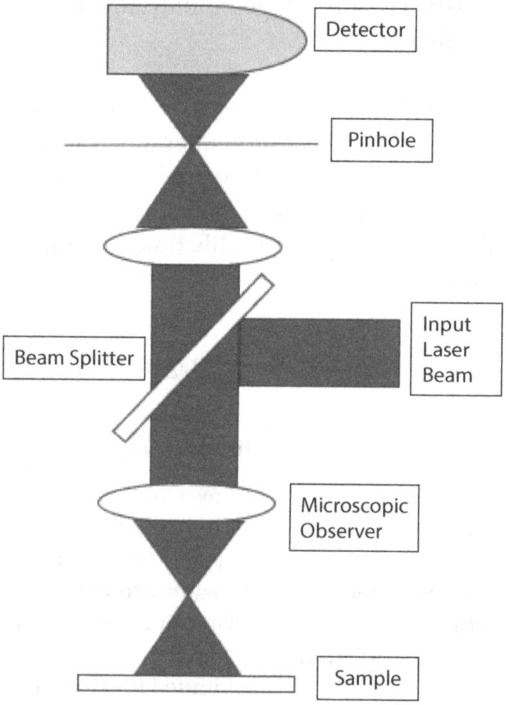

Figure 11.3 Created "*Working mechanism of confocal microscope*" by Biorender.com (2023).

plane (in focus) to enter the detector. The fluorescence or reflected light that passes through the pinhole is detected by the photomultiplier tube or photodetector, creating an image pixel by pixel [11]. The working mechanism of confocal microscope is illustrated in Figure 11.3.

Features of a Confocal Microscope

Confocal microscopes typically use lasers as the light source. These lasers emit focused and high-intensity light beams at specific wavelengths (colors). Different lasers can be used for various fluorophores or markers within the specimen. The objective lens focuses the laser light onto the specimen and collects the emitted or reflected light from it. High-quality objective lenses with a high numerical aperture (NA) are crucial for achieving high resolution. The scanning system directs the laser beam to scan across the specimen point by point in a raster pattern. This scanning process allows for precise control over the illuminated regions of the specimen. The selective detection enhances image contrast and resolution. The detector, often a photomultiplier tube (PMT) or avalanche photodiode (APD), captures the emitted fluorescence or reflected light from the specimen. It records the intensity of light at each scanned point. Confocal microscopes can capture multiple optical sections at different depths within the specimen, creating a series of images known as a Z-stack. This allows for the reconstruction of three-dimensional (3D) images and the examination of complex, multi-layered structures [12]. The advantages and disadvantages of stereomicroscope discussed in Table 11.3.

Application: Confocal microscopes have several valuable applications in forensic science due to their ability to provide high-resolution, three-dimensional imaging and optical sectioning. Trace evidence analysis, tool

Table 11.3 Advantages and disadvantages of confocal microscope.

Advantages	Disadvantages
➢ Improved Image Quality ➢ Optical Sectioning ➢ Reduced Photobleaching and Phototoxicity ➢ Fluorescence Imaging ➢ 3D Imaging ➢ Real-Time Imaging ➢ Highly Specific Imaging	➢ Cost ➢ Complexity ➢ Slow Image Acquisition ➢ Laser Bleeding ➢ Limited in Some Applications ➢ Specimen Preparation ➢ Cost of Maintenance

mark analysis, gunshot residue analysis, bloodstain pattern analysis, document examination, firearm and ballistics analysis, fingerprint analysis, tire tread and footwear impressions, materials analysis, biological evidence analysis, drug analysis, and entomology [13].

11.2.5 Fluorescence Microscope

A fluorescence microscope is a specialized type of optical microscope used in scientific research and various fields. It is designed to visualize and study specimens that emit fluorescence when exposed to specific wavelengths of light [14]. Fluorescence microscopy allows researchers to selectively target and observe specific structures or molecules within a specimen, providing valuable insights into their distribution, behavior, and interactions.

Principle: The high-intensity light source produces excitation light at specific wavelengths that correspond to the absorption spectrum of the fluorophores within the specimen. When the excitation light interacts with the fluorophores, it excites their electrons to higher energy states. As the excited electrons return to their ground state, they emit light at longer wavelengths, a process known as fluorescence. This emitted fluorescence contains valuable information about the specimen's composition and structure. Filters, including the excitation filter, dichroic mirror, and emission filter, ensure that only the desired wavelengths of light are used for excitation and detected as fluorescence. These filters eliminate unwanted background light. The emitted fluorescence is collected by the objective lens and directed to the detector. The detector records the intensity of fluorescence at each point, creating an image that represents the distribution

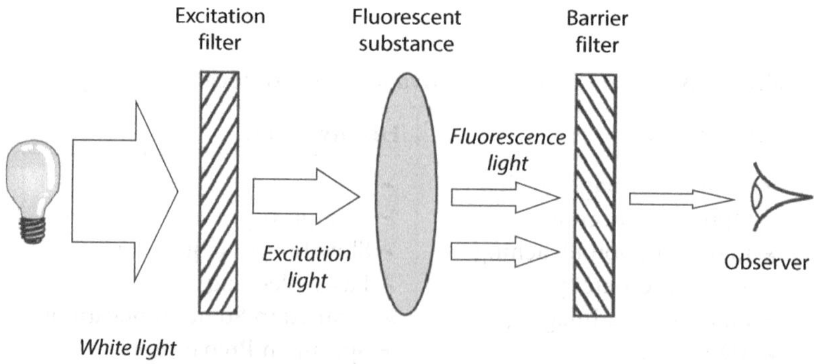

Figure 11.4 Created "*Working mechanism of fluorescence microscope*" by Biorender.com (2023).

of fluorophores in the specimen [15]. The working mechanism of fluorescence microscope is depicted in Figure 11.4.

Features of Fluorescence Microscope

Fluorescence microscopes use a high-intensity light source, often a mercury or xenon arc lamp, or modern light-emitting diodes (LEDs), to produce excitation light at specific wavelengths. This light source excites fluorophores (fluorescent molecules) within the specimen. The excitation filter, placed between the light source and the specimen, selectively transmits the excitation wavelength of light. This filter ensures that only the desired excitation light reaches the specimen. Positioned within the microscope's optical path, the dichroic mirror reflects the excitation light toward the specimen while allowing the emitted fluorescence to pass through. High-quality objective lenses are used to focus the excitation light onto the specimen and collect the emitted fluorescence. These lenses play a crucial role in image resolution and quality. The emission filter is positioned in front of the detector (e.g., a photomultiplier tube or a charge-coupled device camera). It selectively transmits the longer-wavelength emitted fluorescence while blocking any residual excitation light. The detector captures the emitted fluorescence and converts it into an electronic signal, which is then processed to generate an image. Detectors can range from traditional photomultiplier tubes (PMTs) to digital cameras and image sensors [14, 15]. The advantages and disadvantages of stereomicroscope discussed in Table 11.4.

Application: Fluorescence microscopy is a powerful tool used in forensic science to detect and analyze various types of evidence that fluoresce or emit light when exposed to specific wavelengths of light. Blood and

Table 11.4 Advantages and disadvantages of fluorescence microscope.

Advantages	Disadvantages
➢ Selective Labelling ➢ High Sensitivity ➢ Multiplexing ➢ Three-Dimensional Imaging ➢ Live Cell Imaging ➢ Quantitative Analysis ➢ Wide Range of Applications ➢ Fluorophore Selection	➢ Photobleaching ➢ Phototoxicity ➢ Sample Preparation ➢ Cost ➢ Complexity ➢ Background Autofluorescence ➢ Limited Tissue Penetration

Body Fluid Detection, Fiber and Hair Analysis, Gunshot Residue Analysis, Drug Analysis, Latent Fingerprint Examination, Counterfeit Document Detection, Trace Evidence Analysis, Biological and Pathological Analysis and Arson Investigation.

11.2.6 Polarizing Microscope

A polarizing microscope, also known as a polarized light microscope or a polarimeter microscope, is a specialized optical microscope used in various scientific and industrial applications to examine and analyze the optical properties of materials, particularly those that interact with polarized light [16]. It's like a regular microscope but with special filters that control the direction of light waves. This helps scientists see things like stress patterns, mineral characteristics, and other important details in different kinds of samples, such as minerals, crystals, and even biological tissues. It's a tool that helps scientists study the hidden properties of various materials by using light in a special way. The working mechanism of Polarizing microscope is illustrated in Figure 11.5.

Principle: The principle of a polarizing microscope is based on the manipulation and analysis of polarized light as it interacts with materials. Ordinary light, like sunlight or light from a lamp, vibrates in all directions perpendicular to its direction of travel. However, in a polarizing microscope, this unpolarized light is converted into polarized light, where the vibrations occur in a specific orientation. The first component of the microscope is a polarizer placed below the sample. This polarizer allows only light waves vibrating in a particular direction to pass through, blocking light waves vibrating in other directions. This results in the illumination of the sample

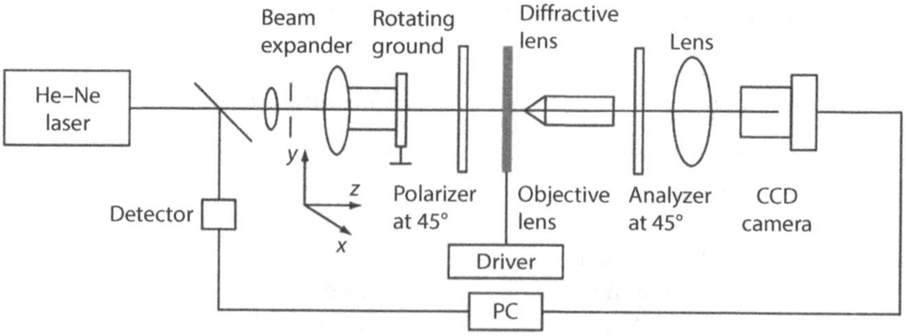

Figure 11.5 Created *"Working mechanism of Polarizing microscope"* by Biorender.com (2023).

with polarized light. When polarized light passes through a sample, it interacts with the material's optical properties. Some materials have a property called birefringence, where they split the polarized light into two different paths with different velocities. This occurs because the material's molecular structure affects the speed of light in different directions. The second polarizer, known as the analyzer, is placed above the sample. It can be rotated to control the orientation of its polarization. When the analyzer's polarization direction is the same as the polarizer's polarization direction (parallel), the light that passes through the sample is allowed to pass through the analyzer, and you can see the sample. When the analyzer is turned perpendicular to the polarizer (crossed), it blocks the light that has passed through the sample. When the analyzer is set at an angle between parallel and perpendicular to the polarizer (typically at 90 degrees), it allows some light to pass through the sample, creating interference patterns. These patterns provide valuable information about the sample's optical properties, including birefringence and stress patterns. In some cases, compensators, such as quarter-wave plates or full-wave plates, are added to the microscope to modify the polarization of light and enhance the visibility of certain sample features or to determine optical properties more precisely [17].

Features of Polarizing Microscope

Polarizing microscopes have two polarizers: the polarizer and the analyzer. The polarizer is located below the specimen and polarizes the incoming light, typically using a polarizing filter or a polarizing prism. The analyzer is positioned above the specimen and can be rotated to control the polarization of the transmitted light. Compensators are optical devices that can be introduced into the optical path to manipulate the polarization of light further. They are used to measure birefringence or to determine the optical properties of materials more accurately. The microscope stage holds the specimen, which is usually a thin section of a material, a mineral, or a biological sample. The stage may be equipped with a rotating stage for precise sample orientation. Polarizing microscopes are equipped with specialized objective lenses designed for use with polarized light. These lenses are optimized to minimize optical aberrations and provide high-quality images. To observe birefringence, the polarizer and analyzer are typically set at right angles to each other (crossed polarizers). When the polarized light passes through the specimen, it interacts with the material's optical properties, revealing features such as birefringent minerals, stress patterns, and other optical characteristics [18]. The advantages and disadvantages of stereomicroscope discussed in Table 11.5.

Table 11.5 Advantages and disadvantages of polarizing microscope.

Advantages	Disadvantages
➢ Reveals Optical Properties ➢ Identification of Minerals ➢ Material Analysis ➢ Biological Application ➢ Quality Control ➢ Research and Education ➢ Photography and Imaging	➢ Complex Setup ➢ Limited Depth of Field ➢ Higher Cost ➢ Sample Preparation ➢ Not Suitable for All Samples ➢ Limited Magnification Range

Application: A polarizing microscope is a valuable tool in forensic science for examining various types of evidence and providing critical information that can aid in criminal investigations and court proceedings. Fiber Analysis, Hair Analysis, Glass Analysis, Drug Analysis, Gunshot Residue Analysis, Paint Analysis, Trace Evidence Analysis, Tool Mark Analysis, Forgery Detection and Biological Evidence.

11.2.7 Electron Microscope

An electron microscope is a type of microscope that uses a beam of electrons instead of visible light to magnify and observe extremely small objects at a much higher resolution than is possible with optical microscopes. Electron microscopes are powerful tools widely used in various scientific fields to study the fine details of a wide range of materials and biological specimens. There are two main types of electron microscopes: transmission electron microscopes (TEM) and scanning electron microscopes (SEM).

Principle: The principle behind electron microscopes, both transmission electron microscopes (TEM) and scanning electron microscopes (SEM), is based on the use of electrons rather than visible light to magnify and image specimens. A series of electromagnetic lenses, similar to optical lenses in conventional microscopes, are used to focus and control the electron beam. These lenses manipulate the path of the electrons to ensure they converge and remain in focus as they interact with the specimen. In a TEM, the electron beam is transmitted through a very thin specimen, typically a thin section of the sample. In SEM, specimens need to be prepared as thin sections to allow electrons to pass through. The thickness of the specimen is typically in the range of tens to hundreds of nanometers, depending on the specific application and the type of specimen being studied. When a focused beam of high-energy electrons is directed at the thin specimen, these electrons interact with the atoms in the specimen [19]. In TEM, electrons that successfully pass through the specimen are focused onto a fluorescent screen or a detector. The electrons create an image by forming a pattern of light or electrons on the screen, which is then magnified and recorded to produce the final image. In SEM, the emitted secondary electrons or backscattered electrons are collected by detectors. The intensity and position of these electrons are used to construct an image of the specimen's surface. This process is repeated as the electron beam scans across the specimen, resulting in a detailed three-dimensional image. Electron microscopes can achieve much higher magnifications than optical microscopes because the wavelength of electrons is much shorter than that of visible light. This high magnification allows for the visualization of fine details and structures at the nanometer scale, providing exceptional resolution [20].

11.2.8 TEM

TEM stands for Transmission Electron Microscope. It is a powerful type of electron microscope used in scientific research and various fields to examine the internal structure and fine details of materials at the nanometer level. TEM operates on the principle of transmitting a beam of high-energy electrons through a thin specimen to create highly magnified and detailed images. The working mechanism of TEM illustrated in Figure 11.6.

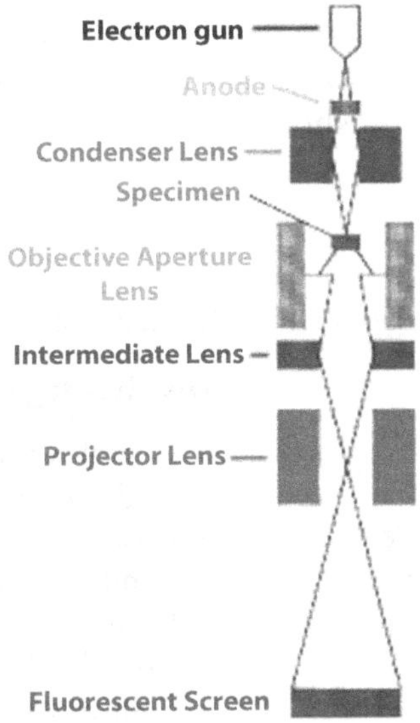

Figure 11.6 Created "*Working mechanism of TEM*" by Biorender.com (2023).

Features of a Transmission Electron Microscope (TEM)
TEMs are equipped with an electron source, which can be a heated tungsten filament or a more advanced field emission gun (FEG). A series of electromagnetic lenses, similar to optical lenses but operating with magnetic fields, are used to focus and control the electron beam. These lenses ensure that the electron beam remains in focus as it passes through the specimen. The thin specimen to be examined is typically prepared by sectioning it to a thickness of around 100 nanometers or less. This thin sample is mounted on a specialized specimen holder, which is placed in the TEM for analysis. The sample stage allows precise positioning and movement of the specimen within the microscope. It enables researchers to select specific areas of the specimen for analysis. After passing through the specimen, the transmitted electrons are focused onto a fluorescent screen or a detector. These electrons create patterns of light or electrons on the screen or detector. The patterns created on the screen or detector are magnified and recorded to produce the final image. These images reveal detailed information about the internal structure and composition of the specimen. TEMs can achieve extremely high magnifications, often in the range of 50,000x to over 1,000,000x, allowing for the visualization of individual atoms and atomic structures. The resolution of TEMs is also exceptional, typically in the range of 0.1 to 0.2 nm [21]. The advantages and disadvantages of stereomicroscope discussed in Table 11.6.

Application: Transmission Electron Microscopy (TEM) has several applications in forensic science, particularly in the examination of trace evidence and the analysis of materials at the nanoscale. Forensic Trace Evidence Analysis (hair, Fiber, Gunshot Residue), Biological and Pathological Analysis, Forensic Materials Analysis (Glass, Paint and Drug), Counterfeit

Table 11.6 Advantages and disadvantages of TEM.

Advantages	Disadvantages
➢ High Resolution ➢ Magnification ➢ Internal Structure ➢ Crystallography ➢ Elemental Analysis ➢ Wide Range of Applications	➢ Complex Sample Preparation ➢ High Vacuum Environment ➢ Cost ➢ Limited Field of View ➢ Beam Damage ➢ Complex Operation ➢ Limited Depth Information ➢ Sample Size

Currency and Document Analysis, Forensic Nanotechnology and Tool Mark Analysis [22].

11.2.9 Scanning Electron Microscope (SEM)

SEM stands for Scanning Electron Microscope. It is a significant type of electron microscope that uses a focused beam of high-energy electrons in order to scan the surface of a specimen, creating detailed three-dimensional images of the specimen's topography and morphology. SEM is a valuable tool in various scientific fields, including materials science, biology, geology, and nanotechnology. The working mechanism of SEM is illustrated in Figure 11.7.

Principle: The electron beam is focused and directed toward the specimen's surface. When the high-energy electrons strike the specimen, various interactions occur, including the emission of secondary electrons and backscattered electrons. Detectors capture these emitted electrons and other signals, generating images that provide information about the specimen's surface features and composition [23].

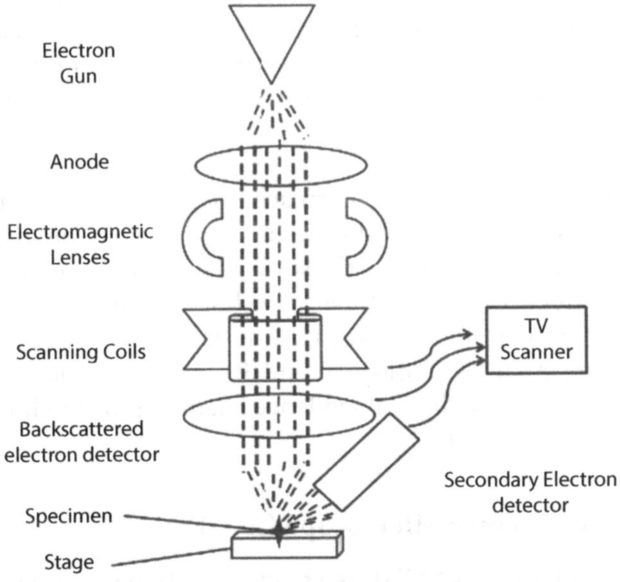

Figure 11.7 Created *"Working mechanism of Scanning Electron Microscope (SEM)"* by Biorender.com (2023).

Table 11.7 Advantages and disadvantages of SEM.

Advantages	Disadvantages
➢ High-Resolution Imaging ➢ Three-Dimensional Imaging ➢ Versatile Sample Analysis ➢ Elemental Analysis ➢ Quick Imaging ➢ Non- Destructive Imaging	➢ Sample Preparation ➢ High Vacuum Requirement ➢ Beam Damage ➢ Complexity ➢ Limited Depth Information ➢ Cost ➢ Limited Field of View

Features of Scanning Electron Microscope (SEM)
SEMs typically use a tungsten filament or a field emission gun (FEG) as the electron source to generate a focused electron beam. Electromagnetic lenses are used to focus and control the electron beam's path, allowing it to be scanned across the specimen's surface with high precision. The specimen is mounted on a specialized stage that can be tilted, rotated, and adjusted to position the sample accurately within the microscope. Scanning coils are responsible for deflecting and scanning the electron beam across the specimen's surface in a raster pattern. SEMs are equipped with various detectors that capture signals generated by interactions between the electron beam and the specimen's surface. The images reveal the surface morphology and texture. SEMs have a greater depth of field compared to optical microscopes, allowing for the imaging of 3D structures on the specimen's surface. The advantages and disadvantages of stereomicroscope discussed in Table 11.7.

Application: Scanning Electron Microscopes (SEMs) have several valuable applications in forensic science due to their high-resolution imaging capabilities and the ability to analyze the surface morphology of various materials. Trace Evidence Analysis (fiber, gunshot residue), Material Analysis (Glass, paint) Tool Mark Analysis, Counterfeit Currency and Document Analysis, Drug Analysis, Biological and Pathological Analysis, Ballistics and Forearms Analysis, Physical Evidence Examination and Biometric and Microscopic Analysis [24, 25].

11.2.10 Atomic Force Microscope (AFM)

Atomic force microscopy (AFM) is a high-resolution variation of scanning probe microscopy, which is referred as scanning force microscopy (SFM).

The gadget scans the sample surface using a cantilever with a pointed end [26]. The Van Der Waal forces, which can also include electrostatic and hydrophobic/hydrophilic forces, attract or repel the tip from the sample when the probe passes over its surface, causing the cantilever to deflect. By reflecting off the cantilever gadget scan the sample surface using a cantilever with a pointed end into the photodiodes, and a laser is utilized to measure the deflection [27]. The elevation of the tip, as it moves across the surface, is then controlled by a scanner using the information that is then provided to it. An image of the sample's topography in three dimensions can then be produced using the height variance of the scanner [28].

Principle: An AFM examines a sample surface by applying a cantilever with a very sharp tip. As the tip approaches the surface, the cantilever deflects in the direction of the surface due to the close-range, attractive force among them. As the cantilever is brought closer to the surface, it will begin to deflect away from it until the tip meets the surface. This is due to the growing repelling force that is active. A laser beam detects cantilever surface deflections in either direction. Due to the incident beam's tendency to reflect off the cantilever's flat end, any cantilever movement will induce a slight change in the trajectory of the reflected beam. A position-sensitive photo diode (PSPD) can be used to track these variations. As a result, the reflected beam's direction changes as an AFM tip passes over a raised surface feature, and the PSPD captures this change in direction as well as the cantilever deflection that results. The morphology of a sample surface is captured by an AFM by moving the cantilever over a desired area. The raised and depressed characteristics on the sample surface have an effect on the cantilever's deflection, which is measured by the PSPD. The AFM may create a precise topographic map of the surface features by utilizing a feedback loop to control the tip's height above the substrate and maintain a stable laser position [27].

Features of Atomic Force Microscope (AFM)

The AFM probe consists of a sharp tip attached to a flexible cantilever. The tip typically has a radius of a few nanometers and can be made from materials like silicon or silicon nitride. A laser beam is directed onto the back of the cantilever, and the reflected laser light is detected by a position-sensitive photodetector. The deflection of the laser beam caused by the cantilever's bending provides information about the forces between the tip and the sample. The sample is mounted on a precise stage that allows for accurate positioning and scanning. AFMs use feedback control mechanisms to maintain a constant force or setpoint between the tip and the sample during scanning. As the tip encounters variations in the surface,

Table 11.8 Advantages and disadvantages of atomic force microscope.

Advantages	Disadvantages
➢ High Spatial Resolution ➢ Non- Destructive ➢ Versatility ➢ Topographical Mapping ➢ Mechanical Property Measurement ➢ Multiple Modes ➢ Biological Applications	➢ Slow Scanning Speed ➢ Sample Preparation ➢ Limited Depth Information ➢ Complex Operation ➢ Cost ➢ Environmental Control ➢ Risk of Tip Damage

the system adjusts the tip-sample distance to maintain the set force. As the tip scans the sample surface, the variations in tip-sample interaction are recorded, and this information is used to generate images of the sample's topography, surface roughness, and other properties. The advantages and disadvantages of stereomicroscope discussed in Table 11.8.

Application: Atomic Force Microscopy (AFM) has found several applications in forensic science due to its high-resolution imaging and probing capabilities at the nanoscale. Surface Analysis of Trace Evidence, Toolmark, and Firearm Analysis, Fingerprint Analysis, Document Examination, Drug Analysis, Biological and Tissue Analysis, Physical Match Analysis, Surface Contamination Analysis, Material Characterization and Forensic Geology.

11.3 Forensic Application of Microscopy

11.3.1 Biological Samples

Microscopy is crucial to forensic research, especially when investigating biological samples. In forensic microscopy, a range of microscope types are used to analyze evidence related to criminal investigations. The following is a list of some significant forensic applications of microscopy in the analysis of biological materials:

- ➢ Hair analysis: Microscopy is routinely used to investigate hair samples that have been found at crime scenes. Forensic experts can determine the source's species (human or animal), match hair samples to recognized norms, and assess a variety of characteristics like color, length, and shape to pinpoint a specific source or person [29].

- Textile fibers found on clothing, at crime scenes, or in other pieces of evidence are analyzed using a microscope. Fibers can be traced back to their source and linked to a particular location or person by comparing their optical properties and shape [30].
- Microscopy is used to investigate bloodstains and, in specific, to determine the path of blood spatter, that can provide important details about the sequence of events during a crime. The blood types can also be identified via microscopy, and patterns can be studied to reconstruct crime scenes [31].
- For the purpose of identifying and detecting semen during sexual assault, microscopy is used. Sperm cell existence can be confirmed through this examination, and DNA can be retrieved for DNA profiling, that can be used to determine or rule out potential suspects.
- Microscopy can be used to ascertain whether forensic material contains saliva by performing a salivary amylase test. The level of stress experienced by a person at the time of the event can also be determined by measuring and analyzing the salivary amylase activity [32].
- Microbial analysis is the process of identifying and describing microorganisms, such as bacteria, fungi, or parasites, in a range of forensic materials using a microscope. When there is sickness or contamination, this is helpful.
- Fingerprint analysis: Though not a biological specimen, microscopic examination is commonly a part of fingerprint analysis. The evaluation of the ridge patterns, minute points, and other fingerprint characteristics by forensic experts using microscopes allows them to match particular fingerprints to particular people [33].
- Tissue and Organ Examination: In cases involving violent crimes, autopsies and histological examinations of tissues and organs are carried out under a microscope to determine the cause of death and identify any wounds or illnesses.
- Trace Amounts of Biological Fluids or Tissues on Items at Crime Scenes: Microscopy can be used to study small amounts of biological fluids or tissues on items like weapons, clothing, or objects, assisting in the establishment of links between the evidence and suspects or victims.

11.3.2 Fibers

Microscopy is an essential tool in forensic science for examining fibers connected to or found at crime scenes. In order to gather significant evidence for criminal investigations, fiber analysis involves examining both natural and synthetic fibers. Important forensic applications of fiber analysis with microscopy include the following:

Cotton, wool, silk, and synthetic fibers like polyester or nylon can all be identified and distinguished from one another using microscopy. This might aid in identifying the fabric or attire present in any pieces of evidence [34].

Comparative Fiber Analysis: By using microscopy, forensic experts can assess the similarities and differences between fibers from a crime scene and those from a suspect's personal items, such as clothing, a car, or a house. If the fiber type, color, or other qualities match, it may be possible to establish connections between the suspect and the murder scene. Microscopy is useful in identifying fiber interaction or transfer between people, things, or environments. For instance, it can show whether fibers from a suspect's clothing were transferred to a victim's clothing as a result of physical contact. Analysis of fiber dyes can benefit from microscopy since it can show how the fiber's dyes are made up. In circumstances when the color of the threads is significant, such as when attempting to identify fibers from a suspect's clothing after a hit-and-run accident, this can be quite helpful.

Environmental Fiber Analysis: In cases involving environmental crimes or pollution, microscopy can help in identifying and analyzing fibers that may have been discharged into the surroundings as a result of illegal conduct, such as improperly disposing of hazardous trash.

Materials for Packaging and Binding: Using a microscope, it is possible to study the fibers on packaging materials, ropes, bindings, or duct tape used in crimes like abductions, bombings, or homicides. This can demonstrate the means by which items were obtained or used for illicit purposes. High-resolution images of fibers are utilized as evidence and are documented using microscopy. Using these images as vital visual evidence in court can aid juries and judges in comprehending the findings.

11.3.3 Explosives and Gunshot Residues Analysis

In forensic science, the examination of explosives and gunshot residue (GSR) relies heavily on microscopy. Investigations involving explosions, weapons, and related incidents use these analyses heavily [35]. In order to analyze explosives and gunshot residue, forensic microscopy is used in the following ways:

Explosives

Characterization of Particles: Using microscopy, explosive residue and particle collections from crime scenes or people are analyzed and categorized. These granules might include fragments of other explosives or nitrocellulose, nitroglycerin, or other exploding materials. Using microscopy, forensic experts can determine the size, shape, and morphology of explosive particles. From this information, it is possible to deduce the explosive type that was used as well as the explosion method [36]. Microscopy greatly facilitates the detection of explosive residue on surfaces, clothing, or other objects. This can aid in reconstructing an explosion or bombing's timing sequence.

Environmental Analysis: The presence of explosive residues in environmental samples like soil, trash, or air can be examined using microscopy. It can be used to find out who makes the explosives that are utilized in illicit operations. The detection and identification of small quantities of explosive residues on people's goods, vehicles, and other items associated to suspects is done using microscopy. This evidence could implicate specific people in explosives-related crimes. Explosive Device Inspection: In cases containing explosive devices, microscopy can be useful for examining parts, wires, and bits to determine how the device was created and what trigger mechanism it used.

Gunshot Residues

Microscopy is used to identify and analyze GSR particles, which can be detected on the hands, clothing, or objects of people who may have discharged weapons and are composed of components such as lead, barium, and antimony. Their presence can be a sign of recent gunfire [37].

Particle Morphology: Using microscopy, forensic professionals can determine the type of firearm by analyzing the morphology and properties of GSR particles. Microscopy can be used to determine how GSR particles are distributed on a person's hands or clothing, which can provide information about how far and in which direction the gun will fire when it is discharged. Gunshot primer residue can be distinguished from other types of particles that are typically seen on hands or clothing using microscopy. Finding out if a person has recently shot a gun requires this discrimination. ***Evidence for cross-examination:*** GSR particles can be recorded and seen on evidence thanks to microscopy. These images might be presented in a courtroom as visual evidence during a trial. Criminal investigations involving explosions, shootings, and related incidents require both explosives and GSR examination with microscopy. They offer useful information that can identify suspects in relation to particular criminal actions and help identify the explosives or weapons used [38].

11.3.4 Glass

Glass evidence found at crime scenes or linked to criminal conduct is extensively investigated by forensic science using microscope. Glass analysis is useful in criminal investigations. Glass fragment comparison: Using a microscope, glass shards from a crime scene are contrasted with those from a potential source, such as a smashed window or glass object. Refractive indices, thickness, color, and physical characteristics can all be closely compared to link specific pieces of evidence to a specific source [39]. Microscopy is used to identify the type of glass, whether it is laminated, tempered, soda-lime, borosilicate, or another form. Use of this information can be necessary to reconstruct how a crime or accident happened. Fragments of glass found in the path of a bullet or projectile are examined using microscopy in cases involving gunshot wounds. The direction and firing order of the rounds can be ascertained through this research, which can also help pinpoint the gunfire's origin. Measurement of Glass Density and Thickness Glass samples' densities and thicknesses can be evaluated using microscopy. Variations in these factors can reveal information about how the glass was made and its intended application. Examining Laminate Glass: Microscopy is used to investigate laminated glass found in windscreens or windows in circumstances involving auto accidents or vandalism. It can aid in establishing the order of impacts and if safety glass features were compromised. Microscopy is used by forensic professionals to examine the color, coatings, or layers that are present on samples of glass. This knowledge may be useful in situations involving windows with unique qualities, mirrors, or vehicle glass. Glass Transfer Analysis: Glass transfer evidence on clothing, tools, or other items connected to suspects or victims can be examined using microscopy. Glass fragments can connect people to certain places or occasions.

11.3.5 Paint

Forensic scientists use microscopy as a crucial tool when analyzing paint evidence discovered at crime scenes or connected to criminal activity. Criminal investigations can benefit from the information that paint analysis can provide. Paint chip samples taken from suspects, items, or vehicles are compared to paint chips or fragments found at crime scenes using a microscope. In-depth comparisons of layers, colors, pigments, binders, and other physical characteristics may reveal parallels that aid in identifying the origins of the evidence. Microscopy is used to analyze the layer structure of a paint sample. By observing how different types of paint have varied layering patterns, it might be possible to determine the type and location of the paint. Identification of Paint Binder and Pigment: Forensic experts analyze paint samples using microscopy to identify the binder and pigment components. This information might be crucial for determining the type or brand of the paint and possibly linking it to a particular producer or item. Paint samples can be examined cross-sectionally using a microscope, revealing the arrangement of the paint layers and any potential alterations. In cases of forgeries or vandalism, this information may be crucial for locating additional or altered paint layers. Damage Assessment: When paint evidence is linked to damaged objects, such as cars involved in accidents or vandalism, microscopy can be used to identify the type and origin of damage. This can help explain how the events took place. Microscopy can be used to determine whether paint has been handled or transported between objects, persons, or locations. This could be useful when paint evidence links a suspect to a crime scene or a victim. Environmental Analysis: Microscopy can be used to investigate paint samples collected from the environment, such as vandalism or paint spills. This investigation can identify the kind of paint which was used, which may also help identify the source. Analysis of antiques and artwork: In cases of art fraud or theft, microscopy can be used to look at the paint and pigments used in the artwork. This method can be used to determine whether paintings and other forms of art are real. Microscopy can be used to identify the automotive paint on vehicles involved in crashes or hit-and-run incidents. This information can be used by investigators to determine the brand and model of the cars. Documentation and imaging: High-magnification microscopy is used to record and capture paint evidence. These pictures can be used as visual proof in trial and help jurors and judges understand the findings. Investigators and forensic scientists can use forensic microscopy in paint analysis to reconstruct crime scenes, correlate evidence to specific sources, and provide vital information for criminal investigations and legal actions [40].

11.3.6 Questioned Document

The forensic examination of contested documents, which includes evaluating various characteristics of handwriting, ink, paper, and other features to establish the validity and provenance of documents, heavily relies on microscopy. Analysis of Handwriting: Using a microscope, one may examine the finer details of handwriting, such as the amount of pressure applied by the pen, the clarity of the lines that are and the distinctive characteristics of the letters and numerals. This method aids in the identification or exclusion of suspects through the comparison of the questioned handwriting to known handwritten samples. In order to determine the composition, age, and other details of the ink used in documents, forensic experts use microscopy. By identifying the number of entries or changes that were made over time, ink comparison can spot fabrication or manipulation. Microscopy makes it simpler to analyze the paper or substrate used in documents, including its texture, watermark, color, thickness, and other properties. These characteristics can change or display anomalies that can reveal information about the origin or legitimacy of a document. Microscopy is helpful in revealing grooves and impressions on paper caused by the pressure used when printing or writing on top an additional sheet. Erasures and modifications: Microscopy is employed to detect alterations, erasures, or obliterations in textual materials. It might reveal altered or obscured text. Different features of the ink or paper could be visible when magnified. Because some inks or alterations are more obvious when viewed in the infrared region, it is possible to examine papers with infrared technology. You can use this technique to locate information that has been changed or concealed. Microscopy can be used to examine seals, stamps, and other imprints on documents to determine their validity and identify any modifications or forgeries. Analysis of Security Features: Microscopy can be used to examine security features like microprinting, UV rays, and watermarks in order to verify authenticity in cases involving counterfeit cash, checks, or identification documents. The use of labels and other adhesive materials, such as tapes, to secure objects to documents can be examined using microscopy. Through this examination, it is possible to learn details about the attachment's origin or time frame [41].

11.3.7 Soil and Materials

Microscopy is a valuable tool in forensic science for the analysis of soil and various materials found at crime scenes or associated with criminal activities. These analyses can help establish connections between evidence, suspects, and crime scenes. When comparing soil samples from a crime scene with those from the suspect's clothes, footwear, or cars, microscopy is utilized. An in-depth study can highlight parallels in the mineral composition, size of particles, form, and other physical properties, assisting in the establishment of connections between the evidence and a particular site. The arrangement and arrangement of soil particles at the scene of a crime are examined using microscope by forensic experts to develop soil profiles. The course of events or the movements of people or vehicles can be inferred from these profiles. Microscopy is used to find and identify traces of soil on suspects' clothing, shoes, or tools. People and particular surroundings or crime scenes can be connected by certain soil types. Microscopy is useful in determining whether soil has been transferred or in contact with people, things, or places. When soil evidence connects a suspect to a specific crime scene, this can be helpful.

Geological and Mineralogical Analysis: Using microscopy, it is possible to determine the geological and mineralogical features of soil samples, which can shed light on the area or place from whence the soil originated. Microscopy is used to compare the materials collected at a crime scene to standards or materials connected to suspects. A particular material's origin, such as that of glass, paint, fibers, or plastics, may be ascertained through this study.

Material Characterization: Using microscopy, forensic professionals can identify a material's physical and chemical characteristics, such as its morphology, color, composition, and texture. This knowledge can be used to determine the kind and country of source of materials. When components are associated with damaged objects like shattered glass, torn fabric, or damaged metal objects, microscopy can be utilized to examine the type of damage and its origin. This can clarify how a crime's events developed. Microscopy can be used to determine whether substances like fibers, polymers, or paint have been transported across individuals, things, or locations. This can be very helpful in retracing the movements of persons or objects during a crime. Microscopy is useful for analyzing and identifying foreign compounds that are discovered in food, medicine, or other products. Evidence of tampering or contamination may be revealed by this analysis [42].

11.3.8 Fingerprint Identification

Microscopy is used to analyze the distinctive ridge patterns and minutiae (ridge features) present in a fingerprint in order to identify it. To identify and compare fingerprints to known people, suspects, or database records, forensic experts examine these qualities. Comparative Analysis: Using a microscope, it is possible to compare unknown fingerprints—those taken from people or things at crime scenes—with known fingerprints. In order to evaluate if there is a match or exclusion, forensic examiners use this comparison methodology.

Latent Fingerprint Development: Latent fingerprints, which are invisible to the naked eye, are developed with the help of microscopy. Latent prints on materials like glass, metal, or paper are enhanced and visualized using a variety of ways, such as powder, chemical, or physical procedures [43].
Enhancement of Fingerprints: To make fingerprints more distinct for analysis and comparison, forensic professionals use microscopy to improve the clarity and contrast of the prints. Digital image processing, lighting modifications, and contrast enhancements are some examples of enhancement methods.
Sequence of Prints: Microscopy can help identify the order of partially imprinted or overlapping fingerprints obtained at a crime scene. This can be quite useful in retracing the movements and behaviors of those involved. Loops, whorls, and arches are just a few of the fingerprint patterns that may be recognized and categorized using microscopy. Identification of the common fingerprint type is aided by the occurrence and direction of these patterns.
Latent Print Recovery: Latent prints from a number of materials, including paper, plastic, or fabrics, can be retrieved using microscopy. Recovered prints can be analyzed, compared, and matched to known fingerprints [44]. Microscopy is used to record and take pictures of fingerprint evidence that has been magnified. To aid jurors and judges in comprehending the conclusions, these images are utilized as visual evidence in court [45]. Microscopy is crucial in all of these applications because it provides important data and evidence for forensic investigations, assisting law enforcement authorities and the legal system in resolving crimes and delivering justice [46].

Conclusion

In conclusion, microscopic techniques play a pivotal role in forensic science, serving as a standard and indispensable tool for investigators and analysts in various aspects of criminal investigations. Microscopic techniques enable forensic experts to examine physical evidence at a microscopic level, allowing for the detection of subtle details that may be imperceptible to the naked eye. This includes the analysis of trace evidence such as fibers, hair, paint, and glass fragments. Microscopy allows for the identification and comparison of unique characteristics in evidence samples. This is particularly crucial in fingerprint analysis, firearm examination, and toolmark analysis, where the distinctive features can link a suspect to a crime scene or weapon. The advancement of microscopy techniques, including electron microscopy, fluorescence microscopy, and scanning probe microscopy, continues to expand the capabilities of forensic science. These technologies enhance the precision and accuracy of evidence analysis. Microscopy bridges the gap between various forensic disciplines, allowing experts in different fields to collaborate and corroborate evidence. This multidisciplinary approach strengthens the overall investigative process.

References

1. Morris J.D., Payne C.K. (2019). Microscopy and cell biology: new methods and new questions. *Annu. Rev. Phys. Chem.*, 70:199–218.
2. Albuquerque PC, Fonseca BPF, Girard-Dias W, Zicker F. *et al.* (2019). Mapping the Brazilian microscopy landscape: A bibliometric and network analysis. *Micron.*, 116: 84–92.
3. Hooke R. (1665). Micrographia: or, some physiological descriptions of minute bodies made by magnifying glasses. 1st ed. London: J. Martyn and J. Allestry.
4. Usaj M.M., Styles E.B., Verster A.J., Friesen H., Boone C., Andrews B.J. (2016). High-Content Screening for Quantitative Cell Biology. *Trends Cell Biol.*, 26: 598–611.
5. Inoué S. (2002). Polarization microscopy. *Curr. Protoc. Cell Biol.*, Chapter 4: Unit 4.9.
6. Sanderson M.J., Smith I., Parker I., Bootman M.D. (2014). Fluorescence microscopy. Cold Spring Harb Protoc.
7. Tsien RY. The green fluorescent protein. *Annu. Rev. Biochem.*, 1998; 67: 509–544.
8. Bayguinov P.O., Oakley D.M., Shih C.C., Geanon D.J., Joens M.S., Fitzpatrick J.A.J. (2018). Modern Laser Scanning Confocal Microscopy. *Curr. Protoc. Cytom.*, 85: e39.
9. Verdaasdonk J.S., Stephens A.D., Haase J., Bloom K. (2014). Bending the rules: wide field microscopy and the Abbe limit of resolution. *J. Cell Physiol.*, 229: 132–138.

10. Milestones in light microscopy. (2009). *Nat. Cell Biol.*, 11: 1165.
11. Liu Z., Lavis L.D., Betzig E. (2015). Imaging live-cell dynamics and structure at the single-molecule level. *Mol. Cell.*, 58: 644–59.
12. Harris J.R. (2015). Transmission electron microscopy in molecular structural biology: A historical survey. *Arch. Biochem. Biophys.*,581: 3–18.
13. Bhella D. (2019). Cryo-electron microscopy: an introduction to the technique, and considerations when working to establish a national facility. *Biophys. Rev.*, 11: 515–519.
14. Arms L., Smith D.W., Flynn J., Palmer W., Martin A., Woldu A., *et al.* (2018). Advantages and Limitations of Current Techniques for Analyzing the Biodistribution of Nanoparticles. *Front. Pharmacol.*, 9: 802.
15. Botstein D. (2012). Why we need more basic biology research, not less. *Mol. Biol. Cell.*, 23: 4160–4161.
16. Furrer P., Gurny R. (2010). Recent advances in confocal microscopy for studying drug delivery to the eye: concepts and pharmaceutical applications. *Eur. J. Pharm. Biopharm.*, 74: 33–40.
17. Iannetti E.F., Smeitink J.A., Beyrath J., Willems P.H., Koopman W.J. (2016). Multiplexed high-content analysis of mitochondrial morphofunction using live-cell microscopy. *Nat. Protoc.*, 11: 1693–1710.
18. Renaud J.P., Chari A., Ciferri C., Liu W.T., Rémigy H.W., Stark H., *et al.* (2018). Cryo-EM in drug discovery: achievements, limitations and prospects. *Nat. Rev. Drug Discov.*, 17: 471–492.
19. Bullen A. (2008). Microscopic imaging techniques for drug discovery. *Nat. Rev. Drug Discov.*, 7: 54–67.
20. Federico S., Lassiani L., Spalluto G. (2019). Chemical Probes for the Adenosine Receptors. *Pharmaceuticals (Basel)*, 12: 168.
21. Johnson R.M., Higgins A.J., Muench S.P. (2019). Emerging role of electron micros copy in drug discovery. *Trends Biochem. Sci.*, 44: 897–898.
22. Waaijer C.J., Palmblad M. (2015). Bibliometric mapping: eight decades of analytical chemistry, with special focus on the use of mass spectrometry. *Anal. Chem.*, 87: 4588–4596.
23. Viégas F.B., Wattenberg M., Feinberg J. (2009). Participatory visualization with Wordle. *IEEE Trans. Vis Comput. Graph*, 15: 1137–1144.
24. Richert-Pöggeler K.R., Franzke K., Hipp K., Kleespies R.G. (2019). Electron microscopy methods for virus diagnosis and high resolution analysis of viruses. *Front. Microbiol.*, 9: 3255.
25. Saadat S., Pandey G., Tharmavaram M. (2020). Microscopy for forensic investigations. In: *Technology in Forensic Science: Sampling, Analysis, Data and Regulations*: 101-127.
26. DelRio F.W., Cook R.F., (2017). Quantitative scanning probe microscopy for nanomechanical forensics. *Exp. Mech.*, 57.
27. Ellen D. (2006). Scientific Examination of Documents Methods and Techniques. Boca Raton, USA: CRC Press.

28. LiancLinacre A., Ottens R. (2016). DNA: Hair Analysis, Encyclopedia of Forensic and Legal Medicine. 2nd ed. Elsevier. 337-342.
29. Saverio R.F., Margot P. (2001). Identification of gunshot residue: A critical review. *Forensic Sci. Int.*, 119:195-211.
30. Bartelink, E. J., Wiersema, J. M., & Demaree, R. S. (2001). Quantitative analysis of sharp-force trauma: an application of scanning electron microscopy in forensic anthropology. *J. Forensci Sci.*, 46(6), 1288-1293.
31. Jones, B. J., Downham, R., & Sears, V. G. (2010). Effect of substrate surface topography on forensic development of latent fingerprints with iron oxide powder suspension. *Surface and Interface Analysis: An International Journal devoted to the development and application of techniques for the analysis of surfaces, interfaces, and thin films*, 42(5), 438-442.
32. Jones, B. (2019). Microscopy in Forensic Sciences. *Springer Handbook of Microscopy*, pp.2-2.
33. Korda, E. J., MacDonell, H. L., & Williams, J. P. (1970). Forensic applications of the scanning electron microscope. *J. Crim. L. Criminology & Police Sci.*, 61, 453.
34. Meng, H. H., & Caddy, B. (1997). Gunshot residue analysis—a review. *J. Forensci Sci.*, 42(4), 553-570.
35. Li, F., Liu, S., Qi, R., Li, H., Cui, T. (2017). Effective visualization of latent fingerprints with red fluorescent La2(MoO4)3:Eu3+ microcrystals. *J. Alloys Compd.*, 727:919-924.
36. Locard, E. (1920). Enquête criminelle et les méthodes scientifiques. Paris : Ernest Flammarion.
37. Andrea Martiny, Andrea P.C. Campos, Marcia S. Sader, Maj André L. *et al.* (2018). SEM/EDS analysis and characterization of gunshot residues from Brazilian lead-free ammunition. *Forensic Sci. Intl.*, 177:9-e17.
38. T. Jalanti, P. Henchoz, A. Galluser, (1999). *MS Bonafanti Science & Justice* 39:48-52.
39. Neri, M., Turillazzi, E., Riezzo, I., Fineschi, V. (2007). The determination of firing distance applying a microscopic quantitative method and confocal laser scanning microscopy for detection of gunshot residue particles. *Int. J. Leg Med.*, 121 (4):287-292.
40. Kilty JW. (1975). Activity after shooting and its effect on the retention of primer GSR. *J. Forensic Sci.*, 20(2): 219-230
41. Elspeth Lindsay, Michael J. McVicar, Robert V. Gerard, E. Dale Randall & Jenny Pearson (2011) Passive Exposure and Persistence of Gunshot Residue (GSR) on Bystanders to a Shooting: Comparison of Shooter and Bystander Exposure to GSR. *J. Can. Soc. Forensic Sci.*, 44:3, 89-96.
42. Jones B.J., Downham R., Sears V.G. (2010) Effect of substrate surface topography on forensic development of latent fingerprints with iron oxide powder suspension. *Surface and Interface Analysis*, 42 438.
43. Jasuja O.P., Singh G.D., Sodhi G.S. (2008). Small particle reagents: Development of fluorescent variant" *Sci. Justice*, 48:141-145.

44. Sodhi G.S., Kaur J. (2002). Unconventional reagents for detecting latent fingerprints: A review" *J. Forensic Med. Toxicol.*, 19:18-20.
45. Shahi P.K., Singh P., Singh A.K., Singh S.K. *et al.* (2017). A strategy to achieve efficient dual-mode luminescence in lanthanide-based magnetic hybrid nanostructure and its demonstration for the detection of latent fingerprints" *J. Colloid Interface Sci.*, 491:199-206.
46. Lister G. (2009). Forensic Applications of Microscopy. *Australian J. of Forensic Sciences.*, 21(1): 13-25. doi: https://doi.org/10.1080/00450618809410773

12

EDX and X-Ray Technique in Forensic Science

Muskan Dhawan, Rhea Sharma and Gayatri Sharma*

Centre for Medical Biotechnology, Amity Institute of Biotechnology, Amity University Uttar Pradesh, Noida, India

Abstract
X-Ray Diffraction (XRD) is an analytical technique used in various applications in the forensic science field. It is used to determine the crystalline properties of an investigative sample that has some degree of crystal nature. The Energy Dispersive X-ray (EDX) technique has emerged as a valuable tool in the realm of forensic sciences. This analytical method enables the qualitative and quantitative analysis of the elemental composition of various materials, proving instrumental in diverse forensic investigations. By utilizing the interaction of high-energy electrons with samples to generate characteristic X-rays, EDX allows for the identification of trace elements in evidentiary samples. In forensic contexts, XRD and EDX find applications in gunshot residue analysis, paint chip examination, fiber identification, and the determination of cause of death through toxicological analysis. The non-destructive natures of XRD and EDX preserve crucial evidence, making them indispensable assets in deciphering intricate forensic puzzles.

Keywords: X-ray diffraction, energy-dispersive x-ray analysis, body fluid analysis, fire debris, toxicological analysis

12.1 Introduction and Overview

X-Rays are a type of ionizing electromagnetic radiation that are placed on the electromagnetic spectrum between the high-energy gamma radiations and relatively less energetic non-ionizing ultraviolet (U.V.) rays [8, 9].

**Corresponding author*: gshappy34@gmail.com

Priyanka Chhabra, Divya Bajpai Tripathy, Anjali Gupta, Rajeev Kumar, Kajol Bhati and Shruti Shukla (eds.) Advances in Analytical Techniques for Forensic Investigation, (339–362) © 2024 Scrivener Publishing LLC

By the term 'ionizing', one implies that the electromagnetic waves of X-rays carry an amount of energy in them that is sufficient enough to break molecular bonds and produce 'ions' by the removal (or knock-off) of tightly-bound electrons from atoms and molecules of the material substance. This change at the atomic level alters the properties of that material. This ionizing effect can also cause substantial damage to living cells [9, 10].

X-rays were accidently discovered in 1895 by a German physicist named Wilhelm C. Roentgen, who was working on a cathode ray tube at the time of discovery [23]. He named them 'X' rays after the mathematical sign to denote an unknown value or quantity. X-Ray Diffraction (or simply XRD) is a type of analytical technique that is used to quantitatively analyze the crystallographic properties of a substance. It is a less popularly used technique in traditional forensic studies and has rather specialized applications. It is quite useful when one has to gather information about the material of a forensic sample, in terms of its crystalline structure and composition, without causing any physical or chemical damage to the investigative evidence. Thus, when it is vital to preserve the gathered evidence, especially when it's acquired only in trace amounts, a non-destructive technique of analysis is essentially required. Here comes the X-ray diffraction method to provide a versatile and non-destructive way of analyzing the crystallographic structure and chemical composition of a forensic sample.

In a brief description of the working of the XRD technique, X-rays are primarily produced then directed at a sample that is crystalline in nature. The rays therefore undergo diffraction upon interaction of the X-rays with the crystal lattice of that sample, thus producing a unique pattern of diffracted beams. This unique pattern is produced based on the order of atomic arrangements in the crystalline material. That pattern is recorded and further analyzed or deduced to provide insights into the atomic and molecular arrangement of specifically that crystalline substance.

Energy-dispersive X-ray analysis (EDX) microanalysis plays a pivotal role in various biomedical domains due to its remarkable sensitivity in identifying elemental constituents within tissues. It frequently partners with scanning electron microscopy (SEM) to furnish intricate insights into both the surface and subsurface of specimens. Notably, the EDX technique is of significant value in investigating drug delivery systems, where its capacity to detect nanoparticles proves crucial. These nanoparticles are commonly employed to enhance the therapeutic effectiveness of certain chemotherapeutic agents. Moreover, EDX holds a vital place in environmental studies, especially concerning the identification of heavy metal pollutants [1].

The EDX spectrum encapsulates both semi-qualitative and semi-quantitative information, rendering it an indispensable tool in drug research, including drug delivery investigations where nanoparticle detection is pivotal. Collaborating with SEM, EDX is employed to ascertain the elemental composition and quantity at the surface or near-surface regions of nanomaterials [2]. However, it is noteworthy that as X-rays are generated within a depth of about 2 micrometers, EDX is not optimally suited for precise surface characterization. During EDX analysis, the electron beam traverses the sample, generating an elemental image, offering insights into the elemental composition.

12.2 Importance of XRD and EDX Technique in Forensic Science

12.2.1 Importance of XRD

X-ray diffraction technique is widely used in the fields of physics, chemistry, geology, and material science in order to determine certain physical properties of a substance that has some degree of crystallinity. X-ray diffraction can be used to determine the crystal structures of metals, minerals, and other types of complex molecules. It is utilized to study the stress and strain in crystalline materials. It helps in performing quantitative studies and identifying the various crystalline forms of compounds in materials (also known as the 'phases' of that compound) [12]. For example, it can be used to identify phases in materials like pharmaceutical drugs, metals and alloys, geological samples, minerals, polymers, glass, plastics, ceramics, construction material like cement, soil samples, as well as archaeological artifacts.

In the field of forensic science, X-ray diffraction technique has vital importance because of its wide range of applications in investigations like:

- for the determination of sample crystal structure and atomic arrangement (it helps to provide information like bond angles, unit cell dimensions, atomic position of crystal lattice, etc.)
- for the characterization of sample material by identification of its phases
- to study phase changes in the compound with respect to changes in its conditions like temperature, pressure, time, etc.

- to check the quality and consistency of materials. For example:

  - A large volume of investigative criminal cases come associated with illegal drug activity. These drugs and their adulterants, if any, can be analyzed in their solid forms (crystalline) in forensic laboratories to determine the drug composition and purity [11]. Thus it helps identify quality of drugs and the presence of cutting (bulking) agents in them.
  - Additionally, XRD can help identify the crystal structures of APIs (active pharmaceutical ingredients) used in drugs in order to study their behavior and activity in the drug. In the pharmaceutical industry, this is also done to check the quality and efficacy of the drug being manufactured.

X-ray diffraction is particularly important in forensic science to study and characterize trace crystalline substances found at the crime scene. These samples could be blood residues, gunshot residues, illegal drugs, chemicals of explosives, or any other type of unknown powders. The unique diffraction patterns produced by these substances help forensic scientists link the evidence to sources, solve crime mysteries, identify unknown substances and prevent exposure or mismanagement of potentially dangerous substances.

12.2.2 Importance of EDX

Energy-dispersive X-ray spectroscopy (EDX) stands as a potent instrument applied in both medical and forensic domains for discerning and quantifying the elemental constitution of materials. Renowned for its non-invasive nature, this technique avoids detrimental impact on the scrutinized specimen, rendering it exceptionally suitable for applications where evidence preservation is paramount [27].

In forensic applications, EDX finds a broad spectrum of uses, notably in tracing minute evidence like gunshot residue, paint fragments, and fibers. Moreover, it serves to unravel the root cause of fatalities, encompassing scenarios such as poisonings or drug overdoses. Furthermore, the technique's prowess is harnessed for identifying disease indicators, like cancer or tuberculosis, as well as for analyzing the composition of biological tissues, including bone, muscle, and blood.

Within the medical realm, EDX proves indispensable for diverse objectives, including cancer diagnosis. Given the distinctive elemental composition often exhibited by cancerous cells, EDX facilitates their detection and aids in gauging the disease's progression. Additionally, the technique is harnessed for identifying the presence of toxins and drugs in biological samples, thus contributing to the determination of the cause of death or poisoning. Furthermore, EDX serves as a conduit for comprehending how diseases impact the body, nurturing the development of novel medical interventions [1].

In instances where trace materials like glass fragments, paints, or gunshot residues occur in minute quantities, precision becomes essential. Analytical methodologies of heightened sensitivity are requisite to derive meaningful outcomes from such limited samples, while simultaneously ensuring the preservation of the material for possible future use. Among these methodologies, scanning electron microscopy paired with energy-dispersive X-ray spectrometry (SEM–EDX) emerges as a non-destructive cornerstone. Noteworthy for its ability to investigate object morphology and elemental constitution, SEM–EDX holds considerable prowess in the forensic context [41].

12.3 Instrumentation for XRD and EDX Techniques

12.3.1 Principle, Working and Instrumentation for XRD

Crystals are made up of a uniform atomic arrangement [16]. X-rays have a wavelength like the spacing between the atoms of a crystal [22]. So, the angle of the diffracted ray is determined by the interatomic spacing of the material, whereas rays with a larger wavelength are not affected by the spacing between atoms. This is the reason why x-rays are used for determining crystal sample properties [22]. The sample atoms scatter the x-rays when they fall on the crystal lattice. The x-rays pass through the sample, bouncing off atoms and deviating from their original path of travel. They change directions by a certain angle, known as θ (theta), and reflect as 'diffracted rays.' When these scattered waves interfere with each other, they cancel each other out and it is called 'destructive interference'. However, the waves sometimes have similar wavelengths and constructively interfere in some directions, which creates a diffraction pattern. This occurrence is called 'constructive interference' and it forms the principle of X-ray diffraction. Constructive interference is when two waves of similar wavelength join to create a wave of greater amplitude than their individual ones, and

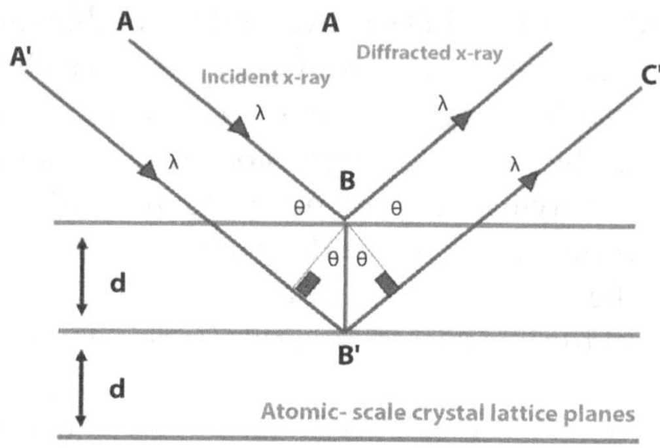

Figure 12.1 Constructive interference shown by diffracted x-rays when distance between paths ABC and A'B'C' differs by an integer number of wavelengths (λ), displaying Bragg's Law [20].

this creates a strong signal that is detected in the form of a pattern [22] (Figure 12.1).

The composition and structure of a crystalline sample can be determined by calculating the distance present between the atomic planes of the crystal. This difference can be calculated using a law known as 'Bragg's Law' [16]. Bragg's Law states that $2d\sin\theta = n\lambda$; where (θ) is the angle of diffraction, (λ) is added wavelength, (d) is distance between two atomic planes (path length difference), and (n) is a whole number (of wavelengths) [20, 22].

X-ray diffraction is carried out in an *X-Ray diffractometer*. Constructive interference happens when a monochromatic x-ray is incident on a crystal lattice. A monochromatic x-ray source produces rays which have the same wavelength, frequency (energy level) and color. This ray source is necessary as diffraction requires the path length difference due to crystal atomic spacing to be same as an integer number of wavelengths [17] (Figure 12.2). In a diffractometer, x-rays are generated by a vacuum X-Ray Tube that contains an electron-rich cathode. The cathode is placed in a high voltage setting which causes acceleration of electrons from the cathode towards a heavy-metal target which is the anode (made of heavy-metal like lead, molybdenum, etc.) [12]. The anode is made thick so as to dissipate the heat produced when high-velocity electrons hit it. The bombardment of electrons on the anode causes generation of x-rays. The generated x-rays further hit the placed crystal sample and scatter by bouncing off the atoms of the crystal lattice. The morphology (crystallinity and amorphousness) of the sample determines how the waves get scattered [12]. Scattering is also dependent upon the difference in phase between the waves, leading to production of 2 scattering types – coherent (x-ray diffraction) and

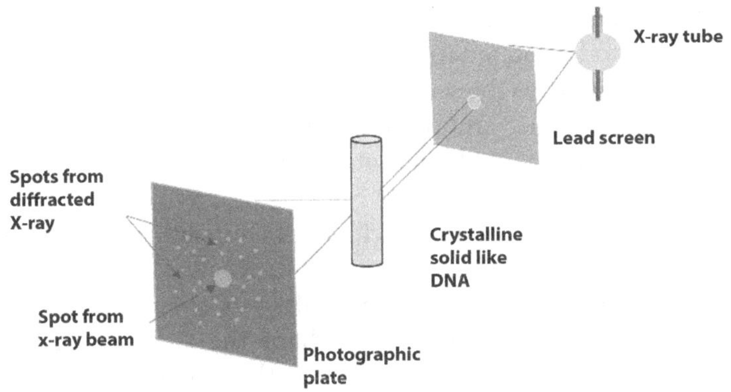

Figure 12.2 X-ray diffraction technique with diffraction pattern [13].

non-coherent (diffused) scattering [12]. In coherent scattering, the wavelength and phase remain the same for incident and scattered (diffracted) rays. It is caused by samples that are crystalline in nature. Whereas in non-coherent scattering, both wavelength and phase change as the incident ray scatters. It occurs for amorphous and partly crystalline samples [12]. Bragg's Law states that scattering will occur only when a monochromatic and coherent x-ray beam are incident on a crystal surface at an angle θ. Crystalline samples produce unique diffraction patterns based on the difference in planar spaces in the crystal. The pattern produced consists of concentric rings which become sharper as the degree of crystallinity of substance increases. Thus amorphous materials show a diffused halo rather than sharp circles. The visual observation and calculative interpretation of the diffraction pattern and its intensity helps determine the morphology and other aspects of the substance such as bond angle and distance, amount of substance crystallinity, crystal region conformations, etc [21] (Figure 12.3).

The forensic X-ray diffraction system consists of several components.

1. An X-ray Source: The heavy-metal anode bombarded by accelerated electrons from the cathode under high voltage produces a monochromatic X-ray beam that has a specific wavelength. It is directed at the crystalline sample.
2. A mount: The sample is placed on a sample holder or mount, that ensures that the material to be analyzed is properly aligned with the incident X-ray beam.
3. A goniometer: A goniometer acts as a high-tech sample holder [14]. It not only holds the crystal sample in the line of

the X-ray beam, but also serves as a turntable that allows the sample to be rotated in a precise manner to desired degrees of rotation. Thus the sample crystal face will get hit by X-rays in various angles and orientations which will allow for collection of substantial amount of data for qualitative analysis [12, 14].

4. A slit arrangement: This includes several slits like the soller slit, divergence slit, anti-scatter slit, receiving slit, and the detector slit. These slits are basically sets of equidistant parallel plates which control and shape the x-ray beam [15]. These narrow openings collimate the x-ray beam into a focused and parallel form, thus ensuring maximum uniformity and consistency in the beam. Sometimes a collimator is used instead which serves the same function.
5. A monochromator: It is function is to isolate x-ray beam of a specific wavelength form a range of wavelengths. A primary monochromator selects a specific x-ray wavelength from the broader spectrum emitted by X-ray source; whereas a secondary monochromator further refines the selected beam and enhances the energy resolution before the beam reaches the detector, so that x-rays of slightly different energies can be easily distinguished from each other. It is often made of quartz.
6. A detector: The x-rays that are diffracted from the crystal get collected by a detector placed at the end of the set-up. It allows one to measure the intensity of the diffracted rays at different diffraction angles.

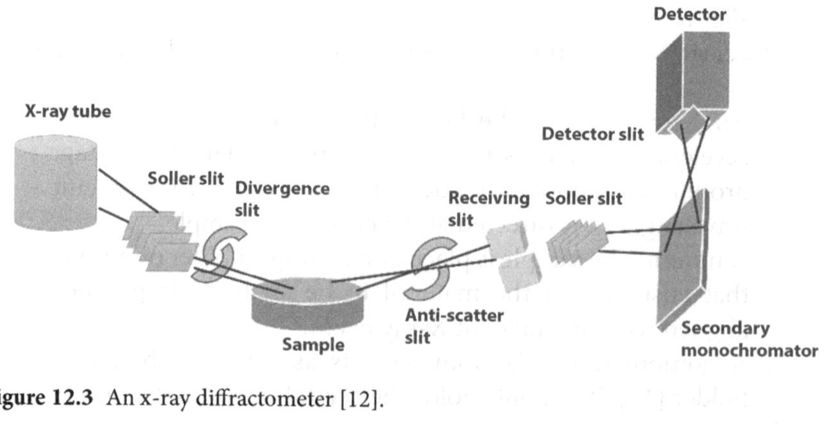

Figure 12.3 An x-ray diffractometer [12].

7. A data analysis software: A software specific for XRD generates a diffraction pattern and enables the computational analysis of the collected diffraction data.

12.3.2 Principle, Working, and Instrumentation for EDX Spectroscopy

Energy Dispersive X-ray Spectroscopy (EDS or EDX) is a microanalytical technique that furnishes both qualitative and quantitative insights into the chemical composition of a specimen, specifically for elements possessing atomic numbers greater than three ($Z > 3$).

Atoms are composed of electrons distributed across distinct energy levels, commonly labelled as K, L, M, and so forth, depending on their proximity to the atomic nucleus, with K being the innermost shell. Upon subjecting a sample to a high-energy electron beam, the electrons within the target atoms are expelled from their inner shells, creating vacancies. This prompts electrons from higher energy levels to transition into these vacancies, liberating energy in the form of X-rays [42] (Figure 12.4).

The X-rays released during this process are distinctive to the involved electron shells. For instance, an electron moving from the L to the K shell gives rise to a Kα X-ray, while a transition from the M shell to the K shell yields a Kβ X-ray [4]. Given that each element possesses a unique electronic configuration and distinct energy levels, the generated X-rays carry an element-specific signature. Through measuring the energy and intensity of these characteristic X-rays, it becomes feasible to ascertain the elemental constitution of a sample.

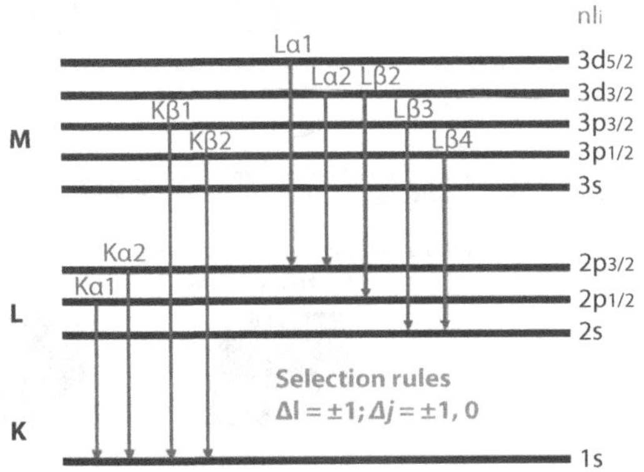

Figure 12.4 Schematic representation of energy levels.

The EDS detector is constructed using a semiconductor device, commonly a silicon crystal. The initial detector developed was the silicon-drifted lithium (Si (Li)) detector, which is now being replaced by the silicon-drift detector (SDD) [43] (Figure 12.5).

A standard EDS detector comprises the following components:

- A collimator, which ensures that only X-rays originating from the interaction point of the primary electron beam with the sample are collected.
- An electron trap that permits X-rays to enter the detector while blocking electrons.
- A vacuum-sealed window that isolates the detector crystal from the microscope chamber, often composed of modern polymers allowing even low-energy X-rays (down to ~0.1 keV) to pass, as opposed to older beryllium (Be) windows which blocked such X-rays [44].
- A semiconductor crystal detector.
- Electronics responsible for detecting the recorded charge in the detector, converting it to a voltage pulse, and transferring it to the pulse processor.

The energy of the incoming X-ray is absorbed by generating electron-hole pairs within the semiconductor crystal.

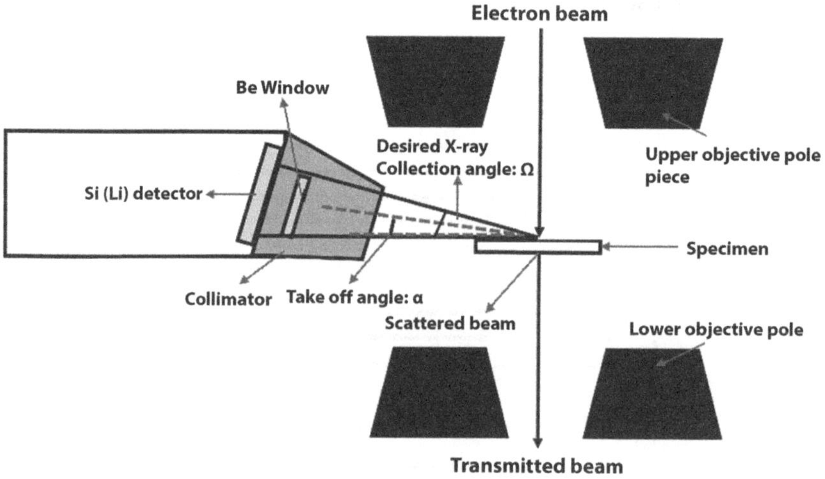

Figure 12.5 Energy dispersive x-ray spectrometer.

- Application of a substantial bias voltage across the crystal prompts the movement of electrons and holes towards electrodes on opposing sides, resulting in a charge signal transmission to the pulse processor.
- The magnitude of this signal is directly proportional to the energy of the incoming X-ray. For instance, around 3.8 eV generates each electron-hole pair in a silicon detector (approximately 2.9 eV for germanium). Consequently, when an Ni Kα X-ray of 7.477 keV energy reaches the detector, it generates 1968 electron-hole pairs, whereas an Al Kα X-ray of 1.487 keV energy induces the production of 391 electron-hole pairs.
- The original energy of the X-ray can be deduced by quantifying the generated current for each X-ray photon. This information allows for the computation of an EDS spectrum, essentially a distribution showcasing the count of X-rays recorded at various energy levels [45].
- To mitigate electronic noise, it is imperative to cool the detector. Si(Li) detectors necessitate cooling to liquid nitrogen temperatures and are connected to dewars necessitating regular refilling. On the other hand, the SDD can operate at -25°C, which can be easily achieved with Peltier cooling, notably minimizing anode noise contribution. EDX can be combined with SEM to analyse materials (Figure 12.6). SEM provides the imaging component, while EDX provides the detection component while SEM using the electrons provide the image component of the material.

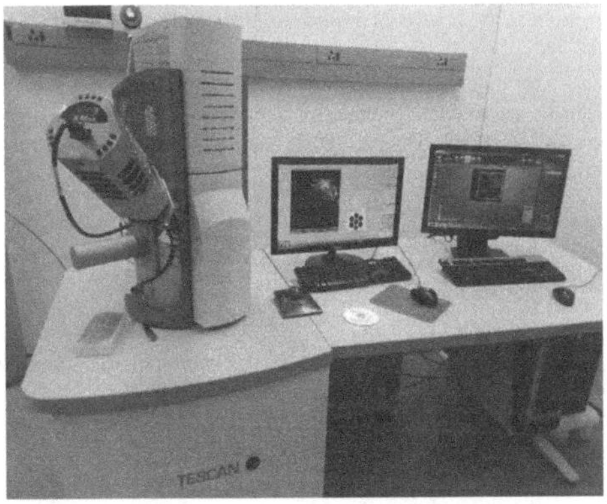

Figure 12.6 Setup of EDX microanalysis with SEM.

12.3.3 Sample Preparation

12.3.3.1 Sample Preparation for XRD

In forensic science, any analytical technique that can be useful for criminal investigative purposes generally gets adapted to suit forensic study [15]. XRD techniques have been utilized for a while to study material characterization in a typically non-destructive manner. Among the various types of materials that can be found at a crime scene, the samples studied most commonly under XRD are those which are found in the powder form [15]. Non-powder samples are generally preferred to not be converted into powders in the interest of preserving the integrity of evidence found at the crime scene. The size, form, and limited quantity of the sample acquired at the investigative scene too are factored in before deciding upon the use of XRD for analysis.

The preparation of the sample is a vital process that will determine the accuracy and reliability of the results in the XRD analysis. The flowchart given below states the suggested steps that are followed for obtaining optimal results in an X-ray powder diffraction analysis (Figure 12.7).

After sample preparation and running the XRD system, the x-ray diffraction pattern data is collected and analyzed. The system data software

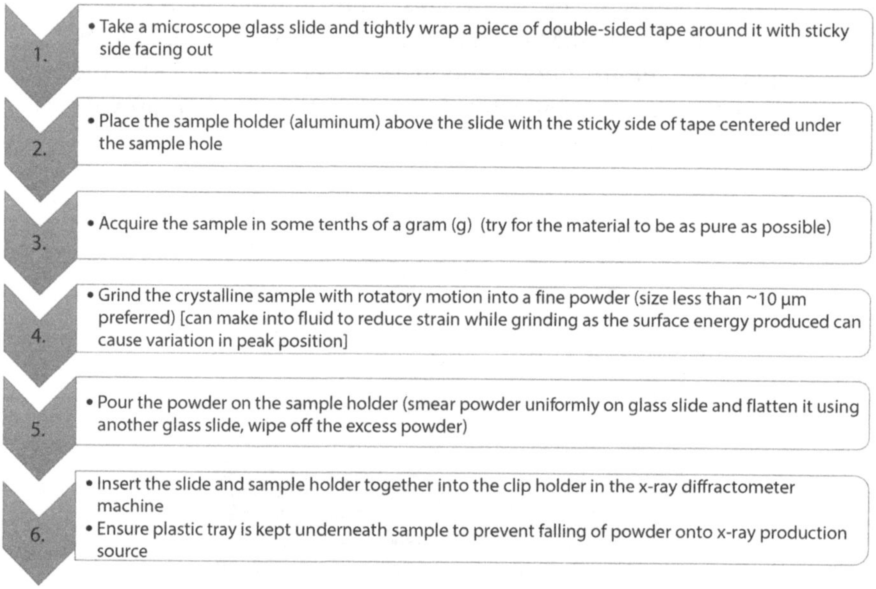

Figure 12.7 Steps for sample preparation in the x-ray diffraction (XRD) process [18, 19].

measures the intensities and scattering angles of the diffracted x-rays. It is observed in the form of an 'intensity vs diffraction angle' graph plot. The diffraction plot (also called a diffractogram) shows peaks produced by constructive interference of the x-rays and crystalline surfaces. The peak positions indicate the phases present, peak heights suggest phase concentrations, peak widths indicate crystallite size or strain, and the background hump suggests the amount of amorphous content present in the sample [12]. A larger number of crystal planes would cause more sharp peaks to form [18]. Different substances show different and unique angles and peak positions, owing to the varying crystalline structures of different materials. This diffraction pattern data collected is further compared to data deposited on a reference database, and that provides information on the identity of unknown sample. This could include information like symmetry of the crystal, unit cell dimensions, crystal lattice parameters, bond angles, atomic positions, etc.

12.3.3.2 Sample Preparation for Biological Specimens Using EDX Technique

The paramount objective in preparing biological specimens for Energy Dispersive X-ray (EDX) microanalysis is to retain the elemental constituents at their physiologically active sites, thereby ensuring precise and meaningful outcomes. In the context of Transmission Electron Microscopy (TEM) sample preparation, the procedure involves fixing specimens in a 4% paraformaldehyde solution followed by post-fixation in 2% osmium tetroxide. Subsequently, samples are treated with a phosphate buffer, dehydrated progressively with varying ethanol concentrations (30%, 50%, 70%, 95%, and absolute), and further dehydrated using propylene oxide. Ultimately, embedding within epoxydic resin finalizes the process. For Scanning Electron Microscopy (SEM) sample preparation, a critical point drying method utilizing supercritical CO_2 is employed to prevent deformation of cell surfaces, albeit the risk of losing diffusible atoms and molecules during these steps [46].

The preservation of elemental distribution mandates low-temperature maintenance following dehydration, and options like freeze-drying or analysis in a frozen-hydrated state are implemented to prevent the mobility of elements. Leveraging cryofixation techniques, originally designed for antigen analysis via immunocytochemistry, emerges as a pivotal strategy. These methods not only prevent element loss or gain during sample preparation but also facilitate the quantification of detected elements using EDX.

However, quantifying elements via EDX is a challenging feat demanding meticulously prepared standard specimens. These standards must closely mirror the composition of the specimen and undergo identical preparation stages. Addressing these intricacies, a novel TEM-EDX analytical protocol has been proposed. This protocol employs archival formalin-fixed paraffin-embedded (FFPE) tissues, leveraging hematoxylin-and-eosin (H&E) stained sections to earmark regions for subsequent EDX analysis. Further steps entail placing embedding beam capsules over the identified regions, which are subsequently detached post-resin polymerization. This innovative approach paves the way for large-cohort EDX investigations on FFPE tissues housed within pathology archives [47].

In the acquisition of EDX spectra, TEM-EDX analysis involves the examination of 100 nm thick unstained ultrathin sections, while SEM-EDX utilizes unstained dried samples. It's worth noting that the introduction of heavy metal staining agents like U, Pb, or Au could potentially compromise the integrity of the analysis. Collectively, these measures and methodologies underscore the meticulousness intrinsic to EDX microanalysis in biological applications.

12.4 Applications of EDX and X-Ray Technique in Forensic Science

12.4.1 Drug Analysis

The rapid screening of toxic chemicals, pharmaceutical drugs, illegal drugs, corrosive and metallic poisons is important in the fields of forensic toxicology EDX is a simple elemental analysis method which detects various elements without special sample preparation. The importance of the technique was highlighted in the case study of the person who had no prior medical history was found dead in the house. He had a strange greenish color fluid with odor in his mouth. The taxological examination by GC/MS and EDX on stomach contents indicated ingestion of methomyl, which is a component of carbamate insecticide [33].

The illegal drugs like cocaine are often processed to avoid detection. The recent study concluded that techniques such as color tests and MIR spectroscopy are only presumptive and can give false positive results. Hence, the confirmatory analysis with GC-MS and GC-FID and SEM-EDX analyses should be performed to quantify and obtain additional characterization [38].

Death due to electrocution is extremely difficult to identify because autopsy results are nonspecific in this case. Electrical current marks may not be clearly identified. Whenever an electric current passes from a metal conductor into the body, electrolysis follows and metallic ions get implanted under the skin, which is termed as metallization. Metallization is a characteristic feature because of passage of electric current in the skin and can be used to diagnose electrocution. Iron (Fe) and copper (Cu) are the only metallic elements that can be detected by histochemical examination. The study conducted by Tananaka *et al.*, 2020 reported that metallic elements like Al, Sn, and Zn in the skin of respective current exposure groups can easily be detected with EDX [34].

Another study using EDX analysis indicated presence of bromide in cardiac blood from medico-legal autopsy cases provides a chemical proof that drowning in seawater is a cause of death [37].

In the recent study, XRD and EDX techniques have been assessed for their efficiency in determining biological age and sex from human dentition, particularly in fire- or heat-affected dental remains. The Carbon (C), phosphorus (P), and calcium (Ca) in unburned roots showed significant changes that were the opposite of those observed in the crowns. The unburned roots of males had significantly higher quantities of oxygen (O), (P), and Ca than females [40].

12.4.2 Fire Debris

In most of the crime cases involving weapons, bullets, cartridge cases, projectile fragments, the evidence from firearm discharge residues are gathered during investigation. This evidence is investigated in forensic labs to provide important investigative information, including to identify a suspected shooter, determine firing ranges, or differentiate between a potential homicide, suicide, or unintentional shooting, among other things. Gunshot residues (GSR) and this data shows a substantial association. Basic components in gunshot include inorganic and organic residues. Most of the organic constituents originate from propellant and lubricant materials while inorganic constituents arise from primer, propellant, ammunition barrel, case, and core of the jacket. The identification of components based on morphological characteristics is crucial for locating GSR particles. The elemental inorganic constituents can be determined by EDX method. The use of morphological and elemental indications makes it possible to distinguish between different types of ammunition as well as the types of firearms used to discharge a round, case, and bullet composition. Sometimes organic components provide additional information about the sample and are useful in differentiating between the GSR and environmental residues [29]. Some research was also performed using SEM/EDX for the analysis of gunshot residue along with glass fragments from the hands of shooters [30].

Gentile *et al.*, 2020 [35] explained processes to conduct SEM/EDX analysis on corpses suffering from various injuries, including blunt force trauma, ligature strangling, electrocution, sharp force trauma, gunshot wounds, and drunkenness. Sharp force trauma can be differentiated from blunt force trauma by the presence of metal microtraces (Fe, Cr, Al, Ti). Blunt force trauma may be caused by deposition of microparticles of that results due to interaction of the blunt instrument with the victim. Exogenous microtraces may be detected in the cutaneous furrow following ligature strangulation. The presence of metals like Cu, Zn, or Fe can be considered as the "electric mark" in electrocution. In the gunshot wounds, the particles Pb, Ba, Sb are detected. Finally, residues of harmful compounds may be found in the examination of intoxicants. The authors draw the following conclusion: SEM/EDX analysis can offer crucial data to support the medicolegal inquiry of death [39].

EDX is a good diagnostic tool for the detection of the osseous origin of samples exposed to different temperatures. In all of the samples that were tested, the Ca/P ratio stayed within the osseous normal range of between 1.6 and 2.58. This showed that even when exposed to high temperatures, bone's overall gross elemental composition and atomic fraction of elements remained consistent, leaving a distinct "fingerprint" for osseous material [36].

12.4.3 Body Fluid Analysis

Body fluids are among the most critical parts of evidence acquired from a crime scene. In serological analysis, evidence is sampled and analyzed for the presence of body fluids. The detection and identification of various body fluids including blood, semen, saliva, vaginal fluid, sweat, and urine collected from a crime scene provide background information for forensic casework such as event timeline, scene reconstruction, and involvement of possible individuals. In investigations, it's crucial to find and identify the source of body fluids to positively identify a person by additional scientific testing, including DNA analysis. The traditional test used for the analysis of various body fluids are generally categorized into presumptive and confirmatory tests. Presumptive tests are preliminary indicators which can establish the likelihood of the presence and/or absence of a certain body fluid. Confirmatory tests are utilized to conclusively specify a certain biological material/substance in the body fluid. SEM/EDX is a part of presumptive test which is used in the chemical analysis of various body fluids for example, the relative concentrations of sodium, phosphorus, sulphur, chlorine, potassium, calcium, and other metal trace elements in the semen, saliva and vaginal samples can be detected. In the saliva sample tests, potassium has the largest peak and can be used as a basis of identification. Chlorine was the largest peak detected in the semen samples, but calcium is used as basis of identification [28].

12.4.4 Paint and Polymer Analysis

Paint is a liquid of complex composition which is generally used to provide good appearance to the surfaces and to protect them from corrosion and degradation. The paint formulas are made up of a huge number of different chemical components. These can be divided into four major classes based on their functions:

(a) Binders (or film formers, resins)
(b) Solvents (Organic or Water)
(c) Pigments (Organic or Inorganic), Dyes, Extenders
(d) Additives (or modifiers)

The combination of the binder and solvent is referred to as the paint "vehicle." Pigment and additives are dispersed within these vehicles. Pigment free paint formulations are derived by drying oils and resins in organic solvents and are referred as varnishes. The thermoplastic solution paints or varnishes dry through ordinary evaporation of solvents. In general paints with non-volatile is converted to a solid film on the surface substrate by oxidation or polymerization. Paint evidence is common in hit-and-run incidents and other crimes where it may prove to be important evidence. When two objects contact with an intensity, material will be transmitted, stay, and can be retrieved. If contacting objects are coated, it is possible to leave its own paint and/or on the surface of the other object as traces in the form of multidimensional flakes, chips, streaks, or powder. The physical components (color, layer thickness, surface and layer features, and contaminants) and chemical components (pigments, polymers, additives) of these evidences can provide important information about the origin of the criminal action or the course of events related with crimes (most common example includes hit-and-run accidents), damage to property (e.g., breaking and entering, vandalism), capital crimes (e.g., terrorist attacks, murder, etc.), and other offences involving the use of painted objects. In forensic paint analysis, in order to determine whether two paint samples have a common origin, physical and chemical features of a paint trace—a suspect, ambiguous, or questioned sample—and a control paint sample—a reference or known sample—are compared. The primary challenge in comparative material analysis is in the interpretation of matched analytical data. Paints are mass-produced items that are frequently produced in large annual capacities. In order to draw the proper conclusions about the value of the evidence, the forensic scientist must be able to differentiate between batches of paint, be aware of how material aging affects analytical results, and be able to deal with application errors and material flaws.

The comparative analysis of paint evidence with its control paint known source is carried out with the sequence of techniques. This sequence depends on the number of factors including quality and quantity of evidential paint available, on the availability of equipment in the laboratory and on the choice of the forensic scientist. At every stage of the sequence, if the questioned and the known samples result undifferentiated, one continues with the other tests in the sequence. Although even after the differentiation of trace and its control with any given techniques of the sequence, the differentiation remains unexplained, a common origin can be excluded. The broad spectrum of microscopic techniques combined with procedures of instrumental microanalysis and spectroscopic methods are earliest approaches in the sequence analysis. The technique of choice for characterizing the morphology and the elemental composition of paint samples is scanning electron microscopy and energy dispersive X-ray spectroscopy (SEM/EDS or SEM/EDX). A wide range of inorganic components as pigments and extenders can be identified by this technique. Although organic pigments cannot be identified, but their presence can be suggested by the existence of elements as chlorine and bromine or nickel, manganese, and copper. Atomic Absorption Spectroscopy (AAS) [24, 25]. Inductively Coupled Plasma Atomic Emission Spectrometry (ICP-AES) [26], and Neutron Activation Analysis (NAA) are some other comparable techniques which provide elemental analysis, but EDX has the advantages of being non-destructive, a qualitative as well as quantitative method, multi-elemental, fast, and cost-effective.

In a study conducted in India, experts studied the layers of automotive paint fragments collected from Maruti Suzuki, which is one of the leading automotive brands. EDX results reported the presence of specific elements in different color samples of automobile paint. Hence, this proved that profiling of chemicals and elements of the sample by EDX may lead to identification of the automobiles from the specific brands [32].

12.4.5 Fiber Analysis

One of the most frequent and significant types of trace evidence obtained during a crime scene investigation are fibers. They generally get transferred from one surface to another whenever two individuals have physical contact. This has relatively high evidence qualities to link the suspects to the crime scene. The forensic examination of fibers, consist of two different areas: fiber identification and fiber comparison. The fiber identification gives information even in the case of non-availability of suspect's fiber and in case it is available, it is regarded a part of fiber comparison. The identification of the suspect's fiber and the fiber from a known origin that are transferred and/or cross-transferred between each other at the crime scene is revealed by the fiber comparison. The fiber identification gives an idea about the fiber type and characteristic properties of the fibers. This analysis can be easily carried out by several kinds of microscopic, spectrophotometer and spectrofluorometer instruments. The tagging in organic elements added by manufacturers to differentiate their product from others, metals from the dyes for example, amide fiber, wool, is dyed by acid mordant dyes, chromium is used in the coloration process are investigated by scanning electron microscopy with energy dispersive X-ray microanalysis (SEM-EDX). The other advanced techniques such as Fourier transform infrared spectrometry (FTIR) and pyrolysis gas chromatography–mass spectrometry (Pyr-GC–MS) are used for the analysis of the polymer composition of man-made fibers.

In this aspect, a unique case which was cited by Zhoas' group is related to medical malpractice [31]. A patient had received surgical treatment for cardiac problem. At later age 53, this patient again underwent surgery in different hospital; she was recovering well but suddenly passed away due to hematemesis. The autopsy reported presence of long surgical gauze in the mediastinum. A SEM/EDX analysis was conducted to compare materials of gauze. The exam showed a morphologically exogenous fiber in the gauze didn't match with the control samples taken from the hospital where second surgery was performed. This indicates importance of EDX to detect the medical negligence even after long period of time.

12.5 Future Aspects and Conclusion

XRD contributes to several aspects in forensic science and will continue to play a significant role in investigative studies. As XRD technology evolves, its sensitivity and ability to analyze even smaller quantities of trace samples will improve and thus help investigations solve sooner and better. XRD has the useful ability to analyze complex materials, which could be enhanced in the future to accurately identify newer materials, thus aiding in solving crimes that involve unknown substances. Further, as the XRD diffraction pattern databases expand and pattern recognition software/algorithms improve, it'll be more helpful to understand and match unknown substances with known patterns, thus speeding up the process of investigations.

Transmission Electron Microscopy (TEM) boasts superior imaging capabilities, while Scanning Electron Microscopy (SEM)/Transmission SEM (T-SEM) combined with Energy Dispersive X-ray (EDX) analysis provides a rapid and practical means for nanoanalysis, encompassing morphology, size, and elemental composition. The latest advanced Energy Dispersive X-ray (EDS) detector systems, such as large-area Silicon Drift Detectors (SDD), continue to enhance sensitivity, crucial for accurate characterization of nanoparticles [5].

In recent times, nanoparticles (NPs) have become increasingly prominent in various sectors, including biomedical imaging, diagnostic testing, and drug administration. Understanding the biological reactions to nanoparticles is crucial for ensuring their safety. The rapid advancement of nanotechnologies has led to the widespread use of products like silver nanoparticles (AgNPs) and gold nanoparticles (AuNPs). AgNPs, known for their antimicrobial properties, find applications in textiles and wound dressings [6]. AuNPs, with their easy synthesis methods and bioconjugation capabilities, are gaining attention for biological purposes such as diagnostics, cell tracking, drug release, and cell imaging. AuNPs are employed with anti-epidermal growth factor receptor (EGFR) antibodies, allowing targeted binding to cancer cells with elevated EGFR expression [7]. This strategic use enables the illumination of cancerous cells, offering a promising avenue in cancer treatment. The integration of nanotechnology into cancer biology has sparked optimism, driving the development of innovative strategies for addressing cancer. The proliferation of these nanomaterials is expected to continue growing in the near future [3].

References

1. Scimeca, M., Bischetti, S., Lamsira, H. K., Bonfiglio, R., & Bonanno, E. (2018). Energy Dispersive X-ray (EDX) microanalysis: A powerful tool in biomedical research and diagnosis. *Eur. J. Histochem. : EJH*, *62*(1), 2841. https://doi.org/10.4081/ejh.2018.2841

2. Bell, D. C., & Garratt-Reed, A. (2003). Energy dispersive x-ray analysis in the electron microscope. In *Garland Science eBooks*, https://doi.org/10.4324/9780203483428
3. Rades, S., Hodoroaba, V. D., Salge, T., Wirth, T., Lobera, M. P., Labrador, R. H., ... & Unger, W. E. (2014). High-resolution imaging with SEM/T-SEM, EDX and SAM as a combined methodical approach for morphological and elemental analyses of single engineered nanoparticles. *RSC Adv.*, *4*(91), 49577-49587.
4. Tommasone, S. (2022, March 10). *Energy Dispersive Spectroscopy (EDS/EDX): An overview.* News-Medical.net. https://www.azolifesciences.com/article/Energy-Dispersive-Spectroscopy-(EDSEDX)-An-Overview.aspx
5. Narayanan, A., Sharma, P., & Moudgil, B. M. (2013). Applications of Engineered Particulate Systems in Agriculture and Food Industry. *KONA Powder and Particle Journal*, 30, 221–235. doi:10.14356/kona.2013021
6. De Jong, W. H., & Borm, P. J. (2008). Drug delivery and nanoparticles: applications and hazards. *Int. J. Nanomedicine*, *3*(2), 133–149. https://doi.org/10.2147/ijn.s596
7. Chaudhry, Q., Scotter, M., Blackburn, J., Ross, B., Boxall, A., Castle, L., Aitken, R., & Watkins, R. (2008). Applications and implications of nanotechnologies for the food sector. *Food additives & contaminants. Part A, Chemistry, analysis, control, exposure & risk assessment*, *25*(3), 241–258. https://doi.org/10.1080/02652030701744538
8. *X-rays*. (n.d.). National Institute of Biomedical Imaging and Bioengineering. U.S. Department of Health and Human Services. https://www.nibib.nih.gov/science-education/science-topics/x-rays
9. *Ionizing radiation*. (2021, June 29). Centers for Disease Control and Prevention. https://www.cdc.gov/nceh/radiation/ionizing_radiation.html
10. *Ionizing radiation*. (n.d.). NRC Web. https://www.nrc.gov/reading-rm/basic-ref/glossary/ionizing-radiation.html
11. Houck, M. M., & Siegel, J. (2010). Illicit Drugs. In *Fundamentals of Forensic Science* (2nd ed.). https://doi.org/10.1016/b978-0-12-374989-5.00013-2
12. Igwebike-Ossi, C. D. (2017). X-ray techniques. *Failure Analysis and Prevention*. https://doi.org/10.5772/intechopen.72447
13. Delhi, I. (2017, February 25). *XRD (X-Ray diffraction) technique & its applications in Forensics*. xrd.co. https://xrd.co/applications-xrd-forensics/
14. Smith, C. (n.d.). *Overview of X-Ray diffraction systems*. https://www.labcompare.com/10-Featured-Articles/128202-Overview-of-X-Ray-Diffraction-Systems/
15. Abraham, J. T. S. S. K. S. a. K. (n.d.). *Research and Technology - Forensic Science Communications - April 2007*. FBI. https://archives.fbi.gov/archives/about-us/lab/forensic-science-communications/fsc/april2007/research/2007_04_research03.htm
16. *What is X-ray diffraction analysis (XRD) and how does it work?*. TWI. (n.d.). https://www.twi-global.com/technical-knowledge/faqs/x-ray-diffraction

17. Ingle, R. (2021, December 3). *What is X-Ray Diffraction (XRD) and What Applications is it Used in?* AZoOptics.com. https://www.azooptics.com/Article.aspx?ArticleID=2076
18. *L Dutrow, B., & M. Clark, C. (2023, August). X-ray powder diffraction (XRD). serc.carleton.edu.* https://serc.carleton.edu/research_education/geochemsheets/techniques/XRD.html
19. *Lisensky, G. (2022, August 29). Preparation of powder x-ray diffraction samples.* https://chem.beloit.edu/edetc/nanolab/XRD/index.html
20. Henry, D., Eby, N., Goodge, J., & Mogk, D. (2016, November 10). *X-ray reflection in accordance with Bragg's Law: Geochemical Instrumentation and Analysis.* Carleton College. https://serc.carleton.edu/research_education/geochemsheets/BraggsLaw.html
21. Rendle, D. (2003). X-ray diffraction in forensic science. *The Rigaku Journal, 19.* http://www.rigaku.com/downloads/journal/Vol20.1.2003/forensic.pdf
22. Libretexts. (2022). X-ray diffraction (XRD) basics and application. *Chemistry LibreTexts.* https://chem.libretexts.org/Courses/Franklin_and_Marshall_College/Introduction_to_Materials_Characterization__CHM_412_Collaborative_Text/Diffraction_Techniques/X-ray_diffraction_(XRD)_basics_and_application
23. Majeed, F. Chapter Six: X-Rays, *Atomic and Molecular Physics*, University of Babylon (n.d.). https://repository.uobabylon.edu.iq/2010_2011/3_25428_65.pdf
24. Walsh, A. (1982). Atomic absorption and atomic fluorescence methods of analysis: their merits and limitations. *The Royal Society Publishing, 305*(1491), 485–498. https://doi.org/10.1098/rsta.1982.0046
25. Walsh, A. (1991). The development of atomic absorption methods of elemental analysis 1952-1962. *Anal. Chem., 63*(19), 933A-941A. https://doi.org/10.1021/ac00019a723
26. Rao, K. S. R. K., Balaji, T., Rao, T. P., Babu, Y., & Naidu, G. R. K. (2002). Determination of iron, cobalt, nickel, manganese, zinc, copper, cadmium and lead in human hair by inductively coupled plasma-atomic emission spectrometry. *Spectrochim. Acta B: At. Spectrosc., 57*(8), 1333–1338. https://doi.org/10.1016/s0584-8547(02)00045-9
27. Wang, P., Zhang, Q., Li, Y., Matsiko, J., Zhang, Y., & Jiang, G. (2017). Airborne persistent toxic substances (PTSs) in China: Occurrence and its implication associated with air pollution. *Environmental Science: Processes and Impacts,* 19(8), 983–999. doi:10.1039/c7em00187h
28. S. Seta, Application of scanning electron microscopy and energy dispersive x-ray microanalysis to the criminal identification of body fluid stains, *Int. Crim. Police Rev.*, 307 (1977) 119–123.
29. Lebiedzik, J., & Johnson, D. L. (2000). Rapid search and quantitative analysis of gunshot residue particles in the SEM. *J. Forensic Sci., 45*(1), 83–92.

30. Collins, P., Coumbaros, J., Horsley, G., Lynch, B., Kirkbride, K. P., Skinner, W., & Klass, G. (2003). Glass-containing gunshot residue particles: a new type of highly characteristic particle?. *J. Forensic Sci., 48*(3), 538–553.
31. Migliorini, A. S., Bailo, P., Boracchi, M., Crudele, G. D. L., Gentile, G., & Zoja, R. (2019). Forensic - Pathological SEM/EDX analysis in prosecution of medical malpractice. *Leg. Med. (Tokyo, Japan), 40*, 43–46. https://doi.org/10.1016/j.legalmed.2019.07.005
32. Kaur, N., Abi, K., Verma, P., & Mahajan, M. (2022). An elemental analysis of Indian automotive paint using SEM-EDS. *Mater. Today: Proc., 48*, 1748–1753. https://doi.org/10.1016/j.matpr.2021.10.046
33. Ameno, K., Lee, S. K., In, S., Yang, J., Yoo, Y., Ameno, S., Kubota, T., Kojima, H., & Ijiri, I. (2001). Blood carbofuran concentrations in suicidal ingestion cases. *Forensic Sci. Int., 116*(1), 59–61. https://doi.org/10.1016/s0379-0738(00)00336-4
34. Tanaka, N., Kinoshita, H., Jamal, M., Ito, A., Yamashita, T., Nagata, K., & Miyatake, N. (2020). Determination of metallization with energy-dispersive X-ray fluorescent spectrometry in experimental electric injury. *Leg. Med. (Tokyo, Japan), 47*, 101768. https://doi.org/10.1016/j.legalmed.2020.101768
35. Gentile, G., Andreola, S., Bailo, P., Battistini, A., Boracchi, M., Tambuzzi, S., & Zoja, R. (2020). A Brief Review of Scanning Electron Microscopy With Energy-Dispersive X-ray Use in Forensic Medicine. *Am. J. Forensic Med. Pathol., 41*(4), 280–286. https://doi.org/10.1097/PAF.0000000000000609
36. Ellingham, S. T. D., Thompson, T. J. U., & Islam, M. (2018). Scanning Electron Microscopy-Energy-Dispersive X-Ray (SEM/EDX): A Rapid Diagnostic Tool to Aid the Identification of Burnt Bone and Contested Cremains. *J. Forensic Sci., 63*(2), 504–510. https://doi.org/10.1111/1556-4029.13541
37. Takahashi, M., Kinoshita, H., Nishiguchi, M., & Nishio, H. (2010). Bromide detection in blood using energy dispersive X-ray fluorescence; a chemical marker supportive of drowning in seawater. *Leg. Med. (Tokyo, Japan), 12*(3), 132–136. https://doi.org/10.1016/j.legalmed.2010.01.006
38. Eliaerts, J., Meert, N., Van Durme, F., Dardenne, P., Charles, S., De Wael, K., & Samyn, N. (2021). Challenges for cocaine detection in smuggling samples. *Forensic Sci. Int., 319*, 110534. https://doi.org/10.1016/j.forsciint.2020.110534
39. Muccino, E., Giovanetti, G. F., Crudele, G. D., Gentile, G., Marchesi, M., Rancati, A., & Zoja, R. (2016). Characterisation of the weapon used in a patricide by SEM/EDS analysis of a microscopic trace from the object. *Medicine, science, and the Law, 56*(3), 221–226. https://doi.org/10.1177/0025802415623094
40. Pate, M. L., Aguilar-Caballos, M. P., Beltrán-Aroca, C. M., Pérez-Vicente, C., Lozano-Molina, M., & Girela-López, E. (2018). Use of XRD and SEM/EDX to predict age and sex from fire-affected dental remains. *Forensic Sci. Med. Pathol., 14*(4), 432–441. https://doi.org/10.1007/s12024-018-0028-1

41. El-Deftar, M. M., Speers, N., Eggins, S., Foster, S., Robertson, J., & Lennard, C. (2014). Assessment and forensic application of laser-induced breakdown spectroscopy (LIBS) for the discrimination of Australian window glass. *Forensic Sci. Int., 241*, 46-54.
42. Abd Mutalib, M., Rahman, M. A., Othman, M. H. D., Ismail, A. F., & Jaafar, J. (2017). Scanning electron microscopy (SEM) and energy-dispersive X-ray (EDX) spectroscopy. In *Membrane characterization* (pp. 161-179). Elsevier.
43. Shaw, R. A., Goodenough, K. M., Deady, E., Nex, P., Ruzvidzo, B., Rushton, J. C., & Mounteney, I. (2022). The Magmatic–Hydrothermal Transition in Lithium Pegmatites: Petrographic and Geochemical Characteristics of Pegmatites from the Kamativi Area, Zimbabwe. *The Canadian Mineralogist, 60*(6), 957-987.
44. Newbury*, D. E., & Ritchie, N. W. (2013). Is scanning electron microscopy/energy dispersive X-ray spectrometry (SEM/EDS) quantitative?. *Scanning, 35*(3), 141-168.
45. Laskin, A., & Cowin, J. P. (2001). Automated single-particle SEM/EDX analysis of submicrometer particles down to 0.1 μm. *Anal. Chem., 73*(5), 1023-1029.
46. Schlossmacher, P., Klenov, D. O., Freitag, B., von Harrach, S., & Steinbach, A. (2010). Nanoscale chemical compositional analysis with an innovative S/TEM-EDX system. *Microscopy and Analysis, 5*.
47. Takadama, H., Kim, H. M., Kokubo, T., & Nakamura, T. (2001). TEM-EDX study of mechanism of bonelike apatite formation on bioactive titanium metal in simulated body fluid. *Journal of Biomedical Materials Research: An Official Journal of The Society for Biomaterials, The Japanese Society for Biomaterials, and The Australian Society for Biomaterials and the Korean Society for Biomaterials, 57*(3), 441-448.

13

Nanotechnology in Forensic Science

Bhoopesh Kumar Sharma[1]*, Megha Walia[1] and Faray Jamal[2]

[1]*Department of Forensic Science, SGT University Gurugram, Haryana, India*
[2]*Central Forensic Science Laboratory, Bhopal, Madhya Pradesh, India*

Abstract

The field of nanotechnology is characterized by its rapid progress and focuses on the manipulation and regulation of matter at the nanoscale. At this particular magnitude, materials demonstrate distinct characteristics and phenomena that can be effectively utilized for a diverse array of purposes inside different sectors. Nanotechnology possesses the capacity to significantly transform several industries and effectively tackle a multiple range of global concerns. The applications of nanotechnology encompass various fields of interest such as medical, energy, electronics, environment, agriculture, and specifically forensic science. It is anticipated that further breakthroughs in this technology will yield substantial enhancements in these domains. The utilization of nanomaterials and nano techniques in several facets of forensic investigations constitutes integration of nanotechnology within the various fields of forensic science. The emerging discipline holds the capacity to completely reshape the investigation procedures in forensic work through the provision of cutting-edge instruments and methodologies capable of increasing the efficiency, precision, and sensitivity of forensic analysis. Nanotechnology has made significant contributions in various domains of crime scene and evidence investigation. Nanomaterials, including nanoparticles and nanofibers, possess the potential to augment the capacity for detecting and analyzing minute traces of evidence, such as DNA, latent finger impressions, and gunshot residue. Moreover, the utilization of nanotechnology pertains to the ongoing progress in the creation and enhancement of sophisticated forensic imaging methodologies. Nanoparticles have the potential to serve as contrast materials in various imaging techniques, including Magnetic Resonance Imaging (MRI) and Computed Tomography (CT) scans, with the aim of augmenting the detectability of pertinent evidence, such as concealed bloodstains or latent fingerprints. This technology has the potential to

**Corresponding author*: bhoopesh_fosc@sgtuniversity.org

Priyanka Chhabra, Divya Bajpai Tripathy, Anjali Gupta, Rajeev Kumar, Kajol Bhati and Shruti Shukla (eds.) Advances in Analytical Techniques for Forensic Investigation, (363–394) © 2024 Scrivener Publishing LLC

assist investigators in the more precise and efficient identification and analysis of evidence. This chapter provides an examination of the characterization, production, and application of nanoparticles within the realm of forensic science and the interpretation of evidence.

Keywords: Nanotechnology, nanomaterials, applications of nanoparticles, nanotechnology in forensic investigations

13.1 Introduction

Nanotechnology in current scenario is playing a substantial role in various domains of scientific and technological advancements. Nanotechnology refers to the utilization of materials at the nanoscale, characterized by their exceptional strength and wide-ranging applicability across diverse fields of study and progress [1]. Nanotechnology encompasses the examination and utilization of matter on a nanoscale, with potential applications across several scientific and technological domains [2]. On the metric system, a nanometer is equivalent to one billionth size of a meter.

In a broader sense, nanotechnology is defined as the process of synthesizing, creating, or developing nanomaterials with dimensions measured in nanometers. In the last few decades, nanotechnology has demonstrated its influence across various scientific domains, including engineering, medical science, plant science, animal science, and environmental science among others [3]. In recent years, the application of nanotechnology and nanomaterials in the field of forensic and criminal investigation has yielded significant results. This technology has proven to be a valuable alternative to traditional laboratory-based evidence analysis, offering cost-effective and real-time analysis of evidence or suspicious materials discovered at crime scenes. Nanotechnology has made significant contributions to various aspects of forensic science. The ability of nanomaterials to detect and analyze crucial evidence at the nanoscale level is attributed to their distinctive properties. Furthermore, nanomaterials possess the capacity to facilitate the identification and retrieval of evidence that was previously challenging to obtain, such as heavy metals, gunshot residues, DNA, and so on. In addition, the utilization of nano-enabled materials has been consistently employed in various domains of forensic science, such as the advancement of fingerprint analysis, identification of toxic substances, detection of illicit drugs, identification of food contaminants, and examination of disputed papers, among others [4].

There are several instrumental techniques used for detection and analysis, but they are costly and time-consuming. Examples of such techniques include High-Performance Liquid Chromatography, Gas Chromatography, Electrophoresis techniques, several spectroscopy techniques, etc. The utilization of nanotechnology is progressively replacing conventional instrumental procedures. Numerous sensors have been devised as alternatives to traditional instrumental approaches in order to address the limitations associated with them. Nanomaterials, including gold and silver nanoparticles, are currently being employed as chemical and biosensors due to their unique and specific chemical composition. The optical characteristics of these nanoparticles are dependent upon their morphology, dimensions, and interparticle interactions. In various branches of forensic research, nanotechnology is increasingly supplanting traditional laboratory-based approaches for forensic analysis [5].

13.1.1 Exploring the Field of Nanotechnology

13.1.1.1 Classification of Nanomaterials

Nanomaterials are mainly determined by their morphology and structure, resulting in two primary classifications: Consolidated materials and Nanodispersions. The classification of consolidated nanoparticles encompasses various distinct categories. The term "one-dimensional nano dispersive systems" refers to the categorization of nanomaterials as nanopowders and nanoparticles. The nanoparticles can be further categorized into many types, including Nanocrystals, Nanoclusters, Nanotubes, and supermolecules, among others [6]. A broad classification of nanomaterials can be well understood from Figure 13.1.

The physical property of size holds significant importance in the context of nanomaterials. Nanomaterials are commonly categorized based on the dimensionality that falls within the nanoscale range. Nanoparticles refer to nanomaterials characterized by all three dimensions being on the nanoscale, with minimal disparity between the longest and shortest axes. Nanofibers are materials characterized by their nanoscale dimensions in two directions. Nanotubes are hollow nanofibers, while nanorods are solid nanofibers. Nanoplates refer to materials characterized by having one dimension in the nanoscale. Nanoribbons are a type of nanoplates characterized by possessing two distinct longer dimensions [7].

Nanomaterials can be further categorized into many categories based on phases of matter they include. These categories include nanocomposite materials, nanofoam materials, nanoporous materials, and

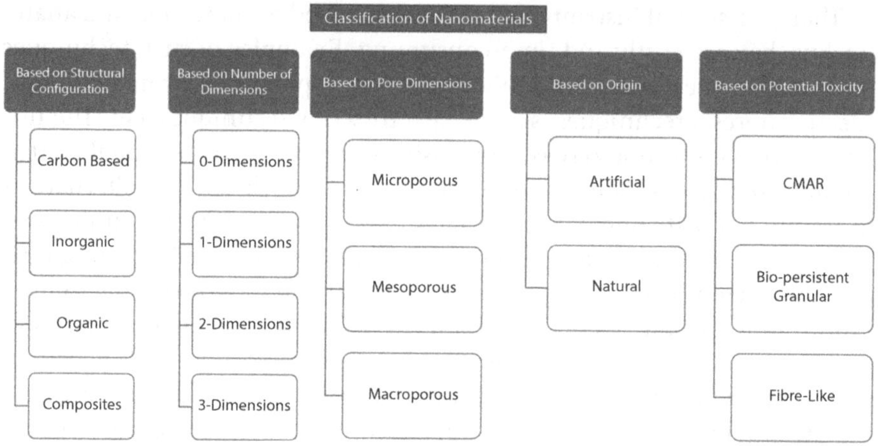

Figure 13.1 Classification of nanomaterials.

nanocrystalline materials. Nano composites are classified as solid materials that possess at least one region with different physical or chemical properties, and at least one region with dimensions in the nanoscale. Nanofoams consist of a matrix, either in liquid or solid form, that is infused with a gaseous phase. Notably, one of these phases possesses dimensions at the nanoscale [8].

Nanoporous materials are defined as solid substances that possess nanoscale dimensions in the form of nanopores or cavities. Nanocrystalline materials are characterized by the presence of crystal grains at the nanoscale [9].

13.2.2 Characterization of Nanomaterials

Numerous techniques have been developed to examine the dimensions, dispersion, morphology, surface charge, and porosity of nanoparticles in various settings [10]. However, the following techniques have been widely used in current scenario for the characterization of nanomaterials:

13.2.2.1 UV-Visible Spectroscopy (Spectroscopic Analysis)

UV/Visible spectroscopy is a commonly employed scientific technique for quantitatively evaluate the absorption and scattering of light by a specific material. The variable known as extinction comprises the collective influence of both absorbed and dispersed light. At its most basic level, the experimental setup involves positioning a sample between a source of light and a photodetector.

The primary objective is to assess the alteration in intensity of a UV/visible light beam as it passes through the sample, which is quantified prior to and during its contact with the sample. The observations are analyzed and compared at various wavelengths to quantify the extinction spectrum of the sample, which varies depending on the wavelength [11]. The standard method for representing the data involves plotting the extinction as a function of wavelength. In order to prevent the inclusion of spectral characteristics arising from the buffer solution in the sample extinction spectrum, a buffer blank is utilized for background correction of each spectrum [12].

Silver and gold nanoparticle's optical characteristics are affected by a number of parameters, including their dimensions, morphology, concentration, aggregation state, and the refractive index (μ) of the surrounding medium in near proximity to the nanoparticle surface. Other parameters that can have an effect on these optical properties include their size, shape, concentration, and aggregation state. As a result, UV/Vis spectroscopy is useful technique that can be employed in the process of identifying, characterizing, and researching nanomaterials [13]. A comparison can be made between the spectrum that was obtained through measurement and the spectrum that was predicted using numerical models. When compared to plasmonic nanoparticles, the size and the concentration of non-plasmonic nanoparticles have less of an impact on the optical properties of the particles than they do on the optical properties of plasmonic nanoparticles. The spectral characteristics of non-plasmonic nanoparticles are not as strongly affected by the dispersion qualities [14].

13.2.2.2 Transmission Electron Microscopy (TEM)

TEM is a measurement technique characterized by its ability to achieve high magnification. It involves the imaging of electron transmission through a sample. Imaging contrast in the transmitted beam is affected by variations in amplitude and phase, which are determined by the sample thickness and the material composition [15]. These fluctuations depend upon the thickness of the sample under examination. Specifically, the electron beam's passage through the specimen is affected by the scattering of electrons, with heavier atoms exhibiting greater scattering and a reduced electron mean free path compared to lighter atoms. Due to the utilization of electrons instead of light for sample illumination, transmission electron microscopy (TEM) exhibits substantially enhanced resolution compared to imaging approaches reliant on light [16].

The effectiveness of nanoparticle imaging through the utilization of Transmission Electron Microscopy (TEM) relies on the distinction between the sample and background. The procedure of sample preparation for imaging involves the elimination of moisture from nanoparticles deposited on a copper grid that has been coated with a thin carbon layer [17]. In this process, the materials with electron densities that demonstrate a significant difference in comparison to amorphous carbon can be easily observed. The materials encompass a wide range of elements, including various metals like silver, gold, copper, and aluminum [18].

Additionally, they consist of several oxides such as silica, aluminum oxide, and titanium oxide. Furthermore, the materials incorporate a variety of nanoparticles including carbon nanotubes, polymer nanoparticles, quantum dots, and magnetic nanoparticles [19]. Transmission electron microscopy is widely recognized as the optimal technique for directly assessing and quantifying a variety of nanoparticle characteristics, including particle size, grain size, size distribution, and particle morphology. Typically, sizing precision is within a range of 3% deviation from the true value [20].

13.2.2.3 Dynamic Light Scattering (DLS)

It is a prominent methodology employed for the study of nanoparticles and other colloidal solutions. The utilization of DLS encompasses the quantification and examination of light scattering that arises from the interplay between a laser beam and a colloidal solution, as depicted in Figure 13.2.

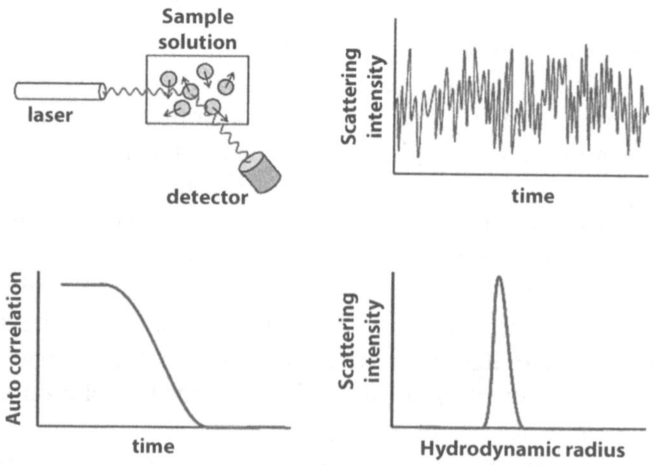

Figure 13.2 Principle of dynamic light scattering (DLS) technique.

By analyzing the temporal correlation of the intensity of scattered light, it is possible to derive useful information regarding the particle size in the solution. This is primarily based upon the observed phenomena of diffusive motion that is exhibited by particles in a solution, commonly known as Brownian motion [21]. The phenomenon of larger particles displaying less mobility and increased light scattering in comparison to smaller particles has been experimentally noted. The estimation of the hydrodynamic diameter entails analyzing the temporal dynamics of scattering intensity measurements, which represents the size of an idealized impermeable sphere that diffuses at a comparable rate to the particles under investigation. The hydrodynamic diameter serves as a valuable adjunct to other sizing techniques, including TEM, as it offers insights into the aggregation status of nanoparticle solutions. On the other hand, colloidal solutions that demonstrate stability and absence of aggregation frequently manifest particles with hydrodynamic diameters that are either similar or slightly larger than their apparent size. Conversely, solutions that are substantially aggregated will display significantly higher hydrodynamic diameters in comparison to their TEM size [22, 23].

13.2.2.4 Inductively Coupled Plasma Mass Spectrometry (ICP-MS)

ICP-MS is a highly sensitive analytical technique used to identify and quantify the elemental composition of various materials. The technique possesses the capacity of detecting and measuring metals as well as some nonmetals within the atomic mass range of 7–250. The detection and analytical limits of ICP-MS are commonly encountered within parts per trillion (ppt) or parts per quadrillion (ppq) size range [24, 25]. The measurement's sensitivity may be reduced when interference effects are caused by the presence of co-contaminants or plasma interactions. ICP-MS devices are equipped with a collision cell those have the capability to mitigate numerous interferences [26].

In Inductively Coupled Plasma analysis, the process involves the nebulization of liquid samples, which are subsequently driven through a high-temperature heat source, such as an argon plasma. This heat source serves to ionize the elements present in the samples by activating the electrons of individual atoms [27]. The process involves the subsequent isolation of ionized atoms from neutral particles within a vacuum chamber through the utilization of an ion guide, followed by their detection using a mass spectrometer [28].

The utilization of the mass-to-charge ratio of ions is employed in order to achieve element separation. On the other hand, the measurement of the concentration of each element relies on the percentage of ion signals in reference to an internal calibration standard [27].

In order to promote ionization, it is necessary for samples in ICP-MS to be in a liquid state, which may need the process of sample digestion. The necessary sample volume can vary due to several factors, including the concentration of the element being studied, the presence of any interfering substances, the sensitivity of the instrument to the specific element, the number of analyses being performed, and the number of elements of interest [29, 30].

13.2.2.5 Dark Field Microscopy (DFM)

DFM is another significant technique utilized in the domain of light microscopy, wherein samples are visualized by means of oblique incident illumination. The observed image exhibits a dark background as a result of the lack of the incident beam passing through the objective lens, except in regions where it has experienced scattering by the material as mentioned in Figure 13.3. The aforementioned method is commonly employed in the examination of plasmonic nanoparticles, wherein the intensity of scattered light emitted by individual nanoparticles is significantly lower in comparison to the incident beam [31, 32].

Numerous other approaches have also been utilized for the purpose of characterization of nanoparticles including Ionization Mass

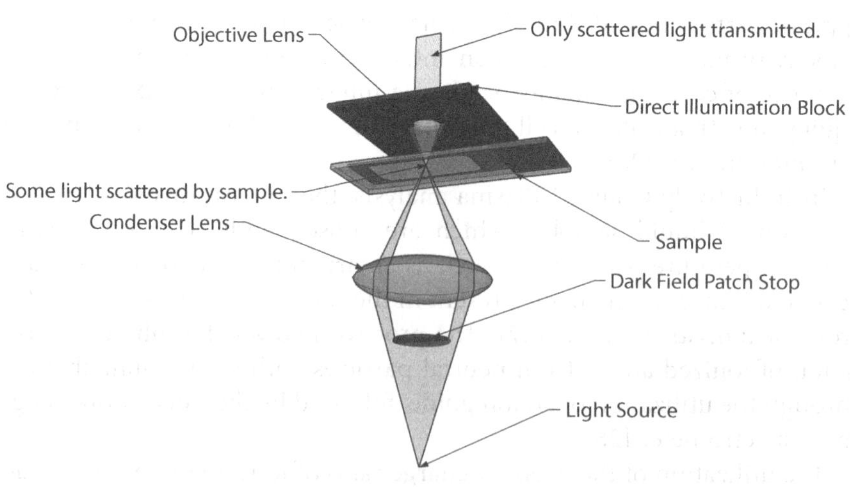

Figure 13.3 Diagram showing the light path in a dark field microscope.

Spectrometry, Scanning Mobility Particle Sizer, Aerodynamic Particle Sizer, Zeta Potential, and others as discussed by several researchers [33].

13.3 Techniques for the Synthesis of Nanomaterials

There exist two predominant strategies utilized in synthesis of most of the nanomaterials: The Top-Down approaches and the Bottom-Up approaches [34, 35].

13.3.1 Top-Down Approaches

13.3.1.1 Mechanical Milling

Mechanical milling is a cost-efficient technique utilized to generate nanoscale products from larger bulk materials. The technique of mechanical milling has gained significant recognition due to its high efficiency in synthesizing composite materials consisting of multiple distinct phases. As a result, it has become a critical method in the production of nanocomposites. Mechanical milling is utilized in the fabrication of aluminum alloys that are strengthened with oxides and carbides, as well as in the formation of spray coatings with enhanced resistance to wear [36]. Additionally, this technique is utilized in the development of nanoalloys comprising aluminum, nickel, magnesium, and copper, alongside various other nanocomposite materials. Carbon nanoparticles produced using ball milling have emerged as a promising and innovative category of nanomaterials. These materials possess the potential to address the pressing needs in environmental cleanup, energy storage, and energy conversion [37].

13.3.1.2 Electrospinning

Electrospinning represents a straightforward top-down approach utilized in the fabrication of nanostructured materials. The process is commonly employed for the fabrication of nanofibers using a diverse range of materials, predominantly polymers. The utilization of coaxial electrospinning represents a notable progression in the domain of electrospinning. Coaxial electrospinning process utilizes a spinneret consisting of two coaxial capillaries. Core-shell nanostructures can be produced with the application of an electric field along with utilizing either of the two viscous liquids or a viscous liquid as the shell and a non-viscous liquid as the core, which are confined within capillaries. The application of coaxial electrospinning has demonstrated itself as a highly effective and uncomplicated technique for generating substantial quantities of core-shell ultrathin fibers. The dimensions of these ultrathin nanomaterials possess the capacity to be extended to lengths that span multiple centimeters [38]. The application of this methodology has been utilized in the production of core-shell and hollow structures composed of polymers, inorganic materials, organic compounds, and hybrid combinations [39].

13.3.1.3 Lithography

Lithography technique serves as one of the valuable method in the production of nanoparticles through the utilization of a concentrated beam of light or electrons. The technique can be classified into two primary categories: Masked Lithography technique and Maskless Lithography technique. Out of these, the masked nanolithography is a technique that facilitates the replication of nanopatterns over a significant surface area by employing a specific mask which is also considered as template. The technique involves a variety of processes, including nanoimprint lithography, photolithography, and soft lithography. Whereas, in maskless lithography technique several other methodologies are employed, such as focused ion beam lithography technique, scanning probe lithography technique, and electron beam lithography technique. Maskless lithography is a technique that allows for the production of diverse nanopatterns without the use of a mask. The achievement of three-dimensional freeform micro-nano-fabrication can be attained through the utilization of ion implantation in conjunction with a focused ion beam, accompanied by the application of wet chemical etching [40, 41].

13.3.1.4 Sputtering

Sputtering is a commonly utilized method in the fabrication of nanomaterials, whereby solid surfaces are exposed to the impact of energetic particles, such as plasma or gas. The utilization of sputtering as a fabrication method for nanomaterial thin films is generally recognized for its great efficiency [42]. The sputtering deposition technique entails subjecting the target surface to high-energy gaseous ions, which leads to the expulsion of tiny clusters of atoms through physical processes. The size of these clusters is dictated by the energy of gaseous ions that collide with them. Sputtering process can be executed through several methods, including the utilization of radio-frequency diode sputtering, magnetron sputtering, and DC diode sputtering. The other two commonly used approaches are "Arc discharge method and Laser ablation method" [43].

13.3.2 Bottom-Up Approaches

13.3.2.1 Chemical Vapor Deposition (CVD)

CVD method plays an important role in the production of carbon containing nanomaterials. It is a method for depositing a thin film onto the surface of a substrate via a chemical reaction involving vapor-phase precursors. To be considered suitable for Chemical vapor deposition (CVD), a precursor must exhibit sufficient volatility along with high chemical purity, excellent stability during evaporation process, affordability, non-hazardous characteristics with an extended shelf life. Additionally, the process of decomposition shouldn't yield any remaining contaminants. During the chemical vapor deposition (CVD) technique for synthesizing carbon nanotubes, a substrate is placed into a high-temperature oven and exposed to higher temperatures. After this, a carbon-rich gas (hydrocarbons) is progressively introduced as a precursor into the system. At elevated temperatures, the gas endures a process of decomposition that releases carbon atoms. Subsequently, carbon nanotubes on the substrate are formed as a result during the process of carbon atoms. Nevertheless, the selection of a catalyst plays a crucial role in determining the form and composition of the resulting nanomaterial. The synthesis of graphene via the chemical vapor deposition (CVD) technique involves the utilization of many catalysts, including nickel (Ni), cobalt (Co), and copper (Cu). The synthesis of multilayer graphene has been observed when Ni and Co catalysts are utilized, while the application of a Cu catalyst resulted in the development of monolayer graphene. In general, chemical vapor deposition (CVD) is widely regarded as a highly effective technique for the synthesis of nanomaterials of superior quality. It has gained significant recognition particularly in the realm of two-dimensional nanomaterial creation [44, 45].

13.3.2.2 Solvothermal and Hydrothermal Methods

Hydrothermal process is widely recognized and actively employed as a significant technology for the production of nanostructured materials. The hydrothermal method entails the synthesis of nanostructured materials by utilizing a heterogeneous reaction occurring in an aqueous environment. High pressure with high temperature conditions near the critical point in a sealed container is required for this reaction to take places. Similarly, the solvothermal technique exhibited as like the hydrothermal approach. The only differentiation exists in the implementation of the procedure is the requirement of a non-aqueous setting [46].

Both the methods are frequently conducted within enclosed systems. The utilization of the microwave-assisted hydrothermal technique has garnered considerable interest in the realm of nanomaterial engineering due to its ability to integrate the advantageous characteristics of both hydrothermal and microwave methodologies. The Hydrothermal and the solvothermal procedures are highly promising and valuable techniques employed in the fabrication of diverse nanostructures, including nanosheets, nanorods, nanowires, and nanospheres.

13.3.2.3 The Sol–Gel Method

The method is a commonly employed wet-chemical technique for the synthesis of nanomaterials. This methodology is employed in the production of numerous classes of superior nanomaterials derived from metal oxides. During the production of metal-oxide nanoparticles, the aforementioned nomenclature is derived from the transformation of a liquid precursor into a sol. This is followed by the transformation of the sol into a network-like gel [47]. It is possible to synthesize nanoparticles using the sol-gel method by following a series of sequential steps. During the initial stage, the metal oxide undergoes hydrolysis in the presence of water or with the aid of alcohol, resulting in the formation of a sol. During the subsequent stage, condensation occurs, leading to a rise in the viscosity of the solvent, thereby forming porous structures that are subsequently allowed to undergo aging. The formation of metal-hydroxo- or metal-oxo-polymer in solution takes place via the condensation or polycondensation mechanism, leading to the generation of hydroxo- (M-OH-M) or oxo- (M-O-M) bridges. During the aging process, the phenomenon of polycondensation continues to occur, resulting in changes to the structure, properties, and porosity. With the progression of the aging process, a decrease in porosity is observed, which is accompanied by an augmentation in the interparticle spacing of colloidal particles. After the progression of the aging process, the second phase is the extraction of water and organic solvents from the gel by a procedure commonly referred to as drying. Finally, the process of calcination is carried out in order to obtain nanoparticles. The variables that influence the resultant product achieved through the sol-gel technique encompass the characteristics of the precursor, the rate of hydrolysis, the duration of aging, the pH level, and the molar ratio between water and the precursor [48, 49].

13.3.2.4 Reverse Micelle Method

This technique is an advantageous approach that is employed for the synthesis of nanomaterials of exact forms and sizes. The formation of an oil-in-water emulsion leads to the formation of typical micelles, where the hydrophobic tails are oriented towards a central region that encompasses oil droplets [50]. Reverse micelles are commonly observed in emulsions characterized by the dispersion of water within an oil medium. Within these structures, the surfactant molecules exhibit an arrangement where the hydrophilic heads are directed towards the interior, resulting in the formation of a central region that is replete with water. The core area of the reverse micelles functions as a nanoreactor for the fabrication of nanoparticles. The primary purpose of this structure is to serve as a storage facility for the research, development, and manufacture of nanostructures. By adjusting the ratio of water to surfactant, the size of the nanoreactors can be altered, thereby influencing the size of the nanoparticles produced by this method. Any decrease in water concentration results in the formation of water droplets with reduced dimensions, thereby producing nanoparticles with smaller dimensions [51, 52].

In addition, the utilization of the reverse micelle method offers a straightforward pathway for the synthesis of nanoparticles that exhibit uniformity in size, which can be precisely controlled. The nanoparticles produced by the reverse micelle method exhibit a high degree of fineness and uniformity in their size distribution [50].

13.4 Role of Nanotechnology in Forensic Investigation

13.4.1 Explosive Residue Detection

The incidence of terrorist actions has witnessed a global upsurge in recent decades, prompting a demand for novel inventions and technologies to aid law enforcement agencies in combating such acts and safeguarding public safety. The majority of terrorist assaults are executed through the utilization of suicide bombing tactics or concealed explosive devices. Currently, a range of detectors and canines that have undergone specialized training are employed for the purpose of detecting concealed explosive materials [53]. However, occasional failures in the detection of some explosives may occur due to the extensive variety of explosive compositions. Moreover, the training expenses associated with dogs are far higher, and there are instances where canines are unable to successfully detect explosives [54]. Advancements in contemporary nanotechnologies have facilitated the detection of diverse compounds with potential application as explosives. Consequently, researchers have successfully engineered a range of sensors utilizing nanomaterials, thereby endowing them with the capacity to perceive and identify distinct chemicals and compounds commonly employed in explosive materials. Highly sensitive antibodies were developed to detect pentaerythritol tetranitrate (PETN) using bioisosteric replacement [55, 56].

13.4.2 Fire Debris Analysis

The utilization of nanotechnology enables the microscopic examination of fire debris. The utilization of nanoparticles has been demonstrated as an effective method for the extraction and identification of particular chemical components found in fire debris, including accelerants and volatile organic compounds (VOCs). The nanoparticles possess the capability to be intentionally engineered in a manner that enables them to specifically adhere to the desired molecules, hence initiating a visual or chemical response upon successful binding.

One such strategy involves the utilization of functionalized nanoparticles that are enveloped with molecules possessing a strong affinity towards the desired chemicals. An illustration of this concept involves the utilization of nanoparticles that have been coated with antibodies or receptor molecules that possess the ability to selectively attach to the target substances present within the fire debris sample. The detection of this binding can thereafter be accomplished through the utilization of diverse methodologies, including fluorescence spectroscopy or electron microscopy.

An alternative methodology involves the utilization of nanosensors capable of identifying the existence of particular chemical components within the remnants of a fire. The nanosensors has the capability to undergo a color change or emit light upon interaction with the specific target chemicals. The alteration in color or emission of light can afterwards be assessed and employed to estimate the concentration of the target components within the remnants of the fire [57].

The utilization of nanotechnology extends to the extraction of minute quantities of certain substances from samples of fire debris. Nanoparticles has the capability to undergo functionalization processes, enabling them to exhibit selectivity in the extraction and concentration of particular molecules from detritus. This approach has the potential to enhance the sensitivity of the analysis, hence facilitating the detection of target molecules even at low concentrations.

In general, nanotechnology presents a highly promising methodology for the examination of fire debris. The utilization of this technology has the potential to enhance the sensitivity, selectivity, and accuracy of detecting and measuring distinct chemical components that are found within the debris. This technology has the potential to assist in forensic investigations and facilitate the determination of the cause and origin of fires [58].

13.4.3 GSR Analysis

The application of nanotechnology enables the microscopic examination of gunshot residue (GSR). Gunshot residue (GSR) consists of minuscule particles that are generated upon the discharge of a firearm. These particles possess significant potential in forensic investigations for the purpose of ascertaining recent firearm discharge by an individual. Nanotechnology can be effectively employed in the realm of nanosensor creation, enabling the detection and identification of specific chemicals present in gunshot residue (GSR). The nanosensors has the capability to be engineered in a manner that enables them to specifically adhere to and identify the distinct chemical constituents of gunshot residue (GSR), including heavy metals and organic chemicals [59]. Upon interaction with GSR particles, the nanosensors have the capability to generate a detectable visual or chemical indication, which may subsequently be quantified and subjected to analysis.

An alternative methodology entails the utilization of nanoparticles that are coated with molecules exhibiting a strong attraction for gunshot residue (GSR) components. The nanoparticles possess the capability to be purposefully engineered in a manner that enables them to specifically adhere to the GSR particles, hence facilitating their retrieval and subsequent examination. The utilization of this technique has the potential to enhance the sensitivity and selectivity of GSR analysis, hence facilitating the identification of minute quantities of GSR [60].

Nanoparticles can be employed in imaging methodologies to facilitate the visualization and analysis of gunshot residue (GSR) particles. An instance of this phenomenon is the utilization of nanoparticles that have been coated with fluorescence dyes, which possess the ability to adhere to GSR particles. Consequently, this enables the viewing of GSR particles through the application of fluorescence microscopy. This methodology can facilitate the detection of gunshot residue (GSR) particles and offer supplementary insights into their distribution and composition.

In general, nanotechnology presents auspicious approaches for the examination of gunshot residue. The utilization of this technology can enhance the sensitivity, selectivity, and accuracy in the detection and identification of gunshot residue (GSR) particles, thereby assisting forensic investigations and offering significant evidentiary support in criminal proceedings [61].

13.4.4 Detection of Fingerprints

The presence of fingerprints at a crime scene constitutes significant evidence. Fingerprints possess the ability to exist in three distinct states: latent, visible, or plastic. Latent fingerprints, which are imperceptible to the unaided human eye, are generated through the deposition of bodily secretions present on the fingertips [62, 63]. These fluids could potentially originate from either sweat glands or sebaceous glands that are found within the skin. There exist multiple powder and chemical techniques for the enhancement of latent fingerprints, including ninhydrin, cyanoacrylate, and silver nitrate, among others. The selection of the appropriate procedure for latent fingerprint development is contingent upon the characteristics of the surface upon which the fingerprint is found, as well as the composition of the fingerprint itself. However, when it comes to aging fingerprints, the fingerprint becomes tainted with environmental substances. In such instances, standard techniques may prove ineffective in the process of fingerprint development. In instances of this nature, the nanomaterial is employed for the purpose of enhancing a latent fingerprint. Various types of nanomaterials, such as zinc nanoparticles, gold nanoparticles, silver nanoparticles, and fluorescent starch-based carbon nanoparticles, have been employed in the advancement of fingerprint development [64–66]. The utilization of silver nanoparticles has been observed to possess the capability of enhancing the visibility of latent fingerprints that have undergone prolonged exposure to sunlight. Furthermore, it has been observed that these nanoparticles had the capability to generate fingerprints on surfaces that are damp. The utilization of zinc nanoparticles has been shown in the enhancement of both recent and aging fingerprints on nonporous surfaces [67, 68]. The use of gold nanoparticles has been found to enhance the visibility and definition of fingerprints. Additionally, when gold nanoparticles are combined with bifunctional reagents, they can be effectively utilized for the development of fingerprints in environments with high moisture levels [69, 70]. Fluorescent carbon nanoparticles derived from starch are employed in the development of fingerprints due to their distinctive fluorescence properties [71]. Metal nanoparticles that are electrodeposited possess the capability to generate fingerprints on surfaces that conduct electricity. The aforementioned technique is utilized on both coarse and polished metallic surfaces [72].

13.4.5 DNA Analysis

DNA is often regarded as the foremost crucial biological evidence that may be obtained in the field of forensic science. The DNA Polymerase Chain Reaction (PCR) is utilized to generate multiple copies of DNA. Recent research has indicated that the utilization of gold nanoparticles in polymerase chain reaction (PCR) has been found to enhance its overall efficiency. The study reported a reduction in reaction time when gold nanoparticles measuring 0.7 and 13 nm were included into the PCR mixture [73].

Blood is a significant form of evidence that is commonly encountered at crime scenes. A range of assays can be utilized to determine the source of the blood specimen. However, ascertaining the age of the blood sample discovered at the crime site is a formidable challenge for the investigators. The Atomic Force Microscope (AFM) holds significant forensic value in the investigation of a diverse array of evidence. Atomic Force Microscopy (AFM) is a commonly employed technique for the purpose of age estimation of desiccated blood samples recovered from crime scenes. The underlying idea of the atomic force microscopy (AFM) technique for estimating the age of dry bloodstains relies on the observed alteration in the elasticity properties of erythrocytes [74, 75].

The acquisition of high-quality PCR products is crucial in the context of DNA typing within forensic investigations. Magnetic nanoparticles, copper nanoparticles, and magnetite nanoparticles are employed in order to enhance the quality of DNA and PCR products derived from various bodily fluids and specimens.

Microfluidic devices are state-of-the-art technology employed for DNA analysis in the context of forensic investigations. These technologies exhibit high speed, possess reduced likelihood of contamination, and can be directly employed at the location of the crime. In a similar vein, microfluidic chips have demonstrated their efficacy and convenience as a valuable instrument in the field of forensic inquiry. The utilization of these chips has been observed in a range of point of care devices [76].

The estimation of the post-mortem interval, also referred to as the time since death, holds significant importance in forensic investigations. However, this stage presents a considerable challenge to forensic experts. There exist several conventional methods for estimating the time since death, which involve assessing several criteria such as rigor mortis, algor mortis, decomposition changes, and ocular changes. These factors have the capability to provide an estimation of the time elapsed since death; nevertheless, it is important to note that they are unable to provide an exact or precise measurement of the time since death. The examination of different bodily fluids, such as blood, pericardial fluid, spinal fluid, aqueous humor, and vitreous humor, is also employed for the determination of post-mortem interval. Among the several bodily fluids, the vitreous humor stands out due to its ability to maintain its composition for an extended period following death, owing to the sluggish nature of its metabolic alterations. Recent research has facilitated the precise estimation of post-mortem interval by the utilization of advanced, highly responsive, and economically viable nanotechnology-based techniques. This method may estimate the post-mortem interval up to 96 hours by establishing a link between the concentration of cystine, an amino acid, and the time elapsed since death [77, 78].

13.4.6 Drug and Toxicology Testing

Nanotechnology is extensively employed in the field of forensic toxicology to facilitate the collection, detection, and analysis of a diverse range of toxic substances present in different biological specimens, such as blood, hair, saliva, and vitreous humor. The utilization of spectroscopic features exhibited by diverse nanoparticles has been employed for the purpose of identifying and detecting substances such as cocaine [79]. Several sensors have been designed utilizing nanoparticles to detect and distinguish different harmful substances and pharmaceutical compounds. Lodha *et al.* developed a sensor capable of identifying clonazepam, a substance commonly associated with instances of date rape, from skeletal and blood samples [80]. Nanoparticles such as Gold nanoparticles, Silver nanoparticles, and titanium oxide nanoparticles have been employed for the purpose of detecting illegal substances inside fingerprint samples [7]. The utilization of nanomaterials is prevalent in the field of narcotics detection and identification. Nanomaterial-enabled sensors, such as electrochemical, Raman, and surface-enhanced Raman scattering (SERS)-based sensors, as well as colorimetric nano sensors, have been extensively employed for the purpose of detecting and identifying narcotics. For instance, the detection of codeine can be facilitated through the utilization of electrochemical sensors, such as silicone/palladium porous nanomaterial. Similarly, the sensing of morphine can be achieved by employing a nano-film of Al2O3, which is created using the sol-gel process. SERS-based sensing technologies have superior capabilities compared to electrochemical sensors in the detection of narcotics due to their non-destructive nature and the absence of direct contact with the sensing material. The utilization of a Raman spectrometer in conjunction with surface-enhanced Raman scattering (SERS) has proven to be valuable in the identification of cocaine within urine samples. Plasmonic nano dome array (PNA) based surface-enhanced Raman scattering (SERS) sensors are employed for the detection of narcotics such as morphine, methadone, and oxycodone. Colorimetric sensors are extensively employed due to their inherent simplicity and user-friendly nature. Numerous sensors utilizing nanomaterials have been designed that effectively interact with drugs, resulting in a discernible alteration in hue. Colorimetric signals have been employed for the purpose of detecting the concentration of different narcotics [81–88].

13.4.7 Detection of Food Adulteration

The prevalence of food adulteration is rising rapidly, posing a significant concern. A variety of foreign substances are incorporated into food products in order to achieve economic advantages. Contaminations of various kinds have been identified as potential sources of numerous health concerns, leading to a significant loss of human lives annually due to the consumption of tainted food. The identification of food adulteration is of paramount importance and is crucial in mitigating any health risks. The identification and analysis of food and drug adulteration constitute a significant area of study within the discipline of forensic science [89]. The typical techniques employed for the detection of adulteration in food materials, such as chromatographic techniques, spectroscopic techniques, and electrophoresis techniques, are characterized by their time-consuming nature and reliance on skilled experts. Contemporary research has led to the advancement of sensor-based technologies capable of promptly detecting adulteration. Numerous research has been conducted to identify and detect a wide range of food pollutants, encompassing biological contaminants such as infections and toxins, as well as chemical contaminants like pesticides and food colorants. Various chemical and biosensors have been devised for the purpose of detecting these adulterations. Milk is a food element that is susceptible to adulteration. The advancement of nano-technology has facilitated the detection of adulteration events even in minuscule quantities [90]. Recent advancements in nanotechnology have facilitated the potential for adulteration through the use of smartphones and paper-based sensors integrated with nanomaterials. The color shift in the sensor of the Smartphone is recorded upon immersion in the milk sample.

This recorded data is then compared with the database maintained in a mobile application in order to assess the degree of adulteration present in the sample [91, 92].

13.4.8 Counterfeiting Prevention and Homeland Security

Computer forensics is a specialized field within the realm of forensic science that encompasses the systematic collection, preservation, and analysis of evidentiary material derived from computing devices. The incidence of cybercrime is steadily rising. Extensive research is being conducted in numerous nations to address these criminal activities [93]. Forensic professionals employ a range of methodologies and specialized software tools to analyze diverse computing systems, including but not limited to the retrieval of deleted or corrupted files, encryption of coded data, and authentication processes. Nanotechnology has been foundational for the development of these approaches. Nanotechnology has made significant advancements in the field of cryptography, which are widely regarded as crucial. Nanotechnology not only provides a means to increase encryption techniques, but also has the potential to render existing standards insufficient [94]. Quantum cryptography possesses the capability to encrypt data in a manner that is exceedingly challenging to decipher. Authentication plays a crucial role in ensuring network security, and recent advancements in nano-technology have significantly enhanced the precision of authentication mechanisms. The field of nanotechnology has made significant progress in enhancing fingerprint detecting devices through the integration of small microchips [95]. This technological advancement has facilitated the implementation of fingerprint authentication in a wide range of devices, including smartphones and personal gadgets, with the primary objective of preventing unauthorized usage. The functionality of this technology is predicated upon the intricate interplay between the ridges and valleys present in a fingerprint and the sensor. The sensor utilizes an analysis of the ridges and valleys present in the fingerprint, hence granting the individual access.

Numerous advancements in nanotechnology continue to be employed within the realm of forensic science and criminal investigations. Numerous portable devices utilizing sensor technology have been developed to aid forensic investigators and law enforcement agencies in crime management. The utilization of digital alcohol breath analyzers has been proposed as a potential solution for mitigating instances of driving under the influence. The breath analyzer employs sensors to ascertain the level of blood alcohol content. The speed gun, also known as a traffic radar, is a portable instrument that is extensively employed by law enforcement agencies to monitor and enforce traffic regulations pertaining to vehicle speed. In summary, nanotechnology is supplanting traditional laboratory-based methodologies with portable, cost-effective, and highly sensitive technologies [96, 97].

13.4.9 Bio Sensors and Nano Trackers

Bio sensors and nano trackers are two developing technologies that possess the capacity to significantly transform diverse domains, such as healthcare, environmental monitoring, and security.

Biological sensors are instrumental devices that employ biological agents, such as enzymes or antibodies, to identify and assess particular substances or biomarkers. The sensors has the capability to be engineered in a manner that enables the detection of a diverse array of chemicals. This includes the detection of glucose for the purpose of monitoring diabetes, the identification of pollutants present in environmental samples, as well as the recognition of disease markers within clinical samples. The integration of nanotechnology enables the miniaturization of bio sensors, facilitating their incorporation into portable devices. This advancement enables the convenient and non-invasive monitoring of several parameters in real-time [98, 99].

Nano trackers refer to minuscule devices or particles that possess the capability to be implanted or affixed onto various entities or organisms for the purpose of tracking their whereabouts, motion, or other pertinent attributes. Nano trackers have the capability to be outfitted with various components such as sensors, communication modules, or other features in order to facilitate the transmission of data or feedback. These devices have several applications, such as monitoring the movement patterns of animals, ensuring the appropriate transit and storage conditions for delicate items, or tracking the whereabouts and actions of individuals for security or surveillance objectives.

The integration of biometric sensors with nanoscale trackers presents enhanced monitoring possibilities. One potential application involves the integration of biosensors into nano tracker devices, enabling the real-time detection and analysis of targeted biomarkers or chemicals. This technology has potential uses in the medical field, particularly in the continuous monitoring of physiological indicators and drug monitoring in patients. Nano trackers with bio sensors have the potential to be employed in environmental monitoring for the purpose of promptly identifying pollutants or toxins in water or air [100–102].

The utilization of biometric sensors and nanotechnology trackers also gives rise to significant ethical and privacy concerns. In order to ensure responsible and ethical deployment, it is imperative to thoroughly address concerns pertaining to data security, consent, and the potential misuse of these technologies.

In broad terms, the utilization of bio sensors and nano trackers has significant promise in augmenting monitoring and tracking capacities across many domains. By harnessing the capabilities of nanotechnology, these technologies have the potential to yield significant data and knowledge, thereby facilitating advancements in healthcare, environmental monitoring, and security [99, 101].

13.4.10 Nanotechnology and Questioned Document

The application of Atomic Force Microscopy (AFM) has been observed in the forensic analysis of questioned documents. This particular microscopy technique possesses the capability to achieve a resolution of less than one nanometer. Operating at the nanoscale, this sophisticated microscope is employed for the purpose of examining the ink crossing on a page by scanning its surface. Atomic Force Microscopy (AFM) is a technique employed to analyze the three-dimensional surface characteristics of a document. It yields crucial insights into the line patterns created by ribbon dye and ballpoint pen, hence enabling the determination of ink penetration depth on the paper. Additionally, AFM serves as a valuable tool for comparing the properties of ink and paper. Additionally, this technique finds utility in the assessment of ink deposition in documents [103–106].

13.5 Conclusion

In summary, the application of nanotechnology in the field of forensic science has significant promise for augmenting the capacities of forensic investigations. Nanotechnology presents a diverse array of instruments and methodologies that have the potential to enhance the processes of evidence collection, analysis, and identification, hence yielding outcomes that are characterized by heightened precision and dependability.

The utilization of nanoparticles, nanomaterials, and nanosensors has the potential to augment the efficacy of fingerprint analysis, DNA profiling, and trace evidence analysis. Forensic scientists have the potential to enhance the visualization and recognition of fingerprints or trace evidence by employing nanoparticles that possess distinctive characteristics, such as heightened fluorescence or magnetic capabilities. Nanomaterials, such as carbon nanotubes or nanoparticles, have the potential to enhance the sensitivity and specificity of DNA analysis, hence resulting in more precise profiling outcomes.

In addition, nanotechnology has the potential to be applied in the fields of drug and toxin detection, identification of explosives or illicit substances, and analysis of gunshot residue. Nanotechnology-based sensors provide the capability to detect and analyze minute quantities of these compounds, hence offering vital evidentiary support for forensic inquiries.

In addition, the field of nanotechnology can be utilized to augment forensic imaging methodologies, including scanning electron microscopy and X-ray imaging. Forensic scientists have the potential to improve the resolution and specificity of imaging techniques by creating nanoscale imaging probes or contrast agents, thereby yielding more comprehensive and enlightening outcomes.

Nevertheless, the application of nanotechnology in the field of forensic research gives rise to ethical, legal, and privacy considerations. The storage and use of nanomaterials necessitate the implementation of specific measures, while also demanding comprehensive consideration of issues pertaining to consent, data security, and potential misuse. Moreover, it is imperative to conduct additional study and engage in further development endeavors in order to comprehensively comprehend the prospective benefits and constraints of nanotechnology in the context of forensic applications.

In general, the incorporation of nanotechnology within the realm of forensic science has significant promise for transforming the discipline, as it presents enhanced methodologies for evidence acquisition, examination, and identification. Through ongoing progress and meticulous examination of ethical and privacy concerns, nanotechnology has the potential to enhance the efficacy and precision of forensic investigations.

References

1. Hulla, J. E., S. C. Sahu, and A. W. Hayes. "Nanotechnology: History and future." *Human & Experimental Toxicology*, 34.12 (2015): 1318-1321.
2. Poole, C. P., & Owens, F. J. (2003). Introduction to nanotechnology.
3. McNeil, S. E. (2005). Nanotechnology for the biologist. *J. Leukoc. Biol.*, 78(3), 585-594.
4. Chauhan, V., Singh, V., & Tiwari, A. (2017). Applications of nanotechnology in forensic investigation. *Int. J. Life. Sci. Scienti. Res.*, 3(3), 1047-1051.

5. Postek, M., & Hocken, R. (2006). Instrumentation and metrology for nanotechnology.
6. Rizwan, M., Shoukat, A., Ayub, A., Razzaq, B., & Tahir, M. B. (2021). Types and classification of nanomaterials. In *Nanomaterials: synthesis, characterization, hazards and safety* (pp. 31-54). Elsevier.
7. Glezer, A. M. (2011). Structural classification of nanomaterials. *Russ. Metall. (Met.)*, 2011(4), 263-269.
8. Sannino, D. (2021). Types and classification of nanomaterials. *Nanotechnology: Trends and Future Applications*, 15-38.
9. Polarz, S., & Smarsly, B. (2002). Nanoporous materials. *J. Nanosci. Nanotechnol.*, 2(6), 581-612.
10. Mudalige, T., Qu, H., Van Haute, D., Ansar, S. M., Paredes, A., & Ingle, T. (2019). Characterization of nanomaterials: Tools and challenges. *Nanomaterials for Food Applications*, 313-353.
11. Kumar, C. S. (Ed.). (2013). UV-VIS and photoluminescence spectroscopy for nanomaterials characterization (pp. 5-7). Berlin, Heidelberg: Springer.
12. George, G., Wilson, R., & Joy, J. (2017). Ultraviolet spectroscopy: a facile approach for the characterization of nanomaterials. In *Spectroscopic Methods for Nanomaterials Characterization* (pp. 55-72). Elsevier.
13. Selvamani, V. (2019). Stability studies on nanomaterials used in drugs. In Characterization and biology of nanomaterials for drug delivery (pp. 425-444). Elsevier.
14. Alessio, P., Aoki, P. H., Furini, L. N., Aliaga, A. E., & Constantino, C. J. L. (2017). Spectroscopic techniques for characterization of nanomaterials. In *Nanocharacterization techniques* (pp. 65-98). William Andrew Publishing.
15. Kumar, C. S. (Ed.). (2013). Transmission electron microscopy characterization of nanomaterials. Springer Science & Business Media.
16. Tanaka, N. (2008). Present status and future prospects of spherical aberration corrected TEM/STEM for study of nanomaterials∗. *Sci. Technol. Adv. Mater.*
17. Deepak, F. L., Mayoral, A., & Arenal, R. (Eds.). (2015). Advanced transmission electron microscopy: Applications to Nanomaterials. Springer.
18. Baer, D. R., Amonette, J. E., Engelhard, M. H., Gaspar, D. J., Karakoti, A. S., Kuchibhatla, S., ... & Wang, C. M. (2008). Characterization challenges for nanomaterials. *Surface and Interface Analysis: An International Journal devoted to the development and application of techniques for the analysis of surfaces, interfaces and thin films*, 40(3-4), 529-537.
19. Zhang, B., & Su, D. S. (2014). Transmission electron microscopy and the science of carbon nanomaterials. *Small*, 10(2), 222-229.
20. Smith, D. J. (2015). Characterization of nanomaterials using transmission electron microscopy. *Nanocharacterisation*, 37, 1-29.
21. Nickel, C., Angelstorf, J., Bienert, R., Burkart, C., Gabsch, S., Giebner, S., ... & Kuhlbusch, T. A. (2014). Dynamic light-scattering measurement comparability of nanomaterial suspensions. *J. Nanoparticle Res.*, 16, 1-12.

22. Murdock, R. C., Braydich-Stolle, L., Schrand, A. M., Schlager, J. J., & Hussain, S. M. (2008). Characterization of nanomaterial dispersion in solution prior to in vitro exposure using dynamic light scattering technique. *Toxicol. Sci.,* 101(2), 239-253.
23. Marucco, A., Aldieri, E., Leinardi, R., Bergamaschi, E., Riganti, C., & Fenoglio, I. (2019). Applicability and limitations in the characterization of poly-dispersed engineered nanomaterials in cell media by dynamic light scattering (DLS). *Materials,* 12(23), 3833.
24. Mozhayeva, D., & Engelhard, C. (2020). A critical review of single particle inductively coupled plasma mass spectrometry–A step towards an ideal method for nanomaterial characterization. *J. Anal. At. Spectrom.,* 35(9), 1740-1783.
25. Su, C. K., & Sun, Y. C. (2015). Considerations of inductively coupled plasma mass spectrometry techniques for characterizing the dissolution of metal-based nanomaterials in biological tissues. *J. Anal. At. Spectrom.,* 30(8), 1689-1705.
26. Zhang, C., Zhang, Z., Yu, B., Shi, J., & Zhang, X. (2002). Application of the biological conjugate between antibody and colloid Au nanoparticles as analyte to inductively coupled plasma mass spectrometry. *Anal. Chem.,* 74(1), 96-99.
27. Gray, E. P., Coleman, J. G., Bednar, A. J., Kennedy, A. J., Ranville, J. F., & Higgins, C. P. (2013). Extraction and analysis of silver and gold nanoparticles from biological tissues using single particle inductively coupled plasma mass spectrometry. *Environ. Sci. Technol.,* 47(24), 14315-14323.
28. Poda, A. R., Bednar, A. J., Kennedy, A. J., Harmon, A., Hull, M., Mitrano, D. M., ... & Steevens, J. (2011). Characterization of silver nanoparticles using flow-field flow fractionation interfaced to inductively coupled plasma mass spectrometry. *J. Chromatogr. A,* 1218(27), 4219-4225.
29. Bolea, E., Jiménez-Lamana, J., Laborda, F., & Castillo, J. R. (2011). Size characterization and quantification of silver nanoparticles by asymmetric flow field-flow fractionation coupled with inductively coupled plasma mass spectrometry. *Anal. Bioanal. Chem.,* 401, 2723-2732.
30. Pace, H. E., Rogers, N. J., Jarolimek, C., Coleman, V. A., Gray, E. P., Higgins, C. P., & Ranville, J. F. (2012). Single particle inductively coupled plasma-mass spectrometry: a performance evaluation and method comparison in the determination of nanoparticle size. *Environ. Sci. Technol.,* 46(22), 12272-12280.
31. Xiao, L., Qiao, Y., He, Y., & Yeung, E. S. (2010). Three dimensional orientational imaging of nanoparticles with darkfield microscopy. *Anal. Chem.,* 82(12), 5268-5274.
32. Badireddy, A. R., Wiesner, M. R., & Liu, J. (2012). Detection, characterization, and abundance of engineered nanoparticles in complex waters by hyperspectral imagery with enhanced darkfield microscopy. *Environ. Sci. Technol.,* 46(18), 10081-10088.

33. Hu, M., Novo, C., Funston, A., Wang, H., Staleva, H., Zou, S., ... & Hartland, G. V. (2008). Dark-field microscopy studies of single metal nanoparticles: understanding the factors that influence the linewidth of the localized surface plasmon resonance. *J. Mater. Chem.*, 18(17), 1949-1960.
34. Abid, Namra, Aqib Muhammad Khan, Sara Shujait, Kainat Chaudhary, Muhammad Ikram, Muhammad Imran, Junaid Haider, Maaz Khan, Qasim Khan, and Muhammad Maqbool. "Synthesis of nanomaterials using various top-down and bottom-up approaches, influencing factors, advantages, and disadvantages: A review." *Adv. Colloid Interface Sci.*, 300 (2022): 102597.
35. Yadav, T. P., Yadav, R. M., & Singh, D. P. (2012). Mechanical milling: A top down approach for the synthesis of nanomaterials and nanocomposites. *Nanosci. Nanotechnol.*, 2(3), 22-48.
36. Chawla, V., Prakash, S., & Sidhu, B. S. (2007). State of the art: Applications of mechanically alloyed nanomaterials—A review. *Mater. Manuf. Process.*, 22(4), 469-473.
37. Dreizin, E. L., & Schoenitz, M. (2014). Reactive and metastable nanomaterials prepared by mechanical milling. Metal Nanopowders: Production, Characterization, and Energetic Applications, 227-278.
38. Lu, X., Wang, C., & Wei, Y. (2009). One-dimensional composite nanomaterials: Synthesis by electrospinning and their applications. *Small*, 5(21), 2349-2370.
39. Lu, X., Li, M., Wang, H., & Wang, C. (2019). Advanced electrospun nanomaterials for highly efficient electrocatalysis. *Inorg. Chem. Front.*, 6(11), 3012-3040.
40. Wang, Y., Fedin, I., Zhang, H., & Talapin, D. V. (2017). Direct optical lithogra phy of functional inorganic nanomaterials. *Science*, 357(6349), 385-388.
41. Colson, P., Henrist, C., & Cloots, R. (2013). Nanosphere lithography: a powerful method for the controlled manufacturing of nanomaterials. *J. Nanomater.*, 2013, 21-21.
42. El-Said, W.A., Akhtar, N., & Kamal, M.M. (2022) 'Fabrication of functionalized nanomaterial-based electrochemical sensors' platforms', Functionalized Nanomaterial-Based Electrochemical Sensors, pp. 445–486.
43. Sharko, S. A., Serokurova, A. I., Novitskii, N. N., Ketsko, V. A., Smirnova, M. N., Almuqrin, A. H., ... & Trukhanov, A. V. (2022). A new approach to the formation of nanosized gold and beryllium films by ion-beam sputtering deposition. *Nanomaterials*, 12(3), 470.
44. Manawi, Y. M., Ihsanullah, Samara, A., Al-Ansari, T., & Atieh, M. A. (2018). A review of carbon nanomaterials' synthesis via the chemical vapor deposition (CVD) method. *Materials*, 11(5), 822.
45. He, C. N., Zhao, N. Q., Shi, C. S., & Song, S. Z. (2009). Fabrication of carbon nanomaterials by chemical vapor deposition. *J. Alloys Compd.*, 484(1-2), 6-11.

46. Li, J., Wu, Q., & Wu, J. (2016). Synthesis of Nanoparticles via Solvothermal and Hydrothermal Methods 12.
47. Nandihalli, N., Gregory, D. H., & Mori, T. (2022). Energy-Saving Pathways for Thermoelectric Nanomaterial Synthesis: Hydrothermal/Solvothermal, Microwave-Assisted, Solution-Based, and Powder Processing. *Adv. Sci.*, 9(25), 2106052.
48. Komarneni, S. (2003). Nanophase materials by hydrothermal, microwave-hydrothermal and microwave-solvothermal methods. *Curr. Sci.,* 1730-1734.
49. Feng, S. H., & Li, G. H. (2017). Hydrothermal and solvothermal syntheses. In *Modern inorganic synthetic chemistry* (pp. 73-104). Elsevier.
50. Arsene, M. L., Răut, I., Călin, M., Jecu, M. L., Doni, M., & Gurban, A. M. (2021). Versatility of reverse micelles: From biomimetic models to nano (bio) sensor design. *Processes*, 9(2), 345.
51. Eastoe, J., Hollamby, M. J., & Hudson, L. (2006). Recent advances in nanoparticle synthesis with reversed micelles. *Adv. Colloid Interface Sci.*, 128, 5-15.
52. Lone, I. H., Radwan, N. R., Aslam, J., & Akhter, A. (2019). Concept of reverse micelle method for the synthesis of nano-structured materials. *Curr. Nanosci.*, 15(2), 129-136.
53. Hesse A, Biyikal M, Rurack K, Weller MG (2015) Development of highly sensitive and selective antibodies for the detection of the explosive pentaerythritol tetranitrate (PETN) by bioisosteric replacement. *J. Mol. Recognit.*, 29(2): 88-94.
54. Rawtani, D., Tharmavaram, M., Pandey, G., & Hussain, C. M. (2019). Functionalized nanomaterial for forensic sample analysis. *TrAC Trends Anal. Chem.*, 120, 115661.
55. O'Mahony, A. M., & Wang, J. (2013). Nanomaterial-based electrochemical detection of explosives: a review of recent developments. *Anal. Methods,* 5(17), 4296-4309.
56. Julian WG, Jehuda Y (2004) Electronic Noses & Sensors for the Detection of Explosives. NATO Science Series II. Springer publishers, Netherlands, pp. 308.
57. Huang, T. Y. (2023). Carbon nanotubes-assisted solid-phase microextraction for the extraction of gasoline in fire debris samples. *J. Chromatogr. A*, 1701, 464063.
58. Mahat, N. A., Shadan, A. F., Juahir, H., & Sukono, S. Uncovering the Fingerprints of Gasoline Residues: A Chromatographic and Chemometric Analyses of Burned Matrices in Malaysia for Forensic Intelligence. Available at SSRN 4374083.
59. Bhatt, P. V., Pandey, G., Tharmavaram, M., Rawtani, D., & Mustansar Hussain, C. (2020). Nanotechnology and taggant technology in forensic science. Technology in Forensic Science: Sampling, Analysis, Data and Regulations, 279-301.

60. Yang, J., Gunn, A., Palmbach, T., Wei, D., & Sinha, S. (2006, January). NanoForensics----Nanoparticles in Gun-Shot-Residue. In *2006 IEEE Conference on Emerging Technologies-Nanoelectronics* (pp. 269-272). IEEE.
61. Venugopal, A., Seth, V., Naik, S. S., Valappil, S., Verma, A., Rajan, S., ... & Munjal, S. (2023). A Mini Review on The Application of Nanomaterials in Forensic Science. arXiv preprint arXiv:2305.09643.
62. Wang, M., Li, M., Yu, A., Zhu, Y., Yang, M., & Mao, C. (2017). Fluorescent nanomaterials for the development of latent fingerprints in forensic sciences. *Adv. Funct. Mater.*, 27(14), 1606243.
63. Prabakaran, E., & Pillay, K. (2021). Nanomaterials for latent fingerprint detection: a review. *J. Mater. Res. Technol.*, 12, 1856-1885.
64. Bhatia, T. (2022). Novel nanomaterials in forensic investigations: A review. *Mater. Today: Proc.*, 50, 1071-1079.
65. Venugopal, A., Seth, V., Naik, S. S., Valappil, S., Verma, A., Rajan, S., ... & Munjal, S. (2023). A Mini Review on The Application of Nanomaterials in Forensic Science. arXiv preprint arXiv:2305.09643.
66. Zhang M, Girault HH. SECM for imaging and detection of latent fingerprints: mini review article. *Analyst*, 2009, 134(1):25–30.
67. Choi MJ, McBean KE, Ng PHR, McDonagh AM, Maynard PJ, Lennard C, *et al.* An evaluation of nanostructured zinc oxide as a fluorescent powder for fingerprint detection. *J. Mater. Sci.*, 2008;43(2):732
68. Cantu A, Johnson JL. Silver physical development of latent prints. In: Lee HC, Ganensslen RE, editors. *Advances in fingerprints technology*, 2nd edn. Boca Raton, FL: CRC Press, 2001;251–84.
69. Tang, H. W., Lu, W., Che, C. M., & Ng, K. M. (2010). Gold nanoparticles and imaging mass spectrometry: double imaging of latent fingerprints. *Anal. Chem.*, 82(5), 1589-1593.
70. Use of gold nanoparticles as molecular intermediate for the detection of fingermarks. *Forensic Sci. Int.*, 2007;168 (2–3):169–76.
71. Li H, Guo X, Liu J, Li F. A synthesis of fluorescent starch based on carbon nanoparticles for fingerprints detection. *Opt Mater* 2016;60:404– 10
72. Qin G, Zhang M, Zhang Y, Zhu Y, Liu S, Wu W, *et al.* Visualizing latent fingerprints by electrodeposition of metal nanoparticles. *J. Electro. Anal. Chem.*, 2013;693:122–6
73. Bonanni, A., & Del Valle, M. (2010). Use of nanomaterials for impedimetric DNA sensors: a review. *Analytica chimica acta,* 678(1), 7-17.23.Kumar I, Kumar S, Singh M, Kumari K, Kumar D, Ansari K, *et al.* Application of nanotechnology in forensic DNA and help to investigation
74. Vikrant, K., Bhardwaj, N., Bhardwaj, S. K., Kim, K. H., & Deep, A. (2019). Nanomaterials as efficient platforms for sensing DNA. *Biomaterials*, 214, 119215.

75. Pandey, G., Rawtani, D., & Agrawal, Y. K. (2017). Future aspects of halloysite nanotubes in forensic investigations. *Journal of Nanomedicine Research,* 6(2), 2.
76. Bruijns B, van Asten A, Tiggelaar R, Gardeniers H. Microfluidic Devices for Forensic DNA Analysis: A Review. *Biosensors (Basel),* 2016;6(3):41.
77. Garg V, Oberoi SS, Gorea RK, Kaur K (2004) Changes in the levels of vitreous potassium with increasing time since death. *J. Ind. Acad. Fore. Med.,* 26(4):136–139
78. Swann L, Forbes S, Lewis S (2010) Analytical separations of mammalian decomposition products for forensic science: a review. *Anal. Chem. Act.,* 682:9–22
79. Harvey JMH (2015) Nanoforensics: Forensic application of nanotechnology in illicit drug detection. *J. Forensic Res.,* 6(5): 106.
80. Lodha A, Pandya A, Sutariya PG, Menon SK (2013) Melamine modified gold nanoprobe for "on spot" colorimetric recognition of clonazepam from biological specimens. *Analyst,* 138(18): 5411- 5416.
81. Lodha A, Alok P, Pinkesh GS, Shobhana KM (2014) A smart and rapid colorimetric method for the detection of codeine sulphate, using unmodified gold nanoprobe. *RSC Adv.,* 4(92): 50443-50448.
82. Lodha, A. S., Pandya, A., & Shukla, R. K. (2016). Nanotechnology: an applied and robust approach for forensic investigation. *Forensic Res. Criminol. Int. J.,* 2(1), 00044.
83. V. Arabali, R. Sadeghi, Surface properties of nano-Al2O3 film and its application in the preparation of 1639 morphine electrochemical sensor. *Ionics,* 19 (2013) 1775-1782.
84. Meng, X. Tang, B. Zhou, Q. Xie, L. Yang, Designing of ordered two-dimensional gold nanoparticles 1650 film for cocaine detection in human urine using surface-enhanced Raman spectroscopy. *Talanta,* 164
85. Kumar, N., & Sharma, A. (2021). Nano-Forensics: The New Perspective in Precision Forensic Science. *Nanotechnology Applications in Health and Environmental Sciences,* 111-134.
86. K. Mao, Z. Yang, J. Li, X. Zhou, X. Li, J. Hu, A novel colorimetric biosensor based on non-aggregated 1653 Au@Ag core–shell nanoparticles for methamphetamine and cocaine detection. *Talanta,* 175 (2017) 338- 1654 346.
87. Costanzo, H., Gooch, J., & Frascione, N. (2022). Nanomaterials for optical biosensors in forensic analysis. *Talanta,* 123945.
88. Kumar, V., Kumar, P., Pournara, A., Vellingiri, K., & Kim, K.-H. (2018). Nanomaterials for the sensing of narcotics: Challenges and opportunities. *TrAC Trends in Analytical Chemistry,* 106, 84–115.
89. Kuswandi, B., Futra, D., & Heng, L. Y. (2017). Nanosensors for the Detection of Food Contaminants. *Nanotechnology Applications in Food,* 307–333.

90. Ameku, W. A., de Araujo, W. R., Rangel, C. J., Ando, R. A., & Paixao, T. R. (2019). Gold nanoparticle paper-based dual-detection device for forensics applications. *ACS Appl. Nano Mater.*, 2(9), 5460-5468.
91. Viswanathan, S., Radecka, H., Radecki, 2009. J. Electrochemical biosensors for food analysis. *Mon. Chem.*, 140, 891e899.
92. Kim, S.J., Gobi, K.V., Iwasaka, H., Tanaka, H., Miura, N., 2007. Novel miniature SPR immunosensor equipped with all-in-one multi-microchannel sensor chip for detecting low-molecular-weight analytes. *Biosens. Bioelectron.*, 23, 701-707.
93. Pandya, A., & Shukla, R. K. (2018). New perspective of nanotechnology: role in preventive forensic. *Egypt. J. Forensic Sci.*, 8, 1-11.
94. McArthur, Douglas, "Fingerprint Identification and Authentication." Sensormag.com, January 2003.
95. Johnson, Colin R., "Quantum Encryption Secures High-speed Data Stream." EEtimes.com, 2002.
96. Bhatt, P. V., Pandey, G., Tharmavaram, M., Rawtani, D., & Mustansar Hussain, C. (2020). Nanotechnology and taggant technology in forensic science. Technology in Forensic Science: Sampling, Analysis, Data and Regulations, 279-301.
97. LaBelle, J. (2013). Trackable Nanobarcode Reading Device.
98. Rahmat, M., Naz, S., & Kiran, S. (2023). Nano-Trackers (Nano-Sensors) for Forensics Investigation. In *Modeling and Simulation of Functional Nanomaterials for Forensic Investigation* (pp. 81-107). IGI Global.
99. Shah, N., Badiye, A., Kapoor, N., & Shukla, R. K. (2022). Nano-biosensors for biochemical analysis. In *Nanobioanalytical Approaches to Medical Diagnostics* (pp. 319-343). Woodhead Publishing.
100. Nadar, S. S., Kelkar, R. K., Pise, P. V., Patil, N. P., Patil, S. P., Chaubal-Durve, N. S., ... & Patil, P. D. (2021). The untapped potential of magnetic nanoparticles for forensic investigations: A comprehensive review. *Talanta*, 230, 122297.
101. Malhotra, B. D., & Ali, M. A. (2018). Nanomaterials in biosensors: Fundamentals and applications. *Nanomaterials for Biosensors*, 1.
102. Solaimuthu, A., Vijayan, A. N., Murali, P., & Korrapati, P. S. (2020). Nanobiosensors and their relevance in tissue engineering. *Curr. Opin. Biomed. Eng.*, 13, 84-93.
103. Din, S. U., Shafique, S., & Khan, F. (2023). Nanotech and Document Security. In Modeling and Simulation of Functional Nanomaterials for Forensic Investigation (pp. 223-242). IGI Global. Kasas, S.; Khanmy-Vital, A.; Dietler, G. Forensic Sci. Int. 2001, 119(3), 290-298.
104. Paikrao, H. M., Tajane, D. S., Patil, A. S., & Dipale, A. D. (2022). Applications of Nanotechnology in Forensic Science. In *Engineered Nanomaterials*

for Innovative Therapies and Biomedicine (pp. 257-276). Cham: Springer International Publishing.

105. Chen YF. Forensic applications of nanotechnology. *J. Chin. Chem. Soc.*, 2011;58: 828–35
106. Chen, S. Z., Tsai, T. L., & Chen, Y. F. (2012). Forensic application of atomic force microscopy——Questioned Document. *J. Chin. Chem. Soc.*, 59(3), 283-288.

Index

aberrations
129, 319
absorbance
95, 98–102, 116, 192
absorption
7, 8, 10, 11, 14–16, 31, 43, 71, 75, 96, 97, 101, 108, 129, 189–95, 197–99, 201, 208–13, 247, 250, 257, 283, 289, 316, 356, 360, 366
accelerants
17, 126, 127, 215, 229, 276, 285, 288, 299, 376
accumulation
77, 103
acetonitrile
39, 256
acetylation
172
adenosine
296, 336
adherence
46, 47, 57
adsorption
218, 241–43, 263
adulterants
19, 123, 259, 261, 277, 288, 342
adulteration
3, 246, 259, 288, 303, 381, 382
amines
288, 303
aminoindane
84
aminophenols
276
amitriptyline
252
amorphous
121, 140, 345, 351, 368
amphetamine
97, 299
anaerobic
180
anesthesia
38
anesthetic
281
anhydride
172
anhydrous
140, 142
anticancerous
211
anticoagulants
39
antidepressants
232, 252, 255, 265, 275, 298
anti-epidermal
358
antigen
351
antimicrobial
256, 358
antipsychotics
232, 294, 304

arsenic
6, 7, 30, 101, 102, 109, 209, 257, 258
arsenical
109
Autofluorescence
317

backscattered
23, 26, 321, 323
Banzodiazepams
85
barbiturates
6, 247, 267, 275
benzaldehyde
296
benzodiazepines
6, 228, 275, 276, 294, 304
benzoylecgonine
295
biodegradation
171, 180
Biodistribution
336
biofluids
73, 122, 133, 144, 146
bioinformatics
144
Biointerfaces
302
bioisosteric
376, 389
biomarkers
4, 73, 134, 295, 383
Biomaterials
362, 390
bioremediation
66
biosensors
365, 381, 383, 391, 392
birefringence
319
blood-spatter
77
cancerous
343, 358
cannabinoids
7, 30, 121, 139, 294, 304
capillaries
297, 371
carboxyhemoglobin
100, 101, 109
cardio-respiratory
281
cardiotoxicity
256, 257
centrifuged
39
chemiluminescence
223
chemometric
30, 65, 74, 77, 82, 89, 132, 133, 146, 282, 389
chromatogram
164, 165, 221, 224, 233, 243, 246, 247, 249, 250, 253, 256, 259, 261, 276, 279, 281, 287, 293
clonazepam
380, 391
Clorazepate
255
criminalistics
1, 63, 86, 215, 216, 226, 236, 268
cross-contamination
40, 41
cryptography
67, 382
crystallographic
27, 340
Cyclotrimethylenetrinitramine
253

deciphering
9, 15, 339
decontamination
44
deconvolution
133, 276

deflections
325
dehydrogenase
103, 110
dehydrogenation
107
demagnetization
131, 145
dichloromethane
44
dispersion
7, 9, 71, 74, 129, 366, 367, 375, 387
dispersive
26, 72, 206, 275, 339, 347, 348, 351, 356–62, 365
Dodecylbenzenesulfonate
289

earthquakes
163
electrocatalysis
388
electrochemical
18, 186, 380, 381, 388, 389, 391, 392
electrochemistry
272
Electrochromatography
298, 305
electrolysis
353
electrolytes
140
electromagnetic
8, 9, 53, 190–92, 198, 199, 290, 320, 322–24, 339, 340
Electrophoresis-Electrospray
305
electrophoresis-mass
296
electrophoretic
296
electrospinning
371, 388
electrothermal
194, 195, 202, 203, 206, 209, 213
energy-dispersive
32, 339, 340, 342, 343, 361, 362
Energy-Dispersive-Spectroscopy
359
Enzymology
303
Epidemiology
185
estrogenic
256

famotidine
262
Faraday-collector
155
fingerprinting
25, 136, 142, 161, 212, 241, 258–60, 284
fluoro-methoxy
285
fluorophores
315–17
Fourier-Transform
116, 117, 291
fractionation
153, 154, 166–68, 171, 277, 387
fragmentation
14, 154, 156, 157, 166, 167, 189, 225, 274, 287, 289, 292
Freeze-thaw
118
FTIR
19, 20, 73, 80, 89, 105, 106, 127, 176, 235, 259, 289–91, 357

Galactosyltransferase
38
Gastroenterologie
110
gastrointestinal
281

Gaussian
247
GC-FTIR
7, 291
GC-IRMS
155
GC-MS
19, 20, 123, 185, 217, 224, 225, 228–31, 234, 240, 255, 272, 273, 275–78, 285, 291, 296, 300, 302, 352
geochemical
163, 207, 214, 360, 362
geochemistry
162, 164, 165, 183
geochemsheets
360
glutamic
103, 110
Glutamic-Oxalacetic
110
glycerin
104
glycol
124, 142, 277

hacking
47
halloysite
32, 391
hallucinogenic
98
handwriting
26, 332
heavy-metal
15, 344, 345
hemechromophore
101
hemoglobin
100, 101, 110
Hepatectomy
110
hepatotoxicity
256
herbalist
258
herbicides
222, 257
heterogeneity
154
heterogeneous
69, 154, 373
hexahydrate
78
hexyl-acrylate-based
298
Histochem
358
histochemical
353
histological
327
homogeneity
206
HPLC–MS
305
HPLC-NMR
20
HPLC-UV
255
HPTLC
18–20, 28, 108, 241–49, 251–54, 258–62, 264–68
hydrophilic
325, 375
hydrophobic
325, 375
hydrophobicity
286, 291
hydrothermal
373, 374, 389
hyperpolarization
134
hyperpolarized
141
hyperspectral
387

Hyperthermia
301
hyphenated
4, 19, 20, 31, 120, 217, 238, 249, 252, 254, 255, 262, 265, 271–73, 291, 299, 300, 302, 303, 305
hyphenation
264, 265, 299
hypodermic
38
hypogastrium
204
hypotension
281
hypothermia
204, 211
hypothesized
7, 291

ICP-AES
206, 356
ICP–MS
210
ICP-SF-MS
202
ignitable
170, 171, 276, 282
illumination
21, 310–12, 318, 358, 367, 370
imipramine
298
Immunoassays
54
insecticides
101, 124, 257, 258
instrumentation
1, 3, 5–8, 31, 116, 154–56, 164, 165, 179, 180, 182–84, 194, 195, 199, 201–3, 219, 237, 241–46, 256, 263, 264, 272–74, 279, 280, 283, 284, 286, 287, 289, 290, 292, 293, 296, 297, 301, 343, 347, 360, 386
interpretation
4, 56, 59, 70, 111, 113, 128, 130–32, 144–46, 160, 179, 180, 213, 239, 262, 273, 275, 303, 345, 356, 364
intoxication
38, 108, 124, 142
invasive
78, 81, 99, 121
invasiveness
83
iodine
50, 51, 102
IR-spectroscopy
285
isobutane
107
isoprene
127
isotope
6, 30, 121, 149–56, 164–81, 183–85, 187

Junkers
143
Jurisdictions
67
juvenile
30

keratin
90
keratinized
294, 304

Lambert
15
lamivudine
262
lanthanide-based
338
light-scattering
386
light-sensitive
309

lipids
82, 145, 258
lipoprotein
77
lithium
348, 362
lithography
372, 388

magnification
21, 22, 308, 309, 311–13, 320–22, 367
m-amino-phenol
277
mass-spectroscopy
14
medications
2, 133, 261, 279
medicinal
65, 133, 203, 255, 258, 262
medicine
20, 21, 29, 96, 99, 114, 134, 136, 141, 202–4, 211, 224, 275, 294, 333, 337, 361
Mesoporous
366
metabolism
6, 30, 263
metabonomics
144, 146, 147
metallization
353, 361
metalloids
202
metal-oxo-polymer
374
methamphetamine
84, 97, 227, 299, 391
methcathione
84
methemoglobin
101, 109
methylenedioxymethamphet-amine
171
Methylenedioxypyrovalerone
275
methylisothiazolinone
256
Methylone
301
microanalysis
340, 349, 351, 352, 356–58, 360
microanalytical
347
microbiological
66
microelectronics
309
microextraction
44, 238, 240, 277, 283, 389
microfluidic
379, 391
Micro-homogeneity
213
microorganisms
56, 78, 157, 327
micro-plastics
183
Microspectrophotometric
111
microspectrophotometry
111
microwave-assisted
44, 203, 374
microwave-solvothermal
389
mineralogical
190, 333
miniaturization
58, 105, 225, 226, 300, 383
mitochondrial
336
multidimensional
74, 88, 120, 143, 178, 223, 224, 238, 240, 264, 265, 355
multi-microchannel
392

nanoalloys
371
nanoanalysis
358
Nano-biosensors
392
Nanobiotechnology
93
Nanocharacterization
386
Nanoclusters
365
nanocomposites
388
nanocrystalline
366
Nanofoams
366
Nanoforensics
390, 391
Nanographene-Armored
303
nanolithography
372
nanomaterials
27, 32, 341, 363–67, 371–76, 378, 380, 381, 384–88, 390–92
Nanomedicine
32, 359, 391
nanoparticles
27, 32, 42, 62, 336, 340, 358, 359, 363–68, 370–72, 374–80, 384, 385, 387–91
nanopatterns
372
nanophysics
309
nanopores
366
nanopowders
365, 388
nanoreactors
375
Nanoribbons
365
nanorods
365, 374
nanoscale
27, 322, 326, 362–66, 371, 383–85
nanoseconds
151
nanospheres
374
nanostructured
371, 373, 390
nanotechnology
1, 4, 27, 29, 57, 93, 323, 358, 363–65, 375–78, 380–86, 389–93
nanowires
374
N-bromosuccinimide
108
Neuropharmacol
301
neurotoxicity
256, 257
Neurotransmitters
303
nitroaromatic
89, 253, 266
nitrocellulose
329
nitrogen
39, 131, 150, 151, 169, 171–75, 177, 184, 218, 220, 221, 234, 243, 274, 283, 349
nitroglycerin
295, 329
N-Nitrosodimethylamine
184
noncellular
78
non-crystalline
206, 295
non-destructive
3, 10, 73, 74, 104, 124, 176, 244, 248, 252, 260, 278, 339, 340, 350, 356, 381
non-hazardous
373

noninvasive
75, 85
non-metallic
81
non-parametric
129
non-plasmonic
367
non-polar
70, 218, 222
non-toxic
80
non-viscous
371
nucleotides
296

o-aminophenol
277
obliterations
332
ocular
23, 25, 309, 380
oculus
308
Odontology
4
Olanzapine
255
one-dimensional
120, 138, 145, 365
opaque
73
organochlorines
258
organophosphorus
124, 251, 258, 265
osemicarbazone
102
O-toluidine
288
oxygenated
142
oxygenates
143
oxyhemoglobin
101, 110

p-aminophenol
277
paracetamol
261, 262
paraffin
282, 298
paraffin-embedded
352
paraformaldehyde
351
paramagnet-doped
122
pentaerythritol
253, 266, 376
peptides
79, 156, 181, 218
petrochemical
217, 222, 223
pharmaceuticals
1, 89, 96, 115, 121, 122, 159, 185, 190, 203, 211, 217, 221–26, 237, 243, 256, 262, 267, 273, 279, 286, 288, 300, 336
Pharmacognosy
184
pharmacological
118
phenothiazines
255
Phenotyping
305
phenylalanine
75, 78
phosphorus
12, 353, 355
Photoacoustic
73
Photobleaching
315, 317

Photography
62, 320
photoluminescence
386
photosynthetic
154
Phototoxicity
315, 317
phytochemical
241
Phytoplankton
305
Plasmas
210
plastic
38, 40, 42, 43, 50, 51, 80, 177, 231, 276, 334, 350, 378
plasticizer
127
poisoning
6, 100, 101, 109, 115, 136, 142, 159, 202, 210, 232, 252, 258, 261, 265, 281, 289, 343
polarization
113, 122, 140, 141, 210, 319, 335
polarized
22, 122, 318, 319
polarizer
318, 319
polyamides
83
poly-butadiene
127
polycondensation
374
polycyclic
238
poly-dispersed
387
polyester
83, 104, 128, 254, 328
polyethylene
231, 276
polyimide
296
polymerase
49, 64, 379
polymerisation
143
polymers
10, 20, 83, 115, 121, 122, 127, 140, 141, 143, 333, 341, 348, 355, 371, 372
polymorph
140
Polymorphic
121
polymorphism
122
polypropylene
38, 39, 128
Polysilicon
237
polystyrene
127
polytetrafluoroethylene
42
porosity
366, 374
post-mortem
6, 12, 42, 115, 162, 204, 261, 267, 281, 294, 298, 299, 302, 304, 379, 380
potassium
99, 102, 256, 262, 355, 391
probabilistic
58
pyrethroid
258
Pyrotechnics
266
pyrrole
75
pyruvate
141

quadrillion
369
quadrupole
157, 275, 287, 303
quantitative-nmr-spectroscopy
137

quartz
104, 197, 199, 346
QuEChERS
65, 275
questioned-document
176

radioactive
151
radiofrequency
12, 157, 200
rape
3, 67, 380
reconstruction
29, 36, 61, 65, 95, 162, 252, 287, 315, 354
recreational
7, 173, 275
reevaluating
236
reproducibility
55, 116, 124, 202, 226, 247, 249, 267
resealable
177
residues
2, 8, 24, 43, 73, 79, 87, 89, 99, 127, 138, 160, 161, 182, 205, 206, 222, 227, 235, 238, 265, 276, 278, 282, 285, 288, 295, 298, 301, 304, 328, 329, 337, 342, 343, 353, 354, 364, 389
resilience
5
resins
84, 127, 163, 260, 355
resistance
371
resonance
11, 19, 20, 89, 113, 116, 133–39, 142, 143, 145–47, 182, 190, 287, 304, 363, 388
retardation
248
retention
16–19, 228, 229, 247, 248, 253, 255, 256, 260, 261, 264, 279, 337
retrospectively
299
revolutionized
20, 58, 149, 217, 225

scattered
21, 26, 27, 71, 343–45, 348, 369, 370
segmentation
65
segregated
6, 13, 273, 286, 287
segregation
72, 246, 289
seismology
163
Simulation
392
spectrofluorometer
357
spectrophotometric
94, 98, 100, 105, 107, 109, 110
spectrum
8, 9, 11–14, 43, 70–73, 75, 78–81, 100, 104–6, 114, 117–19, 121–23, 126, 128–32, 145, 152, 165, 168, 191–93, 197, 199, 201, 225, 231, 256, 274, 281, 283, 286, 287, 289, 290, 292, 293, 296, 316, 339, 341, 342, 346, 349, 356, 367
stabilizers
160
stereomicroscope
24, 259, 310–12, 315, 317, 319, 324, 326
steroids
137, 216
stretching
77, 82
superconducting
116

suspensions
386
synchrotron
7
synergistically
289
taggants
160
tampering
46, 47, 57, 75, 333
taxological
352
Taxonomic
305
teratogenicity
257
terephthalate
128
tetracyclic
275
Tetra-hydrocannabinol
97
tetrahydrofuran
124
tetranitrate
253, 266, 376, 389
tetrazepam
298
tetroxide
351
therapeutic
232, 252, 265, 340
thermodynamic
253, 279
thermoplastic
355
thermospray
13, 287
time-dependent
117, 295
Tomography
363
Topographical
326
topography
323, 325, 326, 337
toxicities
257, 258
toxicological
1, 38, 65, 210, 227, 232, 247, 250, 252, 257, 263, 279, 286, 339
toxins
12, 17, 18, 53, 54, 115, 124, 152, 159–62, 179, 227, 232, 258, 271, 277, 279, 288, 294, 343, 381, 383
transaminase
103, 110
transformation
73, 119, 128, 256, 374
translocation
66
translucent
311
transmission
23, 32, 96, 320–22, 336, 349, 351, 358, 367, 368, 383, 386
transmittance
96, 104, 111, 192
transparency
46, 55
tricyclic
298
triglycerides
288, 303
trimethylsilyl
131
Trimipramine
256
Trinitrotoluene
253
tuberculosis
342
tungsten
194, 199, 322, 324
tyrosine
78, 181

ultrafiltration
143
ultraviolet
10, 18, 89, 108, 190, 255, 302, 339, 386
ultraviolet-visible
10, 53, 101, 107, 111
Uv-vis
11, 28, 53, 93–98, 100–106, 110, 111, 386

vacuum
27, 43, 44, 156, 238, 278, 286, 301, 302, 322, 324, 344, 369
vapor-atomic
208
vaporization
156, 193, 194, 274
varnishes
163, 355
vehicle
49, 98, 234, 330, 355, 383
venipuncture
39
vermilion
257
vibrational
10, 69–74, 80, 81, 86–88, 90, 91, 105, 108, 289
viruses
22, 336
viscosity
296, 374
visualization
57, 64, 82, 87, 132, 288, 321, 322, 336, 337, 377, 384
volatilization
195, 196

water
11, 16, 39, 44, 71, 78, 97, 109, 116, 129, 150, 159, 160, 165, 173–75, 181, 190, 193, 198, 202, 206, 222, 224, 258, 355, 374, 375, 383
watermark
332
weapons
101, 104, 107, 253, 327, 329, 330, 353

Xanthophyll
305
xenobiotics
38, 115, 124, 136, 142
x-ray
26, 27, 32, 84, 85, 206, 214, 268, 339–52, 356–62, 385
x-ray-diffraction
359

Zeta
371

β-sheet
138
λmax
97

Also of Interest

Check out these other related titles from Scrivener Publishing

SECURITY ISSUES AND PRIVACY CONCERNS IN INDUSTRY 4.0 APPLICATIONS, Edited by Shibin David, R. S. Anand, V. Jeyakrishnan, and M. Niranjanamurthy, ISBN: 9781119775621.
Written and edited by a team of international experts, this is the most comprehensive and up-to-date coverage of the security and privacy issues surrounding Industry 4.0 applications, a must-have for any library.

MACHINE LEARNING TECHNIQUES AND ANALYTICS FOR CLOUD SECURITY, Edited by Rajdeep Chakraborty, Anupam Ghosh and Jyotsna Kumar Mandal, ISBN: 9781119762256.
This book covers new methods, surveys, case studies, and policy with almost all machine learning techniques and analytics for cloud security solutions.

ARTIFICIAL INTELLIGENCE AND DATA MINING IN SECURITY FRAMEWORKS, Edited by Neeraj Bhargava, Ritu Bhargava, Pramod Singh Rathore, and Rashmi Agrawal, ISBN 9781119760405. Written and edited by a team of experts in the field, this outstanding new volume offers solutions to the problems of security, outlining the concepts behind allowing computers to learn from experience and understand the world in terms of a hierarchy of concepts.

SECURITY DESIGNS FOR THE CLOUD, IOT AND SOCIAL NETWORKING, Edited by Dac-Nhuong Le, Chintin Bhatt and Mani Madhukar, ISBN: 9781119592266. The book provides cutting-edge research that delivers insights into the tools, opportunities, novel strategies, techniques, and challenges for handling security issues in cloud computing, Internet of Things and social networking.

DESIGN AND ANALYSIS OF SECURITY PROTOCOLS FOR COMMUNICATION, Edited by Dinesh Goyal, S. Balamurugan, Sheng-Lung Peng and O.P. Verma, ISBN: 9781119555643. The book combines analysis and comparison of various security protocols such as HTTP, SMTP, RTP, RTCP, FTP, UDP for mobile or multimedia streaming security protocol.

Books in the series, "Advances in Cyber Security"

CYBER SECURITY AND DIGITAL FORENSICS: Challenges and Future Trends, Edited by Mangesh M. Ghonge, Sabyasachi Pramanik, Ramchandra Mangrulkar, and Dac-Nhuong Le, ISBN: 9781119795636. Written and edited by a team of world renowned experts in the field, this groundbreaking new volume covers key technical topics and gives readers a comprehensive understanding of the latest research findings in cyber security and digital forensics.

CYBER SECURITY AND NETWORK SECURITY, Edited by Sabyasachi Pramanik, Debabrata Samanta, M. Vinay, and Abhijit Guha, ISBN: 9781119812494. Written and edited by a team of experts in the field, this is the most comprehensive and up to date study of the practical applications of cybersecurity and network security for engineers, scientists, students, and other professionals.

DEEP LEARNING APPROACHES TO CLOUD SECURITY, edited by Pramod Singh Rathore, Vishal Dutt, Rashmi Agrawal, Satya Murthy Sasubilli, and Srinivasa Rao Swarna, ISBN 9781119760528. Covering one of the most important subjects to our society today, this editorial team delves into solutions taken from evolving deep learning approaches, solutions allow computers to learn from experience and understand the world in terms of a hierarchy of concepts.

Printed in the USA/Agawam, MA
September 16, 2026

910661.140